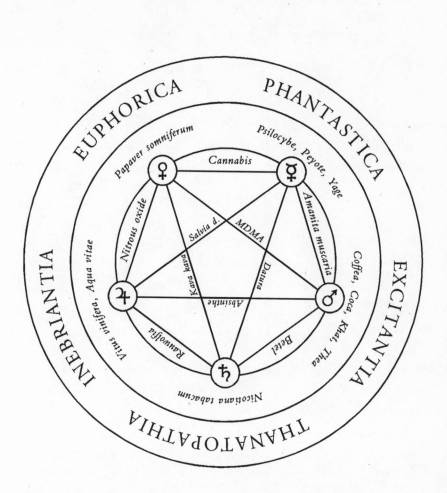

P
H
A
R
M
A
K
O
/
P
O
E
I
A

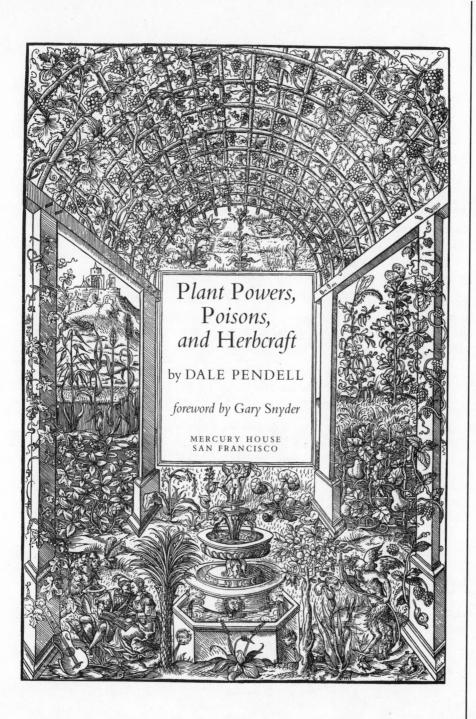

Plant Powers,
Poisons,
and Herbcraft

by DALE PENDELL

foreword by Gary Snyder

MERCURY HOUSE
SAN FRANCISCO

PHARMAKO/POEIA

Manufactured and published in the United States of America by Mercury House, San Francisco, California, a nonprofit publishing company devoted to the free exchange of ideas and guided by a dedication to literary values. Mercury House and colophon are the registered trademarks of Mercury House, Incorporated.

United States Constitution, First Amendment: Congress shall make no law respecting an establishment of religion, or prohibiting the free exercise thereof; or abridging the freedom of speech, or of the press; or the right of the people peaceably to assemble, and to petition the Government for a redress of grievances.

The author and publisher gratefully acknowledge those who have give permission to reproduce their work in this volume. Please see the credits section, beginning p. 282, which constitutes an extension of this copyright page.

Interior design (in Adobe Bembo with Adobe Garamond Titling), art direction, and typesetting by Thomas Christensen. Printed by R.R. Donnelley on acid-free paper.

LIBRARY OF CONGRESS CATALOGUING-IN-PUBLICATION DATA
Pendell, Dale, 1947 –
Pharmako/poeia : plant powers, poisons, and herbcraft / by Dale pendell : foreword by Gary Snyder. – 1st ed.
    P.   CM.
Includes bibliographical references.
ISBN 1-56279-069-2
1. Materia medica, Vegetable.   2. Medicinal plants.   I. Snyder, Gary, 1930–
II. Title.   III. Title: plant powers, poisons, and herbcraft.
RS164.P447 1995   94–48573
615'.32–dc20   CIP

Cover illustration from *Charta Lusoria* by Jost Amman, 1588.

12 11 10 9 8 7 6 5 4 3 2 1

FIRST EDITION

PUBLISHER'S NOTE: A manuscript draft of *Pharmako/Poeia* caused us some concern. The author of this remarkable work was clearly exploring perilous terrain along his "Poison Path." This is a route we strongly advise others not to follow (except through this book, and through other approaches that lead in the direction of wisdom without dangerous self-experimentation).

Did we detect a tongue-in-cheek quality in the manuscript? We could see the depth of botanical knowledge, the extensive scholarly research, the learning, the results of years of alchemical practice and dedicated experience, the poetic beauty, the ingenuity of subtly shifting interior dialogues, the peculiar fascination of strange, beguiling perspectives, the dark wizardry of its authorial persona (wise, but not without a hint of menace) . . .

Pharmako/Poeia makes a contribution to modern poetics and cross-disciplinary study, in the distinguished tradition of the botanical herbal (the tradition launched by Dioscorides in classical times, which reached perhaps its finest flourishing in the early Renaissance); this tradition has influenced our physical presentation of the material.

A companion volume, forthcoming, will explore the remaining hemisphere of the *Pharmako/Poeia* mandala, including plants in the categories *phantastica* and *excitantia*.

CAUTION: This book is an exploration of the "Poison Path." All of the plant substances described in it act on the human body as drugs and thereby as poisons. In many cases there are known and there may also be unknown health hazards involved in their use. *The publisher and the author recommend that dangerous or illegal practices be avoided.*

This is a literary work that takes as its subject the relation that has existed throughout the world since ancient times between "power plants" and shamanic and literary creation. The authorial voice that appears in it should be considered a fictional persona. The inclusion of recipes, preparations, or dosages are an expression of that fictional voice, and should not be regarded as actual recommendations for usage.

Neither the publisher nor the author assume any liability for unwise or unsafe actions by readers of this book.

This book is dedicated to

Isaac Black Elk Goodkind

1970–1993

his friends and his generation

CONTENTS

FOREWORD BY GARY SNYDER
xiii

POWER PLANTS
green allies

Bring Them On, the Power Plants   3
On the Nature of Poison I   4
Plant People   6
Plants As Teachers   8
On the Nature of the Ally   10
13   *The Mad River Plant: Prunus emarginata*
The Great Work   15
Sun Medicine / Moon Medicine   18
21   *Bulrush: Scirpus atrovirens*
Methodology I   23
Ground State Calibration   25
Methodology II   26

THANATOPATHIA
tasting of death

Thanatopathia   29
31   *Tobacco: Nicotiana tabacum*
Phenomenological Taxonomy of
Psychotropes   42
46   *Pituri: Duboisia hopwoodii*
Killing Time   48

INEBRIANTIA
relating to drunkenness

Inebriantia   51
53   *Yeast: Saccharomyces cerevisiae*
58   *Wine: Vitis vinifera*

65   *Beer: Hordeum vulgare*

70   *Aqua Vitae*

The Alcoholic Muse   78

The Poison Path I   81

83   *Æther*

89   *Fossil Fuel*

Mead and the Divine Madness   93

RHAPSODICA
where seeds of song are sown

On the Seduction of Angels   99

103   *Absinthe: Artemisia absinthium*

114   *Calea zacatechichi*

EUPHORICA
plants bearing pleasure

Euphorica   117

119   *Opium: Papaver somniferum*

Heroin and the Nature of Addiction   137

PACIFICA
the peacemakers

The Perfume of Poison   145

146   *Kava kava: Piper methysticum*

EXISTENTIA
the stance of the pre-essential

On Poisoning Wells   155

156   *Ska Pastora: Salvia divinorum*

EVAESTHETICA
sensually pleasing

On Wildness in Plants   177

On Camp Followers   178

179   *Marijuana: Cannabis sativa*
Die Giftküche   208

METAPHYSICA
intimations on the nature of things

Reveries on the Green Man   211
226   *Nitrous Oxide*
The Poison Path II   236

GLOSSARY
241

REFERENCES
248

CREDITS
282

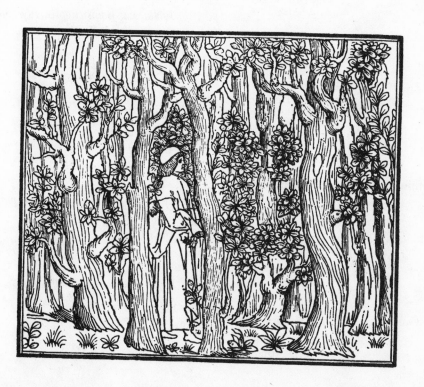

CONTENTS, VOLUME TWO

PLANT ALLIES
a poet's guide

On the Nature of Poison II   .
Divination, Chance, and the Nature
of Power   .

PHANTASTICA
visionary plants

Phantastica   .
Das Mutterkorn   .
          .   *Ayahuasca: Banisteriopsis, Psychotria viridis*
          .   *Teonanacatl: Psilocybe cubensis*

Reflections: Lunar Medicine   .
          .   *Peganum harmala*

Tryptamines and the Spagyric Art   .
The Topology of the Between   .

          .   *DMT*
          .   *Phalaris arundinaceae*
          .   *Arundo donax*
          .   *Desmanthus illinoensis*

The Luminosity of Sentient Dimensions   .
          .   *Lysergic acid amide: Claviceps purpurea*
          .   *Ololiuqui: Ipomoea, Rivea spp.*
          .   *Stipa robusta*

The Great Psychedelic Baseball
Experiment   .
          .   *Peyote: Lophophora williamsii*
          .   *San Pedro Cactus: Trichocereus pachanoi*

The Great Stone and the Bodhisattva
of Excess   .
The Athanor   .

The Vision Quest:
Plant Teachers and Song   .

     .   *The Great Toad Mother: Bufo alvarius,*
           B. marianus

The Divine Signature   .

EMPATHOGENICA
entering the suffering

The Gift of Venery:
Neurotransmitters, Love, and Strife   .

     .   *Terpenes and the kin: Nutmeg, MDMA*

The Garden of Poison: Bias
and Evolution   .

DAIMONICA
here there be dragons

On Goddesses and Consorts   .

     .   *Tropane alkaloids: Datura, Brugmansia,*
           Solandra

     .   *Flying ointments: Henbane, Belladonna*

     .   *Coriaria thymifolia*

     .   *Mescal Bean: Sophora secundiflora*

On the Ground State   .

HYPNOTICA
bringers of sleep

The Poison of Dreaming   .

     .   *Rauwolfia serpentaria*

CHARISMATICA
yearning for grace

The Solar Medicine   .

     .   *Betel: Areca catechu/Piper betle*

Reddening/Yellowing   .

EXCITANTIA
provokers and agitators

Excitantia and Western Culture   .

.   *Coffee: Coffea arabica*

.   *Tea: Thea sinensis*

.   *Cocaine: Erythroxylum coca*

The Genesis of Stoning   .

.   *Chocolate: Theobroma cacao*

Speed/Charisma/Oblivion   .

.   *Khat: Catha edulis and amphetamine*

.   *Misc: Guayusa, Mate*

.   *The Black Drink: Ilex spp.*

TELEPHORICA
bearing a great distance

Wandering: Wildness and Knowledge   .

.   *Tabernanthe iboga*

On Gambling   .

.   *Amanita muscaria*

THE FOOL

Hallucinogenic Properties of Maize   .

The Elementals   .

The Toxicology of Enlightenment   .

The Girl in the Tree   .

The Fool's Journey   .

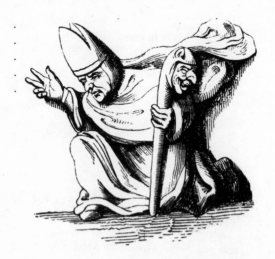

THE BISHOP OF FOOLS WITH HIS BAUBLE

FOREWORD BY GARY SNYDER

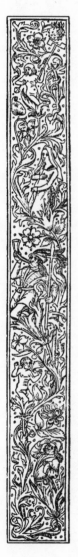

This is a book about plants. Green, sweet, peaceful plants: the harmless beings who give us flowers, nuts, fruits, roots, sap, bark, fiber, and shade. But some aren't so great to eat – sour, bitter, or worse. Plants are all chemists, tirelessly assembling the molecules of the world, and in their transactions with insects, birds, animals, and fungi, they find elaborate ways to defend themselves, to seduce pollinators, to confuse. So it's a book about the interplay of plants, insects, animals, and humans, and suggests a bit how toxins shaped ecological systems. How much we assume about plants, and how little we know them! Pendell playfully says, "Only plants had consciousness. Animals got it from them."

It's a book about people, the plant-women and -men who for millennia investigated the properties of plants and learned to use them for healing, for their effects on the mind, for poisons. These ancient experts and traditional professionals knew and kept plant secrets close for generations. It's a book about knowledge, and secrets.

In recent centuries those who knew plants and their powers have often been stigmatized, as though danger and unpredictability were of themselves evil. This is a book about human cultures, and how those which demonize death or pain or sickness are thus less able to deal with the bitter side of nature, with intoxications; and make themselves doubly sick.

The Buddha taught that all life is suffering. We might also say that life, being both attractive and constantly dangerous, is intoxicating and ultimately toxic. Cupid shoots an arrow which strikes and changes you forever; love is toxic. "Toxic" comes from *toxicon*, Pendell tells us, with a root meaning of "a poisoned arrow." All organic life is struck by the arrows of real and psychic poisons. This is understood by any true, that is to say, not self-deluding, spiritual path.

So Pendell speaks of the "way of poisons." This way (modern and ancient shamanism and herbcraft, verging into ethnobotany and ethnopharmacology) has developed a remarkable body of empirical and scientific knowledge to place against current official ignorance and resistance to the possibility of clear and courageous thinking about the many realms of drugs.

This is a book about danger: dangerous knowledge, even more dangerous ignorance, and dangerous temptations by the seductions of addictions both psychic and cellular. It is a book which requires that one not be titillated by romantic ideas of self-destruction. I hope and believe it will benefit human beings and the plant world too. It is not for everyone – but neither is mountaineering.

Pendell quotes William Blake, "poets are of the devil's party." Poets needless to say are not satanists, so what does Blake mean? I think he is saying that for those who are willing to explore the fullness of their imagination, their mind and senses, there are great risks – at the very least, of massive silliness. Farther out is madness. No joke. But forget about the devil; poets and such travelers also bring a certain sanity back home. Here is a look at half-understood truths and serious territories of remaining mystery. This is a book of imagination and poetry.

Industrial toxins and wastes are in the air and oceans, and buried and heaped up on the land. Our very food now seems suspect. "Better living through chemistry" was brought us by our own entrepreneurial and selectively regulatory societies. The developed world now has to work all these questions out, with vast environmental destruction as the stakes. Who indeed are the crazies of the twentieth century? We desperately need to understand the basics, of plants, of consciousness, of poisons. This book is a tentative map with scribbled reports by scouts from the territory beyond the ranges, and it aims for sanity.

– G.S.

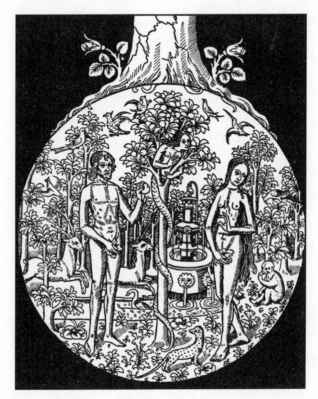

THE ROOT OF EVIL

(hey!)

I hear you.

(any cops around?)

These are just words.

(yeah right . . .
any prospective
employers around?)

I don't want to hear this.

(then why did you call me?)

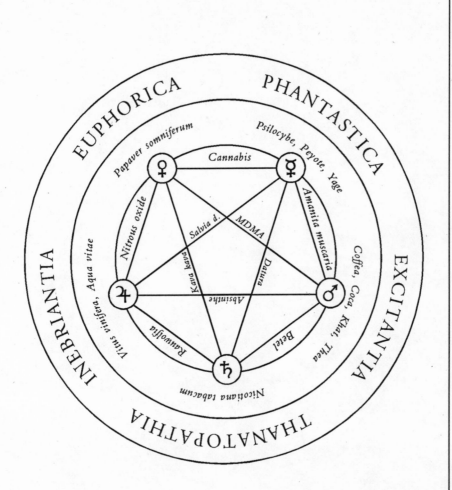

PHARMAKO/POEIA

BRING THEM ON,
THE POWER PLANTS

All the palmate-leaved ones, the
    pinnate, and the pinnatifid, the entire –
Rosy Hawaiian babies, wise Mazatec sages,
    and the old Indian rope trick.
Come on, you indoles, you terpenes,
    you alkaloids, you medicine plants.
Hello, star-eyed betel juice plants, Amazonian
    vine plants, Chihuahuan cacti;
Come, blue-eyed witch plants; come you
    dung-loving fun guys . . .

Come on, O rueful Syrians,
    and all you thick-smelling
    solanaceous plants;
You cultivated-in-rows tobacco and coca plants;
You maligned poppy plants and worshipped
    grapevine plants –
All forgotten plants, and fad plants:
Come forth, you motley troop –
    not a gentleman among you –
Not one that won't lie, cheat, or swindle
    a ride –
Come, all ye ruffians:
Be fruitful, we have need of poison.

POWER PLANTS

ON THE NATURE OF POISON

In poison there is physic.
> – Shakespeare, 2 Henry IV

Our way is the way of poisons. Mercury,
the poisonous changeling.

MERCURY

Some plants
like to lap up to you, doglike.
Others hit you like a mallet.

Once they get in you, they've got you. From then on, the plant-poison is part of you.

Our way is the way of poison. If you want sacredness, highly evolved consciousness, spiritual magnificence, holiness, sweetness, beauty, and truth,

GOOD!
Aspiration is halfway-there.

But our way is the way of poison. The path of sulphur.

Everything is poison, nothing is poison.
> – Paracelsus

SULPHUR

The old doctors were called poisoners.
They were the *lucky* ones. Still today, we will
say to someone, *Good luck.*

Your luck is your power, your poison.

And some lucky people do the bad stuff.

And a lot of doctoring, if you are good, is undoing
the mess
        left by
                the bad shamans.

The bad shamans . . . their weapon
        is the Lie. Sometimes the lies are like arrows
        that go in easily but are very difficult
        to pull out.

Sometimes bad shamans who poisoned for money had to be tolerated, as they were often the only recourse for a person struck by a "dart." Sometimes the doctors who wore animal skins, like maybe grizzly bear skins, got too mean. Then the people would have to get together and kill the bad doctor. Sometimes those bad ones were weeded out in the apprenticeship process.

> *Blind Hall called his medicine "my poison." The Indian word is*
> *"damaagome." Some Indians translate it in English as "medicine" or*
> *"power," sometimes "dog" (in the sense of pet dog, or trained dog).*
>
>   *— Jaime de Angulo, Indians in Overalls*

For our purposes, it is enough to get over thinking "good" and "not good" and to proceed with a scientific, that is to say, poetical, investigation.

> *Let the lover of God understand us right; we do not go upon an historical*
> *heathenish conjecture, nor only upon the light of the outward nature; both*
> *suns shine to us.*
>
>   *— Jacob Böhme, Signatura Rerum*

Start with poison, your own:
     a black drip,
oily and shimmering;

start with poison and let it ferment.

(Put poison on poison. Can you poison poison?
     There, in the place where seeds sprout.)

 Better to start
     with poison your own
than all the laurels of your
     friends or dreams —
the first settles accounts,
     the latter compounds note.

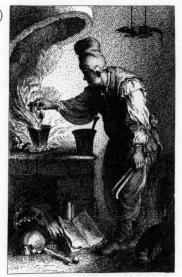

> *In a toad, viper, or adder, or the like poison-*
> *ful beasts, worms, or insects, the highest*
> *tincture is to be found, if they are reduced to*
> *an oily substance, and the wrath of Mercury*
> *separated from them; for all life, both*
> *external and internal, consists in poison and*
> *light . . . all life that is void of the poisonful*
> *Mercury is mort, and an abominate, and*
> *accounted as dead.*
>
>   *— Jacob Böhme, Signatura Rerum*

THE ALCHEMIST, MARTIN
JOHANN SCHMIDT, 18TH C.

No need to mistake any of this for spiritual practice.

(Come, my poisons . . .

PLANT PEOPLE

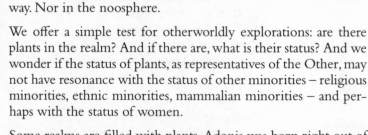

To follow the Way of Poisons, it is essential to learn about plants. As you learn about plants, you will, by the by, meet *plant people.*

Be clear now: most of the plant people you meet are not on the Poison Path, but all the plant people are teachers, nonetheless. They are doctors, though the doctoring of some of them is most subtle.

Almost every gardener is a plant person, as are botanists and horticulturists. Some existentialists are not plant people.

> *I am afraid of cities. But you mustn't leave them. If you go too far you come up against the vegetation belt. Vegetation has crawled for miles towards the cities. It is waiting. Once the city is dead, the vegetation will cover it, will climb over the stones, grip them, search them, make them burst with its long black pincers; it will blind the holes and let its green paws hang over everything.*
>
> – Jean-Paul Sartre, Nausea

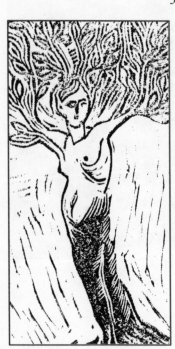

DAPHNE, JACQUELINE BELLON

And, despite the sprouting of fractal ferns and algorithmic roses, there are no plants in cyberspace – not that one could eat, anyway. Nor in the noosphere.

We offer a simple test for otherworldly explorations: are there plants in the realm? And if there are, what is their status? And we wonder if the status of plants, as representatives of the Other, may not have resonance with the status of other minorities – religious minorities, ethnic minorities, mammalian minorities – and perhaps with the status of women.

Some realms are filled with plants. Adonis was born right out of the trunk of a myrrh tree. Buddha, according to tradition, had his enlightenment beneath a tree, and his mother, Maya, is portrayed holding on to the branch of the sacred sal tree as she gives birth. And Jesus, though he once cursed a fig tree to death because it was out of season, died on a tree. That counts for something, in the world of plants. Remember that Socrates once bragged to Phaedrus that he had nothing to learn from the plants of the countryside, and how he was forced to swallow more than his words. That George Washington was said to have chopped down a cherry tree will make more sense in the section on the Mad River plant.

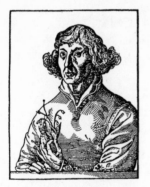

NICOLAS COPERNICUS

In the old times it was not unusual for people to be turned into plants. The old plant doctors knew those stories. The old doctors talked to the plants directly. They knew. That this tree was a girl, that that flower had been a boy. Such things are still true.

In natural, inhabitory societies everyone is a plant person. Sure, there are exceptions – the Eskimos lived entirely by eating other souls – but those are exceptions. To walk through the Amazonian forest with the Waorani- or the Quichua-speaking peoples is to be deluged with plant lore: with names, uses, and legends about plant after plant after tree passing by.

There are those who believe we can live without plants. There is thus some urgency to our task.

A bulldozer grinding and slobbering
Sideslipping and belching on top of
The skinned-up bodies of still-live bushes
In the pay of a man
From town.

   – Gary Snyder, "Front Lines"

I've met plant people in most unplantlike places. One was chief executive officer of a computer corporation. And the noted mycologist Gordon Wasson (who never, incidentally, accepted Keynesian economic theory) was vice president of the J. P. Morgan Trust. Some plant people end up as professionals: as botanists, ethnobotanists, farmers, landscapers. Some plant people change their names to plant names: like Yerba Santa, the spinner and jeweler; or Red Pine, the poet and translator; or Ponderosa Pine, the naturalist. One of poet Gary Snyder's most important books (from which the lines above were quoted) is called *Manzanita*. Robert Aitken, a Zen *roshi* in the Sanbo Kyodan lineage, wrote a book about Zen and ethics called *The Mind of Clover*. D. H. Lawrence titled a book of poetry *Pansies*.

Plant people have a way of being invisible, of blending perfectly with the landscape, or of being visible only to other plant people. Our Way, however, is not about being a plant person. Ours is the Poison Path.

Watching gardeners label their plants
   I vow with all beings
to practice the old horticulture
   and let plants identify me.

   – Robert Aitken, The Dragon Who Never Sleeps

PLANTS AS TEACHERS

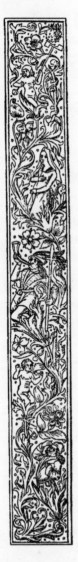

Every plant is a teacher,
  but as in every crowd,
    there are always
      a few loudmouths.

Along the upper Amazon at the base of the Andes, in the Oriente of Ecuador, there are *yachaqs* who learn shamanism directly from the *doctores,* the plant teachers. These *yachaqs* are also called *vegetalistas.* There are other kinds of shamans, seers, and healers in that watershed who are not *vegetalistas* – *yachaqs* who are spirit mediums, or who work with dowsing, or with spells – but the *vegetalistas* are the plant specialists.

Vegetalistas differ in their opinions as to which plants ought to be studied first, which last, even which plants to use as teachers at all. Some *vegetalistas* use only one plant, like tobacco, while others have intercourse with three or four. Some may maintain relations with as many as a dozen, but as there are many more than a dozen possible power plants, even in localized regions, it is clear that different doctors are going to have different teachers and different methods.

Often, it's true, shamanism runs in families or clans, and it is not unusual for shamans who are related by blood or marriage to share lore or plants. But every true *vegetalista* has to meet *Sacha Runa,* the Forest Person, face to face. In the jungle.

Sacha Runa is like us, except that he lives in the forest.
Sacha Runa is the one who takes care of the animals –
  the one who lets them out in the morning.

By jungle I really mean primary forest – forest that hasn't been cleared – that's where Sacha Runa lives. And it's through Sacha Runa that one is introduced to the plant teachers, the *doctoritos.* Sometimes Sacha Runa will come out from behind a ceibo tree and say hello to a person who wasn't even looking for him. But not usually. Usually one has to fast, purify oneself, maintain a strict diet of no salt or domestic meat, and go out into the forest and wait for him, sometimes a long time. I said *him,* but more likely the forest person will be *her,* unless you are female yourself.

Jaguar, crocodile,
  anaconda, puma.

Oftentimes the Forest Woman, *Sacha Huarmi,* will appear in the form of a relative, and if you don't know what you are doing, you will just say "Hello," or "What a surprise to see you here," and go on your way. If you do that you may have lost your chance. Or maybe Sacha Huarmi will look like a friend or an old acquaintance, or, as I once heard from a young *vegetalista,* like a beautiful green-skinned, green-eyed, green-haired woman.

Sometimes the forest person will be sitting in a chair that is really an anaconda, and will ask you if you want to learn. If this happens, just say yes.

> *A brilliant macaw headdress, nine*
> *necklaces of toucan feathers,*
> *twelve bracelets she wears,*
> *a skirt woven of bark, a feathered lance –*
> *a new blowgun, perhaps, for you, and perhaps*
> *a little iron pot filled with medicines . . .*

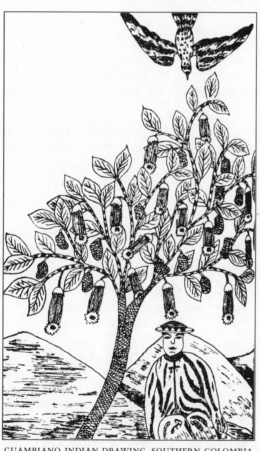

GUAMBIANO INDIAN DRAWING, SOUTHERN COLOMBIA

The forest person will scrutinize you closely. Maybe she will sniff you. Maybe not. But she will size you up, that's for sure. Sacha Huarmi wants to see if you are *complete,* if you have the fiber to see the training through to the end.

Maybe you have not kept the diet and you will be too afraid. That's OK, you can probably get another chance. If you still want to! If you pass, Sacha Runa will clean you with a bundle of *sutu panga* leaves. Then she will give you some handy stuff, like a couple of soldiers perhaps, for protection, and then she will begin the teaching by giving you a plant, and a song.

And more, but we'll get to that.

ON THE NATURE OF THE ALLY

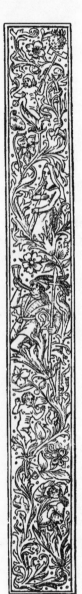

There are many dimensions in alliance space, and the pharmacological axis is only one of many. The old doctors had helpers like

> *mountain lion, owl.*

Maybe the power plant was a conduit, or a call, a sort of whistle. Or the plant was like a delivery service. Not like the plant itself was the ally.

> *maybe the ally lived in the plant,*
> > *or maybe the ally lived in the next world, and the*
> > *plant was like a bridge . . .*

That plants have *virtues,* or "vertues," was known by the ancient herbalists. The virtue of a plant was its truth, its strength. Maybe the best synonym is *integrity.* Or power. Or poison.

And we see how plants are used. If a patient is suffering from heat in the spine, the herbalist will find an herb with a poison that effects exactly those same symptoms and give the patient *a small amount* of that herb.

> *Similia similibus curantur.*

Fighting fire with fire. Thus we have *homeopathy.*

Or a *curandero* applies a particular plant to a skin rash, not because the plant causes a similar rash, but because the juice of the plant alleviates the condition. Maybe the rash is caused by a fungus and the plant contains an herbicide. This is *allopathy.*

And there is another kind of medicine distinct from either of the above. This is the kind of medicine taken by the doctor, not by the patient. Let's ignore the advice of a great poet and make up a word for this kind of healing, *iatropathy.* Here we are in the realm of the *ally.*

The ally is the one who helps you. That is what an ally should do. Allies assist each other in the prosecution of some task.

Allies may also have agendas of their own, however. That is, an ally is not like a fairy-godmother, but is a powerful force in its own right.

An ally is like a half-broken horse, a horse with spirit. A horse that will carry you many days, only to suddenly knock you off on a low branch. Some allies are the subtle type. Maybe you have an ayahuasca ally. She is friendly. She gives you things. She doesn't seem at all malevolent. Or maybe you have an opium ally. She is more than friendly. She'll call you up and invite you over. And she is voluptuous, so you go. She is so good to you it seems like heaven. You get what I mean.

> *The Goddess brought them inside, bade them sit down, and mixed for*
> *them a potion of ground barley, cheese, pale honey, and Pramneian wine,*
> *but added to the mixture the medicines of gloom, that make one utterly*
> *forget his true home.*
>
>   *– Homer, Odyssey*

But if the ally did not have power, why would you be interested?

> *Killers:*
> *a damn lot of them –*

Allies live in the wilderness. That is a good place to find them. Don't get hung up looking for jaguars: mountains can be allies, rain is an ally, minerals are allies. Some are more active and some are more passive. Some you can trust, with some you need to parley; some are so powerful it doesn't matter whether you trust them or not. Go alone.

> *i will go to the mountain to-night!*
> *he will come, he will come!*
> *he will scare me.*
>
>   *– Jaime de Angulo*

We grew up with plant poisons. That plant poisons resemble the chemicals of our own nervous system is not a coincidence. We selected each other – fought great battles on microbial slimes – traded partners and parasites in a primordial orgy.

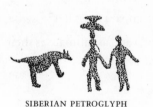

SIBERIAN PETROGLYPH

> *We become trackers, threading through a labyrinth of rocks,*
> *plasma, toxic saps. Nucleic acids,*
> *like a sexual differentiation: iron versus magnesium,*
> *chitin versus cellulose, tracking backwards.*
> *High up in the cliffs find a niche,*
> *wait, fast, find*
> *traces of ochre fading on the sandstone.*
> *Paintings on rocks, yerba santa thick in the air.*

> *It had many legs. It had two heads.*

Once you have an ally, you have to be able to talk to it. Usually an ally understands what you what to know, but it is best to be specific. Sometimes an ally will tell you something that you need to know more than what you asked about. Sometimes it is not pleasant.

> *Name the voices. Don't be judgmental. Be ready to make deals. Try to get*
> *something for yourself.*

They never give anything for free. None of them do, not the most wholly and thoroughly benevolent, not the sun itself.

You think that you can write about this!

Yes.

[Laughter]

If I have to turn my back on you I will do it.

Let's talk about your job.

OK.

Bringing it home a little bit, aren't you?

Look around you!

If this is supposed to be your office, make it at least look like work gets done here.

Right. Guess I screwed up at that meeting today.

No. Stop worrying. Your style is not going to bother them. They don't want some dumbshit, they want you.

Yeah.

One last thing. Don't you think that telling the world about your ally is a little like telling your wife about an affair?

The ally says that it would be wise to come see her from time to time. Like once a week to once a month. And especially when decisions are involved.

But then an ally WOULD say that, wouldn't she? How can you trust her?

Some doctors find their ally ever close at hand. As natural and as intimate as their own breathing.

PRUNUS EMARGINATA

Common Names	Bitter cherry, the Mad River plant.
Related Species	*Prunus serotina,* wild cherry; *Prunus virginiana,* chokecherry; *Prunus ilicifolia,* holly-leaved cherry.
Taxonomy	Rose family.
Part Used	Leaves, dried stem bark.
Pharmacognosy	The chemistry of *Prunus emarginata* is not well studied, but probably is similar to *Prunus serotina,* wild cherry. The presence of cyanide is a likely possibility, so do not ingest the leaves!

Wild cherry, *Prunus serotina,* contains a cyanogenic glycoside called prunasin, which is formed by the partial hydrolysis of amygdalin, common throughout the genus, especially in the almonds. The hydrocyanic acid (HCN) content varies from up to 0.32 percent in the inner bark to practically zero in the trunk bark. The cyanide content seems to depend on the amount of photosynthesis associated with a specific area of bark, the greener areas being much higher in cyanide than the reddish or brown areas. This is significant in that the stems of *Prunus emarginata* are uniformly a deep reddish brown.

Enzymes must act on the glycosides to release the cyanide. In the leaves, this apparently occurs when they wilt or, more importantly, when in the alimentary canal of an animal or a person. Very little HCN remains in leaves that have been dried, however. So while it is possible that pyrolation releases HCN, it seems equally likely that the effects observed through bioassay are due to an as yet unidentified principle.

How Taken — Leaves are stripped from the branchlets and allowed to dry in the air. A few dried leaves are crushed and smoked in a small pipe. A lungful or two is enough.

Smoking the dried leaves was my idea. At Hoopa in northwestern California, the Indians take strips of dried bark in a tea, or keep them directly on the tongue, as a medicinal tonic similar to wild cherry.

Effects — Sedative, without diminishing mental alertness. Or mental stimulant, without bodily agitation.

Prunus serotina, wild cherry, is well known in syrups, where it is considered to be a sedative and an expectorant.

The Ally   The Mad River ally is for impatient artists, for those whose muse pulls them in so many directions at once that they are unable to sit still and actually get something done.

While the Mad River plant does not produce true euphoria, of pleasanter smokes there be not many.

The Plant   I learned about this plant from a basket weaver at Hoopa. She was a plant person through collecting her basket-weaving materials as much as through herbalism. She had several native California plants growing around her home as medicinals, as well as a couple of exotics — one interesting palmate-leaved plant she called *Indian tobacco,* a name I had never before heard applied to this plant of a hundred names.

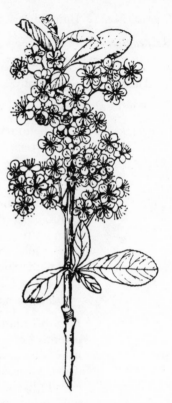

I had told her that I was looking for a plant to relax me, to calm my nerves, and she, after gazing at me for a while, told me about a plant that grew by the Mad River bridge in Humboldt County, California. She made a little drawing of the way the leaves grow on the twigs and told me I would know the plant by the bitter taste of the bark.

> *The bitterness, she said, that's how you know the medicine.*

This genus is best known, poison-wise, for the kernels in the pits. That is where the cyanide is the strongest. Laetrile come from the pits of apricots, another *Prunus* species. My Hoopa teacher told me that apricot pits were "only for shamans." I've never tried them.

PRUNUS EMARGINATA

In the Trinity Mountains I've found *Prunus emarginata* at 4,500 feet, but in the Sierra Nevada it is usually at higher elevations, above 6,000 feet. Sometimes it lives around mountain lakes, other times it is right up on the ridges. It has a distinctive heavy smell, almondy and sweet without being floral. Once you know it, you can detect the plants at some distance.

THE GREAT WORK

The Great Work is accomplished through the *Great Stone.*

Why settle for less?

The Great Stone is the *lapis philosophorum,* the wondrous stone of the Philosophers, and the Grail of our Quest. The stone is something you create, not something you find lying around. The Great Work consists of preparing the Great Stone and then applying it. It is the preparation of the stone that is crucial, alchemically. After all, stones are many, and easy to come by. The application of the stone is the last stage of the process and is called *reddening* by some alchemists and *yellowing* by others. As Paracelsus said, the Philosopher must develop the stone from potentiality into activity. Temper is important here. After the individual application there is the public, marketplace application. It is important not to neglect this political aspect of the process, as the political aspect will certainly not neglect you!

He with ears to hear, let him hear.

In traditional Western alchemy the elements are sulphur and quicksilver – sulphur, quicksilver, and salt forming the alchemical triad. (And the triad is Hegelian in the sense that salt feeds back into sulphur.) Sulphur is said to fix the breath, the spirit, the quicksilver part. Quicksilver, mercury, is *pneuma,* what the Taoists call *yin,* the solvent that dissolves away the fixed part, the sulphur, the part that is stuck. And the process is repetitive: it is like an alembic flask with the long neck bent around and joined to itself, so that the distillate returns to the boiling chamber. That is because sulphur has this fiery, insistent aspect that won't quite go away with any amount of mercury. (Don't try to disprove this!) So Jacob Böhme says:

> *Sulphur is in the outward world, viz., in the mystery of the great God's manifestation, the first mother of the creatures. . . . Mercury is the wheel of motion in the Sulphur.*
>
> – *Jacob Böhme, Signatura Rerum*

As for our mercury, never forget that though it is most essential for our work and much beloved, it contains a subtle poison. Both Böhme and Paracelsus agree on this point. Paracelsus adds that it is the work of the alchemist to separate the poison from the arcanum.

The poison attacks the fixed properties (themselves moribund poisons) and dissolves them. Poison is antidote and antidote poison. When everything fixed and dissoluble is dissolved, continued cooking yields the salt. Salt is the ash, the basic part, the Philosopher's Sal.

The Sal is what was there all along, the part you can't see until you get rid of everything else.

It's your birthright.

Geber called the raising of the dry matter, so that it collects and adheres in the head of its own flask, *sublimation.* Paracelsus said that sublimation is the single and only operation of the Work.

After your cooking, get rid of the salt. Perhaps with mercury. The salt is already tainted, has become something else, become something. There is not really any problem here. The salt takes on a yellow cast because the sulphur is self-engendering. And, as I say, that's not bad. The *process* is what's important, that the transmutation continue. If you let the alembic cool, metaphor becomes superstition.

Psychologists sometimes miss this point.
Poets ought never.

THE WILL within a seed determines the outer
two truths in his work. +Victor Hammer+
form of the plant, a crystal possesses an intellect that creates
will form & order / & with eye & hand try to re-create these
its ordered geometric shapes. Man too must

PLANT & CRYSTAL

WOODCUT BY VICTOR HAMMER, 1938

So what is the mercury, for a plant person? Well, there are so many levels. On one level it is the plant itself. On another level, mercury is the active principle. Then again, clearly, it is liquified consciousness. Or again, it is the *act,* or, more subtly, the *desire* that leads to the act. Now we can see the poisonous part.

In the corporeal realm, mercury is identified with blood and semen. Sulphur is the water in which they burn.

Sulphur is the womb whereinto we
must enter, if we would be new born.

— Jacob Böhme, Signatura Rerum

So sulphur is the matrix, the *material.* That should be plain. Plain, if those alchemists didn't keep using the same word to mean different things in different sentences.

It happened that, meditating on things
as they are, my mind beccoming sublime
and my senses calmed, as one sated
with pleasures or exhausted from
fatigue, a being, of vast and boundless
form, appeared before me and called
my name and asked:

"What is it you want to know? What is it you want to see?"

— Hermes Trismegistus, opening lines of Poimandres

Traditionally, the vegetable work has been considered inferior to the work on metals. There is perhaps some truth to this assertion, especially in regard to the work with *elementals,* as much as such relativism, well, is relevant. But alchemists working with metals can wander off as endlessly into involuted spirals as any *vegetalista,* as history attests. At least in the vegetable work there is a connection to the earth as fertility and life — while the mineral work is subterranean, rooted beneath the deepest mines. I'm of course speaking vulgarly here. Nonetheless, for the purist, I have attempted to maintain alchemical correspondences.

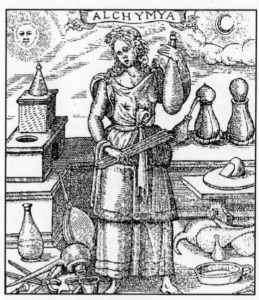

Become one with the work. The true alchemist is no different from the work itself.

THE ROYAL ART

SUN MEDICINE / MOON MEDICINE

On the Poison Path we speak of *sun medicine* and *moon medicine*. And likewise then, there are *sun doctors* and *moon doctors*. For the Great Work neither can be neglected.

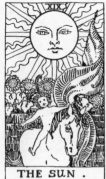

THE SUN .

The life of man is governed by the rhythm of sun and moon. Sun and moon, therefore, became the first symbols under which the human mind tried to understand the universe in which man lived.

– Lama Anagarika Govinda, Psycho-cosmic Symbolism of the Buddhist Stupa

The sun doctor moves easily through the world, unperturbed, seemingly able to open doors anywhere she wishes. A life filled with routines and good health, with attendence to detail and reliability, the sun doctor knows where she stands.

The moon doctor has no need for ground. Realities scatter before him like tarot cards in the wind. He flies to the stars and has his way with the Queen of Heaven in her celestial palace. The moon doctor rides dragons and knows the way through hell. The sun doctor knows how to stay out of hell, and does. To the sun doctor every day is unique, every day happens for the first time. To the moon doctor there are no days. He lives in one instant only, eternally preparing the lunar medicine.

In both the solar and the lunar practices, the medicine comes from the salt. You begin with sulphur and prepare the salt with quicksilver.

As concise a summation of alchemy as you're likely to hear, I daresay.

For poisoners, for the vegetable work, it is most important to have strong sun medicine. Strong sun medicine will allow you to go further in the night – will act as an anchor and a beacon in the realms beyond Arcturus – might save you, even, from an ignoble rebirth. Sometimes it is easier to leave one's body than it is to find it again.

Solar medicine is evident. You can spot it in a person's stance and posture. In style, the sun doctor is conventional or outlandish, but if outlandish, precisely so. Lunar medicine is more subtle. Moon doctors survive where others succumb. In jewels or in rags, or naked and covered with ashes, they will eat worms or a road kill, if worms or a road kill are what is served for dinner. Some say that for the lunar master, solar medicine is unimportant. But not so. You need both of them, together.

> *There are two great Bodhisattvas in this country. The name of one is Radiance of the Sun, and that of the other Radiance of the Moon. . . . They guard the treasury of the right doctrine of this Master of Healing, Azure Radiance Tathagata.*
>
> — *Bhaishajyaguru Vaiduryaprabha Tathagata, Sutra of the Lord of Healing*

Solar sulphur burns, a star with legs. Carbohydrates blossom into oxides: long life, health. Architects plan the City of the Sun; robots roam the earth.

In the lunar realm, sulphur moistens, genitals engorge. The poisonous sulphur struggles with its own inertia. Corporeally, the body lusts. But the static tendency is more like a Pythagorean dodecahedron than like, say, a pencil or any mineral crystal, or any piece of living flesh.

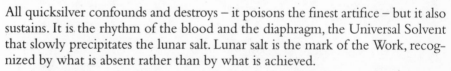

> *Sulphur is the fixer,*
> *Mercury the trickster.*

Solar mercury involves chance, lunar mercury seeks luck. In the solar mercury we find *God's Will,* in the lunar mercury a sorcerer.

> *The Two of Pentacles. Strength. The Magus*

The solar mercury is a tragedian, the lunar mercury wears motley. The lunar mercury dissolves immensities – it is yoga, not philosophy. Mind, body, thoughts, and desires blow away in a whirlwind orgy.

All quicksilver confounds and destroys – it poisons the finest artifice – but it also sustains. It is the rhythm of the blood and the diaphragm, the Universal Solvent that slowly precipitates the lunar salt. Lunar salt is the mark of the Work, recognized by what is absent rather than by what is achieved.

> *Its father is the Sun and its mother is the Moon. The Wind carries it in its belly. Its nurse is the earth.*
>
> — *Hermes Trismegistus, Precepts*

As quicksilver contains the seed of sulphur, and sulphur the seed of quicksilver, solar medicine is partly lunar, and lunar partly solar.

> *In the absence of Sol, Luna thins.*

Sun medicine without moon medicine wreaks havoc on the earth. What is the H-bomb but solar fire stripped of matter?

Radiolarian? Mountain asters? That great flower, so weary of time?

The pure moon doctor is the sorcerer, the necromancer. Slimy and spineless, moon doctors steal to get by. They blow fetid life into old myths and sell them as cures. With hollow eye sockets, they feed on fear, lurkers on the threshold of life. Sometimes they write books. Lunar/solar: one deals in dreams, one meddles in matters; which is the ranker poison?

Let the rain wash away the salt.

In the vegetable work, solar alchemy is associated with carbohydrates and free oxygen, while the lunar alchemy is associated with nitrogen and carbon dioxide.

SCIRPUS ATROVIRENS

Common Name   Bulrush.

Taxonomy   Part of the great sedge family, the Cyperaceae, aquatic plants characterized by triangular stems. Other genera within the family include the sedges, *Carex* spp., and *Cyperus,* tough little ditch plants with long graceful bracts subtending the inflorescence. Papyrus is a species of *Cyperus,* and many other species within the family worldwide are used in mat making and basketry.

Part Used   Rootstock, bulblets.

Chemistry   Unknown, although alkaloids are probably present.

Scirpus atrovirens is a good example of how much investigation still remains to done. Here is a plant, known to be psychoactive, from a very common family, that we know very little about. Its chemistry is uncertain, and few of the hundreds of other species within the genus have ever been studied for psychoactivity. The Tarahumara both revere and fear this plant, claiming that the powers of the plant would drive anyone foolish enough to cultivate it insane.

Scirpus is a widely distributed genus, and while plant chemistry can vary a great deal from species to species, and even among strains of one species, the fact that

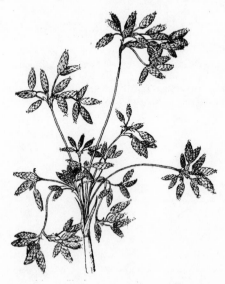

SCIRPUS CALIFORNICUS, "CALIFORNIA BULRUSH"

alkaloids have been discovered in both *Scirpus* and *Cyperus* indicate that local species of both genera are worth some investigation.

How does one investigate? Here we get into methodology. One way is to listen for folklore or ethnic uses of the plant from people who have shared its habitat. Is the plant on any list of medicinals? Does it play a part in any myths? Lists of poisonous plants are also good pointers. *Scirpus americanus* is suspected of producing pulmonary emphysema in cattle in Wyoming. But remember that nobody knows all the plants. There are plant allies waiting that no one has yet discovered.

Effects   The Tarahumara report that the species of rush that they call *bakana* induces brilliantly colored visions, as well as the ability to travel great distances and to speak with the dead.

The Plant   *Scirpus,* or bulrush, is cosmopolitan, but prefers the temperate and subarctic zones. Two species in India are used medicinally, *S. grossus* for diarrhea and *S. articulatus* as a purgative. Montane species of *Scirpus* are generally two or three feet high, but the California tule rush grows to more than fifteen feet in height. Indians used the tule rush to make boats.

> *Floating among the tules on tules . . .*
> *Tule elk. Tule huts, the rushes tied over bent willow ribs.*

The draining of the marshes in the Great Central Valley of California may have been the largest destruction of wildlife in the whole American westward expansion except for the slaughter of the bison.

> *Tule huts. Tule skirts. Tule fog.*
> *Tule mind.*

Related Species   Thousands, worldwide. An Amazonian *Cyperus* called *piri-piri,* in addition to its many medicinal uses, is used as an admixture to ayahuasca. A fungus that reportedly infects every cultivar produces ergot alkaloids.

The *Cyperus* genus is generally shorter than *Scirpus.* They all have the triangular stem characteristic of the Cyperaceae.

METHODOLOGY I

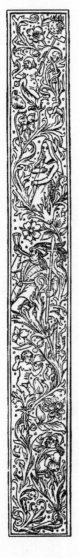

Ethnobotany should be considered a proper subset of our Work. Ethnobotanists are generally both botanists and anthropologists, and it is essential for the owl-chemist to have a basic knowledge of these two disciplines if she is to avoid certain terrible pitfalls of the path, such as clownish foppery or early death.

No mistake here about the seriousness of our endeavor and its concomitant dangers. I remember once seeing a group of edible *Agaricus* in a meadow near an old oak tree. And right in the middle of the cluster was an *Amanita phalloides,* the veil washed off by a recent rain, and the characteristic greenish yellow of the pileus faded to a cream color that just matched the edible meadow mushrooms surrounding it. I remember thinking how if that one mushroom were carelessly dropped into a collecting basket along with the other mushrooms, the stew would contain enough poison to take away not only the collector, but his family and any guest at his table as well.

> . . . *the world's most dangerous sport.*

Ethnobotany, and ethnology generally, are important to our Quest for several reasons. For one, traditionally, poisoners have never lived in a vacuum – which is really a tautology. They worked within a cultural context that, if not actively supporting and encouraging their efforts, at least provided the "special consensus," to borrow Carlos Castaneda's term, necessary for spiritual, social, and psychological integration. Which can be the difference between being an eccentric and being a freak.

Learning about traditional cultures can dispel or correct storybook and Hollywood preconceptions and images relating to posture and stance of poison doctors within their societies. Native and traditional peoples have been studying plants for countless generations: they are the experts. It is best to learn one's plantcraft from the experts. However, unless you are going to *go native,* and live and learn your medicine within an adopted culture, the best place to study ethnology is in a library. An opportunity to do fieldwork should not be passed up, but even fieldwork is not a replacement for library work. Years of work by ethnobotanists is already collected in scientific journals and books.

And getting back to matters of risk – the plants of interest to us, by definition, contain poisons. Certain people and peoples have already conducted extensive tests on these plants – much more protracted studies than could be carried out by the Food and Drug Administration (FDA) in a mere generation. If you can meet, or even read about, people who have been using a particular plant for centuries, that puts some upper bound on the toxicity of the plant in question. (It does not mean that the plant is completely safe; witness tobacco. But then, only a fool would consider any poison to be safe!)

> *The most valuable standpoints are always the last to be found, but the most valuable standpoints are the methods.*
> — *Friedrich Wilhelm Nietzsche*

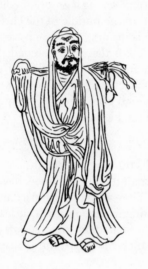

BODHIDHARMA WITH TEA PLANT

GROUND STATE CALIBRATION

Ground state training begins with *nigredo,* and the calibration continues through the *albedo* stage, the sudden flowering of the peacock's tail. *Nigredo* is about coming down. And to come down, all the way down, takes some time. You cannot do it overnight, and you cannot do it by getting high. Nor, as the wise maintain, can you do it by reading or thinking. Body and mind must come to rest.

If you do not know the ground state intimately, how will you be able to separate the signal from the noise, during the phase of amplification?

We speak of a sulphurous ground state and a mercurial ground state. For the sulphurous ground state, attention to diet, even fasting, can be efficacious. And we must interpret *diet* in the largest possible meaning of the word.

We seek the salt, beneath the patina.

By mercurial ground state we do not mean that you have stopped breathing – that would mean you are dead– another matter, as it were. Our mercurial ground state is the "Unground," the source of will and freedom.

The Unground is an eternal Nothing but it gives an eternal beginning, that is, a passion; for the Nothing is a passion for Something.
    – Jacob Böhme, Six Theosophic Points

Just letting the mercury circulate is the whole method. The circulating mercury dissolves the sulphurous corruption. When you attain the Unground you have the salt.

To Sal, all is clear. There is no confusion. You know the true ground state. You know what the stone is, and where it is. You know your own original nature. You know how to proceed. So what I want to know is, since you have this Sal, why are you still interested in poisons?

A fair calibration.

METHODOLOGY II

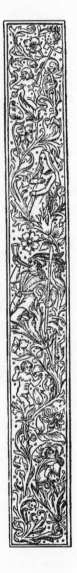

In a dark age such as our own, it is difficult to find the true poison path: difficult to find the living tradition, difficult to find a living teacher. Several religious groups practice in traditional ways: the Native American Church, the *Santo Daime* in Brazil, and the *União do Vegetal,* also in Brazil, are three examples that come to mind. Visit them if you have an opportunity. But otherwise, opportunities are scarce. And "going native," except for certain true misfits, is more often a diversion than a way to harmonic power. Thus we seek for roots and models in the Royal Art – itself at the fringe of things, even in its heyday. The very origins of the alchemical tradition lie in syncretism: Greek religion, Egyptian technology, Jewish *Kabbalah.* Heterodoxy is its nature, and thus it suits our purposes well.

Alchemy involved reading and study, but also experimentation. At some point every alchemist has to try something that hasn't been tested before – something that you can't read about in a book.

The process of extracting the mercury from the sulphur with the alchemical furnace we will call *pyrolation,* and the process of dissolving the mercury in the alchemical flask we will, following tradition, call *ingestion.* Clear enough?

Further, since, as stated most succinctly by the wise Kintpuash, also called Captain Jack, the Modoc chief,

> *Life is sweet,*

when experimenting with an unknown sulphur, go slowly indeed. Search for clues as to the nature of the mercury by scouring for reports in the literature, or reports on its relatives (other members of its family), or folklore.

Do not go into our art blindly. If you, O alchemist, wish to live a whole life – neither ended abruptly by lethal toxins, nor shortened by slow toxins, nor mutated by carcinogens – most certainly, before you experiment,

KNOW THE POISONS!

The more you know about poisons the better chance you have of avoiding them.

> *And it wouldn't take very long to spot an alkaloid test with some Dragendorff reagent, either. We'll talk more about that later.*

So, the alchemist knows the poisons, and knows that his sulphur is within a tolerable dosage. At that point, assuming the material is suitable, I often prefer to begin testing the mercury by pyrolation – again, beginning with a small quantity. If you have good ground state calibration, it is frequently possible to extrapolate

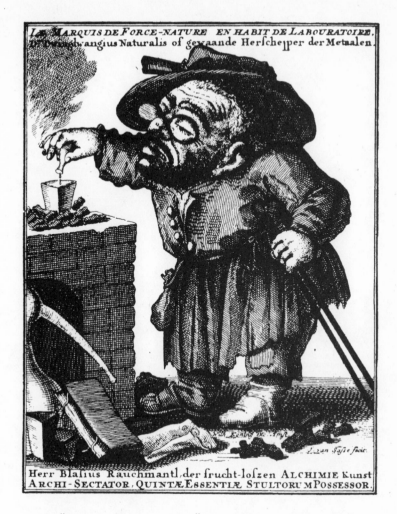

THE "MARQUIS DE FORCE-NATURE" IN HIS LABORATORY DRESS, 1716

the general properties of the substance without recourse to ingestion, which is usually more dangerous.

There. That's about as irresponsible as I can be, in good conscience.

> *With the objective of getting to the bottom of this, I decided on a self-experiment. In order to be cautious I therefore began the planned series of experiments with the smallest quantity with which a definite effect could just barely be expected, considering the activity of the ergot alkaloids known at the time, namely with 0.25 mg lysergic acid diethylamide tartrate. . . .*
>
> *– Albert Hofmann, "How LSD Originated"*

THANATOPATHIA

Here are the gates. Crossroads.

Without hesitation the beautiful goddess replied:
"Zeus-sprung son of Laertes, resourceful Odysseus,
In my house stay no longer against your will,
But before I can send you home, there's one more journey
You must make, to the halls of Hades and dread
Persephone, to hear the truth from Tiresias the blind
Theban seer, whose mind even death has spared."

          – Homer, *Odyssey*

You need a bridge. And barter.

To commune with the Spiritual, the crux of matter. For intercourse with the Other, the heart of issue. At the intersection of the Axes, Origin.

Here is Exú,
midnight Exú
Exú of intersections!
Here are Exú and his wife,
the lovely Pomba-Gira!
He's wearing his black cape
he's wearing his black hat
he's wearing his polished shoes.
With his iron trident in his hand,
Here is Exú,
midnight Exú
Exú of intersections!

        – Macumba song (in Bramly 1975)

Exú likes cigars.

Nigredo   Alchemically, the obvious place to begin. To prepare the material, a lot has to die and slough off. This stage is sometimes called *putrefactio*. In shamanism, this is the stage of initiation: sickness, death, dismemberment. Perhaps a visit to the Lowerworld. *Thanatopathics* are allies that can re-create the initiatory sickness. In varying degrees, *thanatopathics* let you taste death.

The Great Work is healing. If you can figure out how to heal yourself, then you know something for sure. You have expertise. So you have to be sick. And maybe you want to be really good at this healing, so you want to practice. And how can you practice without poison?

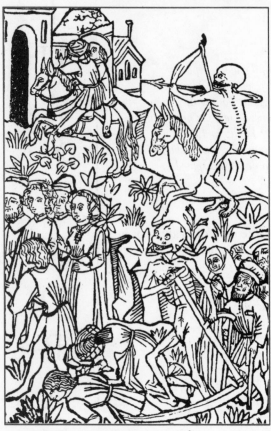

WEAPONS OF DEATH, 1463

Intoxicate means "to poison," "to drug." Greek *toxicon* literally meant "arrow-poison," related to the Sumerian word *tukul,* "a weapon." All *thanatopathics* are weapons – used to kill animals, if not people.

> *A brush with death is stimulating indeed;*
> *A closer taste rather calms.*

Some practitioners rely on the poisons they already have.

> *Beyond that: shadows, rivers, ferrymen.*
> *Eternal peace, or great terror.*
> *Thanatopathia.*

NICOTIANA TABACUM AND RELATED SPECIES

Common Names Tobacco, *petún, piciétl.*

Taxonomy The two cultivated species are *Nicotiana tabacum* and *N. rusticum.* Both of these species are tetraploids, the result of a fertile hybrid between two wild species sometime in antiquity, evidently in the Andean region of South America. Almost all American and European commercial tobaccos are *Nicotiana tabacum.*

There are some five dozen wild species of *Nicotiana,* three-quarters of them native to the Americas. These species include *N. glauca, N. sylvestris, N. trigonophylla, N. attenuata, N. bigelovii,* and *N. petunioides.* Nicotine content is highest in the cultivated species, and is much higher in *Nicotiana rustica* than in *Nicotiana tabacum.*

Part Used Leaves.

Chemistry Alkaloids: primarily nicotine; secondary alkaloids such as nornicotine and anabasine are also present, especially in some of the other *Nicotiana* species. Harman, a harminelike alkaloid, has been found in the smoke of some tobaccos. Expect a lot of variation in the effects among the different species and among different strains of the domestic species.

How Taken Tobacco is ingested by drinking, smoking, snorting, chewing, sucking, licking, by applying it topically as an ointment, and by inserting it rectally as an enema. Drinking a strong decoction is probably the oldest method. Frequently the solution is drunk through the nostrils, said to induce blacknesss and red flashes in the drinker's vision. Tobacco snuffs are also ancient, the tobacco sometimes being mixed with other hallucinogenic plants. There is ancient archaeological evidence for tobacco enemas. Smoking may be a more recent development, though some tubular pipes uncovered in a dig have been dated at three thousand years. Tobacco may be the oldest cultigen in America, going back more than eight thousand years and antedating food plants. Among many Indian tribes, such as the Sinkyone in California, tobacco was the only cultivated crop.

The Plant All the treachery of our beloved poisons is evident in this plant. It is a stimulant, a tranquilizer, a narcotic, and, if we are to believe the ethnobotanical reports, a hallucinogen. It is also the most toxic plant regularly used by human beings. Tobacco is a model of ambiguity: healer and killer, ally and seducer. As poison, it is the type.

> *Spin off, keep them back.*
> *Calm my fears, I will speak.*

Tobacco is the primary shamanic plant of the New World. Within this plant are prototypes of all the lessons of the Poison Path. You could learn them all from this one plant . . . if it didn't kill you first.

> *And it will get you, if you play with it.*
>   *Maybe you chip, nip, lick around the edges,*
> *but it will get you, if you keep it up.*

If you can't kick a tobacco habit you are no *doctor,* and had best not proceed. Face it, you lack the solar salt. And consider, there are even greater dangers ahead. Further, I certainly don't want to get blamed for your demise, which quite possibly would be most miserable. You will cough. You will gasp for breath. You will suffocate at sea level, immersed in an ocean of air.

> *Graffito:* "SMOKING IS A DYING ART."

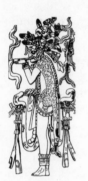

MAYAN RAIN
GOD, SMOKING

Like a drowning man, you will panic and lash out at those around you, curse your own friends and family, and hurt those who love you most. What makes you think you can succeed where so many others have failed? Besides, you are fine just where you are. There is nothing to accomplish by continuing.

> *Turn back now. Freud was never able to quit. The longest he ever stayed off*
> *was fourteen months, "all of it torture."*

And don't think that approaching tobacco as a sacrament gives you any exemption. Andrew Weil suggested that the reason the South American Indians experienced hallucinogenic effects from tobacco, while we do not, is that the Indians only used tobacco on special occasions, as a sacred plant; but I must differ with him. While it is true that in traditional shamanic cultures tobacco is used ritually rather than recreationally, that does not mean that it is used infrequently. The South American shamans have almost all addicted themselves to tobacco, methodically, so that they can tolerate larger and larger doses.

> *When Rocio began her apprenticeship, her teacher gave her infusions*
> *of tobacco to drink every day for a month. She was vomiting up blood.*
> *At the end of a month he took her into the jungle and gave her a draught*
> *of guanto – left her there and told her that the guanto would show her*
> *the way back.*

Tobacco is the great purifier. That is part of its weapon-nature. If you are going to mess with poisons, tobacco is a good plant to be friends with. As an ally, it is fire for fire and earth for earth.

> *Sometimes a plant ally gets uppity, especially some of them. Sometimes*
> *Salvia divinorum grows up through the ground where your feet are resting,*
> *then rushes up through your legs and body. Sometimes the stems get too*
> *numerous: twisting, crossing, leaves sprouting before your face, covering eyes –*
> *at such a time, if you need a respite, a little tobacco will push the ally back*
> *to about arm's length. For a while, anyway.*

In our culture, with our mild tobaccos and our cigarettes, we have forgotten the hammerlike power of *Nicotiana*. We read the early accounts and wonder if it is the same plant we are so frequently bothered by in restaurants. And in most cases, indeed, it is not the same plant.

> *The Indians say that this smoke is very wholesome for clearing and consuming superfluous humors of the brain. Moreover, if taken in this manner it satisfies hunger and thirst for some time. They also commonly use it if they have to discuss some matters among themselves: they draw in the smoke and then speak . . .*
>
> *– André Thevet (in Schleiffer 1973)*

Thevet was a Franciscan friar. It was Thevet, not Nicot, who introduced *Nicotiana tabacum* into Europe in the mid-1500s. Nicot's seeds were evidently *Nicotiana rustica*. Tobacco of the *rustica* species had been known in Spain for several generations before Thevet introduced *N. tabacum* into France, but it had been used almost exclusively as a medicine, not as a recreational drug.

TOBACCO
FLOWER, FROM
AZTEC STATUE
OF THE GOD
XOCHIPILLI

The balance of alkaloids varies among the different species and strains. In some varieties of *Nicotiana rustica* the nicotine content of the leaves approaches 20 percent. Since one or two drops of pure nicotine are a lethal dose, it's clear that, as the gangsters say, we're playing hardball.

> *The Tibetans call tobacco the poisonous dakini killer. They say that tobacco smoke, like the smoke from burning flesh, attracts the wrong spirits, that tobacco grows where menstrual blood drops.*

The smoke from *Nicotiana rustica* is exceedingly strong. Some tobacco shamans have developed a technique of hyperventilating at the same time they are inhaling the smoke from a huge cigar, sucking in air along with the smoke. By doing this they are able get large quantities of the choking smoke into their lungs. They will continue smoking thus until falling unconscious – which after all is the whole point. This method is perhaps slightly safer than drinking tobacco infusions. Drinking, if the initiate does not vomit up the tobacco after losing consciousness, may result in death or permanent injury. The most hazardous technique of ingesting tobacco is the tobacco enema, wherein the danger of overdose is extreme.

Nicotiana tabacum usually contains nornicotine as a secondary alkaloid. Its effects are said to be similar to those of nicotine. *Nicotiana glauca,* the tree tobacco that has naturalized itself in southern California, contains the alkaloid anabasine, an isomer of nicotine. One plant person I know likes tree tobacco and smokes it, but I've always found it rather harsh. Eaten, of course, it can kill just as quickly as does nicotine, and has. Of the wild tobaccos of western North America, *Nicotiana attenuata,* coyote tobacco, is said to be particularly fine. But *Nicotiana acuminata* should also be tried, and in fact there may be some confusion between these two species.

Black tobacco is sometimes made from *Nicotiana rustica*, as are some Turkish tobaccos, but the major industrial use of *Nicotiana rustica* today is in the manufacture of insecticide.

> *I lived for some years in the Sierras in an uninsulated and somewhat drafty cabin. The cabin lay right across what must have been the wasp equivalent of an "elephant walk," because wasps of many varieties were constantly crawling in and out, making their way through, or collecting on the windows. Some of them stayed, and there was a paper-wasp nest right over the loft. At night, when we were in bed, the wasps were in bed also. As they were, at such times, all quiet on the nest, there was never any conflict of interest or great priority to remove the nest. But I do recall the way they would react to any wisp of tobacco smoke if we smoked in bed: instantly the whole nest abuzz – all the wasps stretched up on their thin legs, fanning angry wings . . .*

In the forests of the northwest Amazon *Nicotiana rustica* is made into heavy black cylinders, called *masu* or *mapuchu*. The rolls have the size and heft of a San Francisco sausage. You carve some of the tobacco off with a knife, stuff it in a pipe or roll it in a cornhusk, light it and *watch out!*

Pharmacology Nicotine is structurally similar to acetylcholine, a neurotransmitter active in both the sympathetic and the parasympathetic nervous systems, as well as in the somatic nervous system at neuromuscular junctures. Recent discoveries have also found acetylcholine in the central nervous system (CNS), which gives some neurochemical support for findings that nicotine affects learning.

> *Recognition of the nicotine molecule by cholinergic receptors is possible because the positive charge on its ammonium head and the electronegative charge of its pyridine ring are exactly the same distance apart from each other as are corresponding electrical charges on the acetylcholine molecule.*
>
> *– Johannes Wilbert (1987)*

In the CNS nicotine increases arousal and enhances the learning and performance of simple tasks. Performance of complex tasks has been shown to be impaired in studies by George Spilich (Brower 1993), but the mechanism is not understood and other investigators are skeptical of his results. All agree that dosage is critical to whether performance is enhanced or impaired.

The stimulant/sedative effects of nicotine may be due to the fact that nicotine binds more tightly to the nerve endings than does acetylcholine. Thus, while initially enabling a rush of nervous transmission, the nicotine stays on to monopolize the site, inhibiting further action.

Nicotine's parasympathetic stimulation of the smooth muscles of the digestive tract are well known. Its actions on the sympathetic nervous system are less well understood, but in addition to its direct action by mimicking acetycholine, nicotine stimulates the release of epinephrine (adrenaline) and dopamine, and in lesser amounts norepinephrine, and serotonin. Norepinephrine is a neurohormone chemically related to mescaline. The significance of these neurotransmitters to the alleged hallucinatory effects of tobacco is still inconclusive.

Toxic effects include perspiration, light-headedness, general weakness, tremors, convulsions, and respiratory paralysis.

Tobacco can induce amblyopia, a condition characterized by day blindness but enhanced night vision. Jaguar shamans like tobacco. Heavy tobacco use creates a strong body odor, a raspy voice, and a rough, furred tongue.

CORRESPONDENCES

ACTIVITY	Politics/Diplomacy
ANIMAL	Jaguar, Bison
ARCHETYPE	The Woman-Who-Waits
ART FORM	Theater
BODILY FUNCTION	Respiration
BODY PART	Back of Skull
BUDDHA REALM	Vajra
CHORD	Subdominant
COLOR	Yellow
CRUTCH FOR	Nervousness
DIMENSION	Point
DISCIPLINE	Rhetoric
ELEMENT	Earth
FORM OF ENERGY	Steam
FORM OF IGNORANCE	Artifice
GEMSTONE	Quartz/Zircon
GEOMETRY	Euclidean
GRAMMAR	Deterministic Finite State
HISTORICAL AGE	Paleolithic
IMAGE	The Calumet
LANDSCAPE	Clearings
LOGICAL OPERATOR	Nand

History   At the time of European contact, tobacco was more widely cultivated in the New World than maize. After its discovery by Europeans in the Caribbean, tobacco spread around the world more quickly than any plant in history, before or since. One of the reasons for its rapid spread, undoubtedly, is that nicotine is one of the most addictive substances known. Another reason is that tobacco was a favorite with sailors, and the mariners took it around with them.

> *Tobacco, I do assert, without fear of contradiction from the Avon Skylark, is the most soothing, sovereign and precious weed that ever our dear old mother Earth tendered to the use of man!*
>
> *− Ben Jonson, to Walter Raleigh in the Mermaid Tavern*

Early sailors told of the almost unbelieveable aphrodisiacal qualities of tobacco − how women, after taking tobacco, were more passionate and active . . . Whereas, in our culture, smoking tobacco is more commonly associated with the postcoital state.

> *Howard is a commercial fisherman in Alaska. It's hard to smoke out on the boat, out there, not so much because of the dampness as because you need your hands for work. So he takes "snoose," Copenhagen. A pinch just inside the lip. But you don't swallow the juice, you spit it. At sea on a small boat that is easy, but stateside, in drawing rooms or living rooms, it can present a problem.*
>
> *What he does is to carry around a beer bottle, or a can, and to use it as a spittoon. After a couple of hours such a bottle could collect a surprising quantity of liquid. Sometimes in the course of an evening, especially if there was any partying going on, he would have several bottles in use, leaving them around in different rooms, as he wandered from group to group. Now spitting into the mouth of a beer bottle is a neat trick, but that's not the point of the story. The point is that after enough beers, the dread event would occur. He, or some other guest, promiscuously snatching a beer off the table, would get a slug of snoose juice instead of beer . . .*

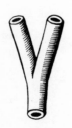

Nicotine is almost as readily absorbed through the skin as through the mucous membranes. I have availed myself of this fact by inserting a nice pinch of snoose between my two little toes. The effect is gentle and sustained. Used to be, if I found myself nodding out at a lecture or a meeting, I would pull out a tiny tin of snuff and snort a dash or two up my nostrils to wake up. Trouble is, at some kinds of meetings, people might think you were snorting coke. (And actually, about a pinhead of cocaine would do the job pretty well.) Anyway, an alternative to snuff at the corporate meeting, if you don't mind getting the reputation of being an eccentric, is to take off your shoe and sock and put a pinch of Copenhagen between your toes. Don't be overly obtrusive, just put your sock and shoe back on. Besides, why worry, if you are reading this you probably *already* have a reputation as an eccentric.

(Myself, however, these days, in such circumstances, I usually just stand up and pace around the room. Pacing is really better than stimulants. Not only does it awaken the circulation, but it also effects presence and breaks conceptual blocks, helping to free one from the confines of others' ideas.)

Snuff is about one hundred times safer than cigarettes. It is estimated that if the 40 million Americans who smoke switched to snuff, the 400,000 annual deaths would be reduced to 6,000. Snuff can cause oral cancer, but the survival rate for oral cancer is 75 percent, whereas the survival rate for lung cancer is only 13 percent.

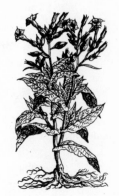

TOBACCO, FROM L'ECLUSE'S
HISTORIA MEDICINAL,
1579

> *Sublime tobacco! which, from east to west,*
> *Cheers the Tar's labor or the Turkman's rest.*
>
> — *Lord Byron, "Sublime Tobacco"*

There were many reactions against the tobacco plant as it conquered Europe. In the seventeenth century possession of tobacco was a capital offense in Russia, was prohibited in many parts of Germany, and was punishable by torture, beheading, hanging, quartering, or crushing in the Ottoman Empire. In England in 1604 King James I published *A Counterblaste to Tobacco,* unsuccessfully attempting to curb tobacco use and, by the by, proving that he was no wimp with the pen:

> *In your abuse thereof sinning against God, harming yourselves both in*
> *persons and goods, and taking also thereby the markes and notes of vanities*
> *upon you: by the custome thereof making your selves to be wondered at by*
> *all forraine civil Nations, and by all strangers that come among you, to be*
> *scorned and contemned. A custome lothsome to the eye, hateful to the Nose,*
> *harmefull to the braine, dangerous to the Lungs, and the blacke stinking*
> *fume thereof, neerest resembling the horrible Stigian smoke of the pit that*
> *is bottomlesse.*

No wimp with the pen, and no wimp with the block either, King James had Walter Raleigh beheaded. Raleigh had probably popularized tobacco smoking more than any other man in England. On his way to the block he stopped and picked up the axe, felt the edge, and remarked: "This is sharp medicine, but it will cure all disease." He refused to give up his pipe. It was in his mouth when the axe fell.

The English settlers at Jamestown had learned about tobacco from Powhatan and Opechancanough. In 1612, the year before he married Matowaka (Pocahontas), John Rolfe managed to obtain some seeds of *Nicotiana tabacum.* It is believed that Rolfe obtained his seeds from the Spanish or Portuguese, since all of the tobacco grown by the Indians in eastern North America was *Nicotiana rustica*. Tobacco became an instant cash crop of astounding success. It is safe to say that the colony would never have survived without it – that the tobacco plant is the father plant of the *United States of America*. (The mother plant, of course, from the northern colonies, would be maize.)

In the nineteenth century, the invention of the cigarette-rolling machine and a new method of curing started the cigarette toward its present dominance of the tobacco market. The new curing produced a milder tobacco that could be inhaled into the lungs even by recreational users, and this method of ingestion proved to be the most quickly addicting of any.

Tobacco Shamanism   Tobacco has to do with energy. Transferring energy, attuning energy. As such, energy being a traditionally godly province, tobacco is the food of the gods. Even gods have to eat, after all. And remember that tobacco is very foodlike. Taking tobacco relieves hunger, much like food does. Further, tobacco grows in gardens, just like food. It likes gardens. It likes rich, sunny soil, and will even volunteer if you prepare a spot for it. We have already stated that tobacco is probably the oldest cultigen in North America. It is quite possible that the cultivation and domestication of plants began with volunteers like tobacco that made themselves at home in the sunny, disturbed ground around dwellings . . . ten to twenty thousand years ago at the dawn of the Holocene.

So we have a plant that looks like food, grows where food grows, allays hunger, but still is not quite food. That is, tobacco allays hunger but only temporarily: eventually you still have to eat real food. And tobacco brings its own hunger, a craving that is analogous to the hunger for food. Given these premises, deducing that tobacco is indeed food, but spirit food rather than human food, is not so far-fetched. Johannes Wilbert, in his excellent book *Tobacco and Shamanism in South America*, notes that the abandoned house sites where adventitious *Nicotiana* plants were common were frequently also used as cemeteries, reinforcing the connection between tobacco and the Other World.

> *A Campa tobacco shaman considers himself the husband of Jaguar Woman and calls his tube of ambil (tobacco paste) "my wife." Human foodstuffs don't satisfy jaguars. To avoid eating any of his own friends or relatives, a shaman hunting in his jaguar form travels great distances.*

The gods' problem is that although they need to eat, just as we do, no food grows in the spirit land. So they have to deal with humans, who have the tobacco monopoly. They have to bargain. In exchange for our feeding them, and enduring the hardships that such feeding entails, they will try to help us out on their side: keeping accidents from happening, diverting disasters, spilling the beans about where certain animals are living or who it was that pilfered the fish traps, and generally acting as diplomats between various, often malevolent, spirits.

> *A deal?*

So the spirits let us know when they are hungry: the craving of nicotine withdrawal is the growling stomach of the hungry spirit. We feed them by taking tobacco ourselves, and a transference takes place. Some shamans smoke tobacco more or less continuously.

> *Sometimes animals in the spirit world drink too much at one of the tobacco pools and get transported into this world.*

Tobacco provides what every shaman must undergo: sickness, death, and rebirth. The symptoms of nicotine poisoning coincide almost perfectly with the stages of shamanic initiation. Nausea and vomiting are followed by tremors, convulsions, and catatonia. This is the shamanic death, the doorway to the realm where the spirits and the gods live. When the shaman recovers consciousness, he has had dreams and visions of the spirit world, has had conversations with the gods, and has learned the secret of traveling between worlds.

> *Tobacco is the muscle. Maybe the mushrooms or the little leaves of the Shepherdess will give you the seeing, but you need tobacco for the muscle, to clean the sickness out.*

And the best part is, for a shaman, that tobacco doesn't waste a lot of time. A busy person needs that, needs an ally who doesn't take all day just to answer a question.

> *You want poison? You got it.*

Divination   Almost all of the early accounts of Indian tobacco use published by Europeans mention its use in divination: in capnomancy, spodomancy, and, through the trance state, oneiromancy. One method of spodomancy involves scrutinizing the shape of the ash on the end of a huge cigar: seeing whether the ash is straight or curved. Capnomancy involves watching the column of smoke from a clump of burning tobacco and seeing in which direction it veers. But by far the most common method of divination is by oneiromancy, by the dreams and visions experienced while under tobacco-induced trances and comas. Those returning from tobacco trances speak with the voices of the gods themselves.

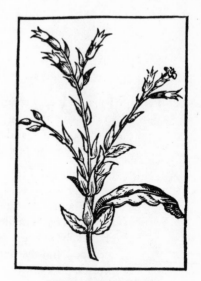

JOYFULLE NEWES OUT OF
THE NEWE FOUNDE WORLDE,
NICOLAS MONARDES, 1577

CORRESPONDENCES

METAL	Iron
METAPHOR	Energy
MINERAL	Slate
MYTH	Theft of Fire
MYTHIC HERO	Raven
NUMBER	Rational/Fractions
OCCUPATION	Warrior
PERIODIC TABLE COLUMN	Alkalai Earths
PHASE OF COITUS	Penetration
PHASE OF MATTER	Crystalline
PHYSICAL CONSTANT	Elementary Charge, *e*
PLANET	Mars
PLATONIC SOLID	Tetrahedron
POISON	Uncertainty
QUARK	Down

Poesis Tobacco is easy to grow, although the germination stage is delicate. The seeds are so tiny that missing a watering can be fatal. Also, many insects seem to be fond of the seedlings, and one slug can consume scores of them in a single night. Once established, the plant is hardy and will probably volunteer every year thereafter.

Preparing good tobacco is another matter. Just drying the leaves results in a surprisingly mild-tasting smoke (not necessarily mild in potency!). Tobacco has to be fermented to have flavor: it has to "stew in its own juices." Jungle tobacco, like *mapuchu,* is made by pouring a hot extraction of some of the leaves over others that have been dried. The whole mass is rolled up into a long cylinder and wrapped tightly with vines. Industrialized countries generally use hydraulic presses.

Breeding high-nicotine tobaccos is difficult. In the 1970s a breeder at the U.S. Department of Agriculture (USDA) was unsuccessful in his attempts. Later, an American tobacco company, Brown & Williamson, obtained some of the USDA seeds and with such advanced breeding techniques as anther culture, tissue culture, and protoplast fusion, were able to breed a strain they called "Y-1" with

6 percent nicotine content, twice the nicotine content of most tobaccos. Even though stronger tobaccos enable a smoker to get the same dose of nicotine with fewer tars, which are by far the most damaging substances in cigarettes, the FDA reacted to the disclosure as proof that the tobacco companies are manipulating the nicotine content of cigarettes to increase their addictiveness. As if that were necessary.

CORRESPONDENCES

QUANTUM FORCE	Graviton
REALM OF PLEASURE	Muscles
RITUAL EVENT	Death
ROCK	Basalt
SEASON	Summer
SENSE	Vision
SEXUAL POSITION	Man Behind
SIN	Avarice
SOCIAL EVENT	General Strike
TAROT KEY	Emperor
TIME OF DAY	Afternoon
TOOL	Hammer
VIRTUE	Prudence
VOWEL	Low Central: *a*

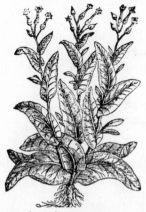

NICOTIANA, FROM L'OVEL'S STIRPIUM ADVERSARIA NOVA, 1576

PHENOMENOLOGICAL
TAXONOMY OF PSYCHOTROPES

Every plant is an individual.

> *Wrong again. We are not individuals at all, we are all connected. We are individuals the way each blossom on an apple tree is an individual.*

Any attempt to force a wild system into the confines of a formal system is inescapably arbitrary. Wild systems and formal systems inhabit separate dimensions. And while there is a hazy, fuzzy-edged intersection of the two planes, the linkage remains metaphorical. Logically (it is so hard to escape logic), the two sets are disjoint. Eddington thought so. Physics is the intersection of a formal set, mathematics, with a wild set, natural phenomena.

Eddington characterized the difference between the scientific domain and the extrascientific not as concrete versus transcendental, but as metrical versus nonmetrical. Those phenomena intrinsically nonmetrical can never be part of science.

> *To put the conclusion crudely – the stuff of the world is mind-stuff . . . something more general than our individual conscious minds; but we may think of its nature as not altogether foreign to the feelings in our consciousness. The realistic matter and fields of force of former physical theory are altogether irrelevant – except in so far as the mind-stuff has itself spun these imaginings.*
>
> *– Arthur Eddington*

Formal systems are well defined; they are describable. In fact, the rules are the system. Chance can be simulated, but it is not clear that chance exists in formal systems: physicists, mathematicians, and Schrödinger's cat are debating the issue. (It's not clear that chance exists in wild systems either, but that's another topic.)

It's like, language is a wild system, whereas generative grammar is a formal system. Generative grammar can describe, more or less, the grammar of wild language, but only more or less. It is this "more or less" that interests us.

Wild systems contain poisons. Formal systems are certainly poisonous, but lack the playfulness of, say, wild coyotes.

> *Coyote is the one who breaks the rules.*

We call this crucial difference the *Coyote Principle.* Stated most succinctly, it goes, "No matter how well you plan it out, Coyote will find some way to fuck it up." Like all poisons, the Coyote Principle is both a bane and a blessing. Sometimes this principle is referred to as the *human factor.*

Botanical taxonomy is not an algebra: it is a lexicon, not a language. Still, all taxonomies have formal structure. Taxonomy wishes to separate the cats from the dogs – not so difficult, you think, until you come to hyenas. We can all recognize roses and grasses and can see that roses may be subdivided into red roses and yellow roses. And we could divide grasses into tall grasses and short grasses, or maybe into grasses with awns (like foxtails) and awnless grasses. And in some way roses are like camellias, while likewise grasses are like sedges. And more, grasses, sedges, and cattails could form a group the way roses, camellias, and peonies form a group. It goes like that. So we try to be rational.

In scientific taxonomy we wish to find those relationships, whether chemical, morphological, or cytological, that express evolutionary developments. It has not always been thus, as is clear from the common names for plants in English and other languages. Older taxonomies were sometimes based on morphological similarity, but often also on other properties, including pharmacological properties. Thus we have "yarrow" and "golden yarrow," related by outward structure, and "sage" and "sagebrush," related by smell. "Dwale-berry" is a pharmacological name, as is *teonanacatl,* "God's flesh."

The point of this long-winded apology is to stress the metaphorical – that is, *magical* – and arbitrary nature of any taxonomic scheme. Our endeavor is to consider the effects of a variety of plants upon consciousness, and to classify the plants thereby. The water here gets murky. For one, the dosage is vital to the results. *Nicotiana* is a stimulant in small doses, but a sedative or deliriant in larger doses.

One might classify the plants on the basis of chemistry, but often a plant will contain a complex mixture of substances, not all of them related chemically, but all contributing to the perceived effect. Further, such classifications would quickly become numerous, and would often fail to reflect experiential similarities between chemically disparate plants.

Pharmacological categories, of course, are ancient, and are still used both in medicine and in traditional herbalism. Some of the pharmacological categories are analgesics, anodynes, sedatives, soporifics, emetics, expectorants, cathartics, cerebral stimulants, analeptics, convulsants, deliriants, etc., etc.

Recently, the Mexican ethnobotanist José Luis Díaz (1979) proposed a system structurally akin to that of Linnaeus, based on an earlier system suggested by J. Dealy and P. Deniker. In this system there are three main classes: *psychoanaleptics,* drugs that produce excitation; *psycholeptics,* drugs that induce depression; and *psychodysleptics,* drugs that produce an alteration. Díaz further divides these classes into "families," the families further subdivided into groups, and the groups into botanical species. Beneath "species," he lists chemical compounds.

DIAZ'S SYSTEM

CLASS	FAMILY
PSYCHOANALEPTICS	Psychostimulants
	Euphoriants
	Antidepressants
	Anxiety Inducers
	Convulsants
PSYCHOLEPTICS	Hypnotic-Sedatives
	Inebriants
	Minor Tranquilizers
	Antispasmodics
	Antimanics
PSYCHODYSLEPTICS	Hallucinogens
	Trance Inducers
	Cognodysleptics
	Deliriants
	Neurotoxins
	Narcotics

As an example, *Salvia divinorum* would be in Class: Psychodysleptics; Family: Cognodysleptics; Group: Terpene Labiatae.

Tree structures are best used to describe evolutionary relationships, relationships based on lineal history. While we will refer to Díaz's system occasionally, our purpose is not genealogical, but shares more with the purpose of a path: that is, to get somewhere. We have begun with the system introduced by Louis Lewin in 1924, the first such system I am aware of relating specifically to mind plants. Louis Lewin's seminal book *Phantastica* divided mind-altering plants into five categories: *euphorica, hypnotica, excitantia, inebriantia,* and *phantastica.* The fivefold scheme is coarse, but has the value of tradition. William Emboden, in *Narcotic Plants,* followed Lewin, but grouped *euphorica* and *hypnotica* together. Lewin had put opium in *euphorica,* and drugs that engendered sleep into *hypnotica.* Emboden broadened the class of *hypnotica* to include sedatives and tranquilizers both, as well as true soporifics, and included the opiates therein.

I have maintained Lewin's fivefold system, but offer a new class, *thanatopathia,* for tobacco. Five is a good number in the plant world, and one that is conspicuously absent from the mineral work.

> *There are things male, and things female –*
> *some reveries are like eating fruits,*
> > *those others like eating nuts,*
> > *these like vegetables, those like grains.*

Or perhaps the altered states of consciousness correspond to planetary metals, or to astrological signs. Or we could devise a scheme based on the organs of the body, or one based upon Jungian psychology. Some would call this last system "scientific."

It is very tempting to create a Cartesian system, with one or more axes, one axis perhaps a continuum from sedative to stimulant. With a second axis, representing heavily somatic to entirely mental, one could have a two-dimensional grid on which to place any number of substances. Roland Fischer, in *Science,* offered a "perception-hallucination" continuum that he claimed correlated to measurable EEG states.

My system is based on Leonhard Euler rather than Descartes. I look forward to someone's organizing plant allies on the enneagram, instead of on the pentagram, as I have done. Or perhaps on the five-element, eight-sided mandala of the I Ching, as Lama Govinda has explored. Or on the Kabbalah.

> *The astute lover of wisdom will contend that my arrangement*
> *is not phenomenological at all, but*
> *Pythagorean.*

> *A nice draught of poison, that one!*
> *We'll let it eat a little hole in our magic circle.*

In any system, numbers emerge: perhaps ten, and twenty-one. Or seven. It's easy to get lost in rationalism: magic and physics are both thick with the Pythagoreans. When the talk is done, however, the ally is there, an objective correlative, as it were, waiting to set things straight. Where "straight" probably means crooked.

> *Striving with Systems to deliver Individuals from those Systems . . .*
> > *– William Blake, "Jerusalem"*

DUBOISIA HOPWOODII

Common Names   *Pituri*, pedgery, pitchery.

Related Species   *Duboisia myoporoides, Duboisia leickhartii.*

Taxonomy   Family: Solanaceae. A shrub, sometimes a small tree. The genus is endemic to Australia.

Part Used   Leaves.

Chemistry   Tropane alkaloids scopolomine and hyoscamine are present in *Duboisia myoporoides* and *D. leickhartii*. Most accounts therefore ascribe the same chemistry to *Duboisia hopwoodii,* but according to Pamela Watson (1983b) *Duboisia hopwoodii* contains nicotine and d-nornicotine. Moreover, the Australian Aborigines apparently did not use the other two species, so there is some confusion in the genus, chemically and perhaps taxonomically.

Chemical studies have shown that there is great variation in both the quantity and the relative proportion of the two nicotine alkaloids among individual specimens of *Duboisia hopwoodii*. It is probable that other alkaloids, such as tropanes, are also present in *D. hopwoodii,* as they are in the other species of the genus. Some species of *Duboisia* are grown commercially for scopolomine.

How Taken   The leaves are roasted and chewed, often along with some ash of burnt acacia. The quid, or chaw, is passed around in a circle, from mouth to mouth, until everyone has had a sufficient chew. The last man in the circle places the quid behind the ear of the first. Pamela Watson points out that the skin behind the ear is rich in capillaries and is close to the brain, and would be an excellent place for transdermal absorption. And, in fact, the Aborigines claim just that – that placing the quid behind the ear strengthens the effects of the drug. Scopolomine patches today are placed behind the ear as a motion sickness preventative.

The leaves were also smoked. Smoking *pituri* may have been a postcontact technique.

Effects   In smaller doses, *pituri* suppresses hunger and thirst and strengthens endurance. In larger doses, *pituri* produces detachment from time and space, hallucinations, and illusions. Its effects mirror those of tobacco in many ways. Like tobacco, in small doses *pituri* is used as a stimulant and mild tranquilizer. And like tobacco, it was a social plant, used in greetings, councils, and diplomacy. But certain effects are reported for *pituri* that are unusual for nicotine alone.

A number of early Australian explorers and scientists were given the opportunity by the Aborigines to try *pituri*. Here is a scattering of reports as to *pituri's* effects:

"Never fails to promote mirth and good fellowship . . . "
"Passed around from one to another as a token of friendship . . . "
"They go off into a daze . . ."
"Produces a dreamy voluptuous sensation . . . "

Pharmacology   Nornicotine is more toxic than nicotine, so the difference between a psychoactive dose and a fatal dose is even smaller than for nicotine. The action is the same as the biphasic action of nicotine: affecting the transmission between nerves. It is not clear that the observed reactions are the result of the pyridine alkaloids alone. There is cause for some fresh analytical study of the genus.

History   As tobacco has completely replaced *pituri* among the Australian Aborigines, ethnobotanists and ethnopharmacologists are dependent on extant written documents for information. All accounts agree that *pituri* was widely traded among the Aborigines. Ancient roads and trails mark the locations of *pituri* trees. The importance of the *pituri* plant is evident in the fact that the only written records kept by the Aborigines were marked sticks having to do with the *pituri* trade.

As poison, *pituri* was used to stupefy emus. Branches of *Duboisia hopwoodii* were bruised and placed in a waterhole. When the emus drank from the spring they were drugged enough to enable the Aborigines to catch them easily.

The Plant   *Duboisia* is a xeric plant, adapted to the arid conditions of central Australia. Freely branching from the base, *Duboisia* grows into a hemisperical shrub three to four meters high. Evidently, although *pituri* grows over a large area of central Australia, only the *pituri* from one particular location was highly prized and traded. This *pituri* was gathered and cured by hereditary *pituri* clans.

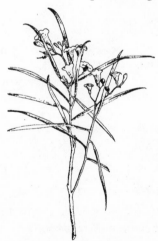

DUBOISIA HOPWOODII

The curing process was the secret of the graybeards – the younger men were not privy. The one sketchy anthropological report states that a fire was built on sand and that when the fire burned low, the coals were raked away. *Duboisia* twigs and stems, picked *just at that moment,* were placed on the hot sand and covered, and left to steam for a very specific length of time. Too much steaming made the herb brittle, while too little left it "musty." The steaming time was known only, as I said, to the elders.

It is likely that the steaming halted enzymatic action, which would have continued degrading the alkaloids in the plant, even after picking. No analysis was ever done on *pituri* prepared in the proper manner. We also know that the natives burned the older branches off of the shrubs, in order to promote growth of new young twigs, which are higher in alkaloids. There may have been some selective propagation as well, favoring plants with the desirable balance of alkaloids and avoiding those too weak or too toxic.

Men returning from the *pituri* expeditions reportedly brought back seventy pounds of cured, dried *pituri* apiece, carried in a specially woven bag.

KILLING TIME

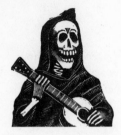

And to kill time while awaiting death,
I smoke elegant cigarettes, thumbing my nose at the gods.
  — Jules Laforgue, "La.Cigarette"

The cigarette is thoughtfulness: reflection and contemplation before action. We smoke to contemplate action, until the smoking and the cigarette become the action. And then that is what we do: we smoke.

I wrap his soul in mine and cradle it
within a blue and fluctuating thread . . .
  — Charles Baudelaire, "The Pipe"

The cigarette is a prop, the flicking tail of a tree squirrel, Chaplin's cane, always ready to twirl.

Or a cool stance: cigarette hanging off the lip in the side of the mouth, sleeveless T-shirt. Sweaty.

Love, lust, loose morals,
a loose white blouse fallen off the shoulder —

Bad girl, bad boy, they break the rules,
they probably fuck, too. Rebellion, allure of the
forbidden.

Only soldiers, convicts, or sorcerers would take up the habit as an adult.

Kids smoke to feel grown up.
Adults smoke to feel like kids.

A cigarette is the perfect type of a perfect pleasure. It is exquisite, and
it leaves one unsatisfied. What more can one want?
  — Oscar Wilde, The Picture of Dorian Gray

A woman is only a woman, but a good cigar is a smoke.

Your loyal alchemist, in the depths of his fuming *athanor*, has by subtle means discovered what is quite possibly the fastest way to addict oneself to tobacco.

Quite a public service.

You need a cigarette holder, a razor blade, and some very strong cigarettes, such as Players Navy Cut. Cut off about half an inch of a cigarette with the razor blade, put it in the holder, and inhale it deeply. Hold the smoke in. For a novice one hit is an overdose.

How can anything so nauseating be so satisfying?

Be sure that you are sitting down if you try this. And have some cushions behind you: it'll knock you down pretty well, if getting knocked down is the sort of thing you enjoy. It lasts about half an hour. Then you get to do it again.

The poor man's crack.

You may think this all Saturnian. But I ask you: who but a fool would deliberately addict himself to nicotine? So we are dealing here with a subset of humanity, the set of fools. Since we are dealing with fools, no amount of wise advice is going to do any good. Legislation and criminal penalties don't even help. So why not just tell it like it is?

Ha ha ha. Now you have to kick.

Cigarette addiction is an expensive ally. The sacred weed costs us more than money: links to early death and illness are well established. It is reported that half a million people die from the direct or indirect effects of tobacco in the United

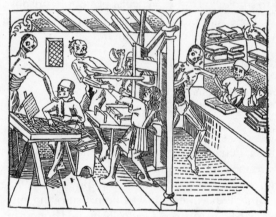

DEATH PRODUCES BOOKS, 1500

States every year. The poor who smoke are able to buy less food, particularly with the rising "sin tax" levied against tobacco. People have to clean up the litter, which is substantial. Forests are cut to heat the flues to cure the leaves.

It's better to kiss cats and to chew on their ears than to smoke cigarettes.

As of 1994, in a double farce, the tobacco companies are still denying that nicotine is addictive, and the federal Food and Drug Administration is just discovering that tobacco may be a drug. In order to achieve uniformity of product, tobacco companies first extract all the nicotine out of the tobacco, and then spray it back on. This practice, supposedly a shocking surprise to those who claim to be protecting us, has elicited charges that the tobacco industry is deliberately lacing their product with an addictive substance.

Why else would anybody smoke it?

Ah, yes,
tobacco, tobacco,
that brings a frown to my brow!

Yes, tobacco,
that brings a grin to my lips.

Inhaled smoke is the most quickly addicting form of tobacco, although perhaps not the most difficult to quit. Snoose, in particular, seems to be even harder to give up than cigarettes.

On a graph of addictions, tobacco is the most tenacious. Almost every junkie gives up narcotics after ten years. Almost everyone gives up cocaine, even crack.

> That magic blend of fire and air, of spirit and death,
> breath made visible:
> this is your life, this is time, time incarnated,
> embodied so that you can watch it.

Still, there are many who are able to play with the fire, to smoke when others are smoking, or when intoxicated with alcohol or marijuana, but never otherwise. These are people deserving study! We can learn more from them than from either the addicts or the abstainers.

> When You Crave a Snack, Reach for a Pack
>   – Lucky Strike advertisement, circa 1920

The poison is habit, the sleepwalker. Smoke deliberately, never "on the side" or out of boredom. It is important to smoke for some particular poisonous purpose, not just because you have nothing else to do. You hold an ancient power, and it should be burned with all the reverence that its lineage implies.

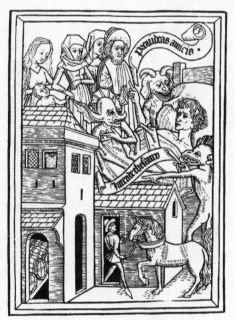

THE ART OF DYING, 1450

> Life is a cigarette:
>   Cinder, ash, fire –
> Some smoke it quickly,
>   Others with savor.
>
>   – Manuel Machado, "Chants Andalous"

I never denied cigarettes. Never recanted my love. Just refined the pleasure: bought samples of various different tobaccos for hand rolling. Bought a rolling machine. Experimented with herbal smoking mixtures. Mixed in tobacco. Gradually limited how many cigarettes I smoked. Finally to one a day. Gradually diminished the amount of tobacco in the smoking mixture. Finally didn't smoke at all. But not because I quit. Just because I haven't gotten around to it.

> Only the revered cigarette, like "last words"
> and the Holy Cross, is privileged to share
> the last rites of the condemned.

Tobacco is the blackness. The darkness.
Close your eyes.

INEBRIANTIA

Only with wine does the true self emerge,
When the mind, like a cave, is empty of doubts.
   – Su Tung-Po

When Mother and Father are away.

Or, if they are home, the inebriants send them upstairs to their rooms, to go to bed like children. Brothers and sisters follow the parents: the whole family scene falling away. Spouses and children. Friends.

The last vestiges of propriety depart.

So initially the inebriants are the rebel's ally: an insurrection in heaven and a return to the blood.

A return to "just do it." A return to what you desire, to beyond what you have been told you want, to what you really want. To do it. Yourself. Now. Leap, leap. License.

> *Sobriety diminishes, discriminates, and says no; drunkenness expands, unites, and says yes. It is in fact the great exciter of the* YES *function in man. It brings its votary from the chill periphery of things to the radiant core. It makes him for the moment one with truth.*
>   *– William James, The Varieties of Religious Experience*

Thomas De Quincey, using a quote from Athenaeus, maintained that "most men are disguised by sobriety, exceedingly disguised," and that it is inebriation that brings out the "true complexion of character." Comparing the inebriation of wine with the euphoria of opium, De Quincey characterized wine as emphasizing the *human* qualities (he said that opium brought out the *divine* qualities).

All inebriants are solvents and general anesthetics. They all lead to unconsciousness. But each inebriant has its own agenda as to who goes to bed first.

With alcohol the superego is the first to go. With nitrous

oxide the first to leave is what we might call the *dimensional gatekeeper,* the mender at the wall who says "good fences make good neighbors."

Dizziness and passing out relate to inebriation, and such inebriation is usually our first glimpse into the liquid, slippery quality of consciousness. We spin around until we fall. We clutch the ground, now itself spinning, and spin around with it: the earth spinning, the horizon heaving, and the sky rocking all together.

> *We spin, we hyperventilate into a bag, we hold our breath, are squeezed by a friend until we pass out. We return to a land utterly strange, evoking memories half myth, half fairy tale. Up out of a tunnel-like darkness, something repeats, pulses: there is Time. Time is the primordial dimension. A strange and incredulous face gazes down at us from above, a face looking like something out of history, out of some past and colorful century. There are past centuries, there is a World, there is us, so there must be an I. I am on the floor. The face becomes familiar. Memory, it has come back. I remember. I passed out. I went away. But so far! To the other side, beyond bodies, planets, and gravity. Beyond immensity!*
>
> *And the returning: a long circular corridor of coupled rings, tubular passageways, each tube a stage in the phylogeny of consciousness. Light, then Form. Body, Time, and Place. Then particulars. Names. Relation, and Self-relation.*

Certain esoteric groups have maintained the ancient initiatory rites of inebriation. Once inebriated, the prospective initiates are closely scrutinized, the adepts watching for particular behaviors, by which they judge the suitableness of the aspirants for the path – whether they are to be admitted to the lesser or to the greater mysteries.

> *Liberation: singing and dancing,*
> *or, at the least, laughing, shaking a fist*
> *at the sun.*

We wander through the inebriants as if visiting the Stations of the Cross, a different member of our party remaining behind in each alcove, our epiphanies ranging from the ecstatic to the terrible. The last stop is Golgotha, the Hill of Skulls.

> *The drunken consciousness is one bit of the mystic consciousness, and our total opinion of it must find its place in our opinion of that larger whole.*
> *– William James, The Varieties of Religious Experience*

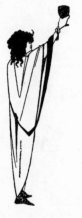

BY AUBREY
BEARDSLEY, 1893

SACCHAROMYCES CEREVISIAE

Common Name	Yeast.
Related Species	Other yeasts, certain bacteria.
Taxonomy	Yeast is a fungus. An ascomycete, to be specific.
Part Used	The excrement.
Chemistry	C_2H_5OH, ethyl hydroxide. AKA ethanol, ethyl alcohol.
How Taken	Through the mouth, as wine, beer, ale, mead, *chicha*, kvass, cider, koumiss, sake, pulque, and as an unbounded number of mixed drinks from the distilled spirits of same, including brandy, cognac, whiskey, rum, gin, vodka, bourbon, tequila, and mescal.
Effects	Analgesic, anodyne, stimulant, sedative, anesthetic, inebriant. Specific reactions seem to vary with body type and psychology, perhaps also with blood sugar level and other hormonal balances. Mesomorphs tend to become boisterous and aggressive, endomorphs expansive, sentimental, or maudlin. Ectomorphs, it is said, just get depressed.
The Plant	Ubiquitous: its conquest of the world is complete. It travels on dust, in the air. In cold climates it can winter over, if need be, in the ground, and then take to the air again in the spring, traveling on anything that flies. Many strains have been domesticated and are carefully nurtured by brewers and bakers. One variety of wild yeast colonizes the wax bloom right on the skins of grapes. Kind of like a message from God. . . .

> *I used to keep a sourdough going in my prospecting days,*
> *even when I was backpacking. I packed a lot of flour and*
> *had fresh bread every night. I mean little loaves of bread,*
> *real bread, not biscuits. I baked them in a sort of reflector*
> *oven rigged up with aluminum foil in front of the campfire.*
> *I never used any store-bought yeast. If I lost my starter,*
> *I just mixed up flour and water in a jar, left it open, and*
> *in a couple of days it would be bubbling and yeasty.*

Fermentation	Alchemically, fermentation is what changes the base metals into the *stone*. In fermentation, we are given a book on spiritual physics, the physics of poisons. All that is required is to see the signature clearly.

FROM DAS GOLDEN
SPIEL, 1472

The food for fermentation is sugar, as it is also our food. The by-products are carbon dioxide and alcohol. If the plant is closed up in a restricted environment, it will die in its own excrement. We can take advantage of that.

And who will take advantage of us?

It would be hard to find an older plant, a plant with a more ancient lineage, or with a simpler poison. The line between the vegetable work and the elementals blurs here.

Many great doctors have studied fermentation: Democritus, Pliny, Priestley, and Pasteur; Rilke, waiting for poems, and Bodhidharma, waiting for nothing.

God made yeast, as well as dough, and loves fermentation just as dearly as he loves vegetation.

– Ralph Waldo Emerson, Essays

The Plant

No leaves. No flowers. No stems. No sexual parts nor gender. Perfect. Or a parasite.

Fermentation is oxidation, fire; it returns carbon dioxide to the atmosphere. The parasite: you build it up, I break it down. The poison called petroleum is from fungi; industrial civilization is the fermenting parasite.

The Preparation

Fermented fruit drinks are generally called wines, while fermented grain drinks are called beer, or ale. At one time the term *beer* referred only to barley drinks to which hops had been added, while ale might be flavored and preserved with any

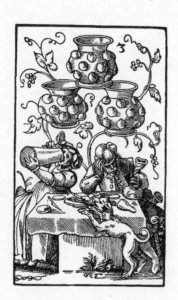

number of other plants. Mead is made from fermented honey, and may be the most ancient of all inebriants. Some etymologists claim the Indo-European root *medhu-*, "mead," is related to similar roots in Akkadian, Hamitic, and other Mediterranean tongues, which would attest to great antiquity indeed.

Fermented drinks are prepared from whatever is at hand: the Siberians ferment koumiss from mare's milk; the Mexican pulque is prepared from agave. It would not be incorrect to refer to these plants and substances as *admixtures,* a term we will use again in the section on ayahuasca.

The admixtures to *Saccharomyces* are a pretty classy lot. They include the leading citizens of the anthropophilic community, as well as many obscure plants with only local reputations. Among the better known are *Vitis* (the grape), *Hordeum* (barley), *Triticum* (wheat), *Malus* (apple), *Rubus* (blackberry, raspberry), *Prunus* (pear, peach, apricot, plum), *Zea* (maize), *Oryza* (rice), *Saccharum* (sugar cane), *Agave* (yucca), *Secale* (rye), *Solanum tuberosum* (potato), *Eleusine* (millet), *Taraxacum* (dandelion), *Manihot* (cassava, or manioc), and *Chenopodium* (lamb's quarters).

FROM JOST AMMAN'S
CHARTA LUSORIA, 1588

CORRESPONDENCES

ACTIVITY	Carnival
ANIMAL	Serpent, Goat
ARCHETYPE	The Vamp
ART FORM	Epic Poetry
BODILY FUNCTION	Digestion
BODY PART	Liver
BUDDHA REALM	Ratna
CHORD	Dominant
COLOR	Sapphire Blue
COSMIC ENTITY	Open Clusters
CRUTCH FOR	Inhibition
DIMENSION	Plane
DISCIPLINE	Poetry
ELEMENT	Water
FORM OF ENERGY	Wood Fire
FORM OF IGNORANCE	Avoidance, Forgetfulness
GEMSTONE	Opal
GEOMETRY	First Order Torus
GOD	Bacchus
GODDESS	Hathor/Ishtar, Ama-Gestin
GRAMMAR	Nondeterministic Finite State
HERO	Gilgamesh
HISTORICAL AGE	Iron Age

The Plant Yeasts are so ubiquitous that other plants have to hide their sugars, either by skin, by bark and cellulose, or by molecular structure (by storing the sugar as starch). Yeast has its own allies, however: enzymes. And at the right temperature the enzyme ally can convert starch into sugar.

Effects *The flowing bowl – whom has it not made eloquent?*
Whom has it not made free, even amid pinching poverty?
     – Horace

In vain I trusted that the flowing bowl
Would banish sorrow, and enlarge the soul.
To the late revel, and protracted feast,
Wild dreams succeeded, and disorder'd rest.
— *Matthew Prior*

Matters of State
and Liberty

A drunkard is not profitable
for any kind of service.
— *Plato*

Laws against drunkenness in public are the oldest of drug laws, and the most widespread. For the Aztecs, drunkenness was a capital crime for members of the aristocracy, since they were then unfit to carry out official duties. Commoners were given more leniency.

The Ally

The ally's secret face is terror. The alcohol ally is like a slime, slow-moving, growing on you, at first only a fine veneer, like a slug trail. But later more layers collect, until you feel unclean. Feel your steps weighted. Feel every hour of the day a tedious distraction and ordeal. You finish as quickly as you can, so that you can return to your place among the rocks where the ally is happy and thrives.

The ally likes darkness. It doesn't like to move around a lot. A little feeding. Mostly it likes you, your body, your brain, your dreams. It likes a chair if you have one.

Once it's fed and watered, it tells you that you can leave your place among the rocks, that you can arise from your mossy boulders and enter the world of humankind, but you seldom do. At such times the growing weight of the layers of film that the ally has coated over you seems to lighten and soften. The mass becomes gelatinous and pliable, and you feel free.

Pain is banished or forgotten.

The world is light. You feel spontaneous. Problems are solvable or ignorable. And you can live like that for a very long time perhaps. For a very long time indeed. Maybe until you die.

Or maybe not.

Maybe the mass of stuff that the alcohol plant has deposited on you begins to harden. Maybe you haven't been able to feed it enough and the veneer has begun to crack. It's like the way the wine itself kills the yeast, its own mother, when the poison is fully formed. Then it is time for your friend across the table to unmask. He does, and you see that he is not there, that he has already departed. In fact, he has not been there for some years, or perhaps it is she. Only the coating, the facade deposited day after day by the poison, has been keeping you company.

In truth, you are totally alone, and frighteningly alone. And tonight, of all nights, you are out of food. A night like this, when you are alone and people that you don't want to talk to are knocking on your doors and windows. You are aware that soon they will abandon civility altogether and just force their way in.

Oh, it's got you now. By the balls, by the short hairs, got your tit in a wringer, it does. It's got the hold on you. It's got tiny wet sucking fingers, green fingers – it's the slime, and it's got you.

It's saying it is time to start paying your dues. It's saying that it is time to start feeling all that pain that has built up on you like a crust. It's saying that it is time to get back to work. To free your words. To face your children, your spouse, your divorce, the ruin of your life, or perhaps its success. That it is time to deal with the devil you have created. For they are all your creations, all of them. It is your own children that call to you.

It's a sneaky kind of plant, a patient kind of plant. It is glad to wait, to let you control it. It is always ready to talk or parley and negotiate. But note, the plant is a shrewd negotiator. It loves to make deals, but it always takes the first night for itself: you say to the ally, "OK, I'll spend tonight with you, but tomorrow night I spend with my family, and you stay locked up in the cupboard." It will always say yes to deals like this, but never to the converse.

It's a nightmare. It's a slime well. Every direction is uphill and it's all ice.

The ally says that it is time to deal with the devil you have created. It is your own creation, it is your art. It is, perhaps, gothic, but nonetheless there is an inner integrity to it. It is your genius, only your genius could have created such an elaborate prison for your own self. The ally is telling you you have built enough. Enough locks, enough doors, enough curtains and shades, bars and obstacles. They are all yours to burn.

Look upon it as the devil's firewood, and now you have a shed-full. Call it your "material" in the alchemical sense. So there is still cause for hope, for now you have a practice, you have a discipline, a path – a true path and an everyday path – probably what you were after from the beginning.

Sun doctors, of course, avoid this wonderful creative opportunity, if they can.

> *Took up with whiskey*
> *to drown my sorrows.*
> *All that's happened is*
> *they've become*
> *better swimmers.*
>
>   *—Steve Sanfield, A New Way*

VITIS VINIFERA

❧

Common Names	Grapevine, wine.
Related Species	Almost any sugary or starchy fruit or berry.
Part Used	The fermented juice of the fruit.
Chemistry	Ethanol, ethyl alcohol.
How Taken	Best drunk with food, but by drunks drunk almost any way.
Effects	The first glass warms and gladdens, the second inspires poetry and seduction. The third glass evokes boasting, the fourth glass stumbling; the fifth glass stupor, and sleep.
The Plant	We choose wine as the symbol for *inebriantia,* and the grape as its type plant. In this we mean no slight to Demeter and her grains. It is likely that beer is the more ancient beverage. But wine has a mythic quality that beer lacks. Jesus' blood is wine, and wine is the blood of Dionysus. Wine is the secret medicine of Osiris. A wineglass is a chalice, and if the Grail once contained mead, surely anything but wine in it now would surprise us. The color of wine is so rich and distinctive that we use it to name other colors, and if we need to refer to the redness of wine by another name we often invoke gemstones. Life is toasted with wine, and life (*vita*) is homophonic to the name of the vine itself.
	Changing water into wine was Jesus' first miracle.
History	The oldest known evidence of wine is from residues found in the area of the southern Caucasus and Anatolia, what is now Georgia, and dates to about 4000 BC. Telltale tartrates from lees, identified by infared absorption spectroscopy, still cling to the bottoms of large jars and urns. By 3500 BC, in early Sumerian times, wine and vinicraft were already well established in Mesopotamia. And in those ancient Sumerian beginnings of the class struggle, the excavations show that wine was drunk only in the wealthier households, beer being the beverage of commonty.
	The words *wine* and *vine* are cognates, as is the Greek-derived *oenology.* According to Eric Partridge, neither the Latin nor the Greek words are of Indo-European heritage. Rather, both seem to share a common root with other Mediterranean Semitic and Hamitic cognates, probably in the Caucasus. In Georgian, a Caucasian language whose only known relative is Basque, the word for wine is *qvino*. And the traditional symbol for Mother Georgia is the grapevine. In Sumerian mythology, the Tree of Life is a grapevine.

As ancient as wine is, however, beer is probably older, as attested by brewers slops found on Neolithic middens. As Edgar Anderson says, man was a brewer before he was a baker. Some believe that brewing was the impetus behind the domestication of grains. The domestication of grains made possible living in cities, and it was living in cities that made possible imperialism, police, and slavery, which, in turn, led to writing, which led to, well, we all know: our present dilemma.

Civilized drinking (drinking in specialized places of business) prompted the first drug laws. Hammurabi made it a capital offense for priestesses to open taverns or to go to them with the intention of drinking. It was likewise a capital crime to operate a drinking establishment where treason was plotted, without reporting it. Stiff stuff, even by modern standards. While the prohibition against priestesses drinking was probably religious, the latter law is clearly more concerned with politics and hegemony than with morality.

Egyptian records of the same period depict guests at banquets vomiting into basins held by servants. There are records of a father warning his son of the evils of following the bottle instead of a career, and of a woman who, being given a reward, asks for eighteen bowls of wine, because she "loved drunkenness." Wine, as well as beer, was sacred to Hathor, the cow-headed goddess who had been slaughtering the race of mortals until Ra pacified her with drink. She was worshipped with a monthly Day of Drunkenness to commemorate the event.

The Egyptians were beer people, but we also know a great deal about their wines, through written records, paintings, and archaeological finds. By the Fifth Dynasty, if not before, they were producing both white wine and red wine, which were named the left and right eyes of Horus, respectively. The white wine was said to be the better. Then, five thousand years ago, as now, wine jars were labeled with distinctive seals.

Winemaking was probably discovered by a woman. In Sumer, the goddess Ama-Gestin was the keeper of the grapevine. Egyptian Isis conceived Horus by eating grapes. In the *Epic of Gilgamesh,* the wild man, Enkidu, is given his first wine by a "temple woman." When Gilgamesh, seeking the Tree of Life, comes to the garden of the gods he finds trees with "fruit of carnelian with the vine hanging from it." Siduri, priestess of Ishtar and the maker of wine, sits veiled in the garden with golden bowls and golden vats, given her by the gods.

> *According to the Persians, wine was discovered by a woman who was looking for poison. King Jemsheed discovered that his grape juice had gone bad, and accordingly labeled the jar as "poisonous." A woman driven to suicide by sick headaches found the jar and drank a large cup, expecting to die. Instead she fell asleep, and awoke refreshed.*

The first wine may have been date wine or raisin wine: wild dates contain enough sugar for fermentation, while wild grapes, *Vitis sylvestris,* do not, unless they are dried. The migration of wine parallels the spread of storage and drinking vessels, whether bronze or pottery.

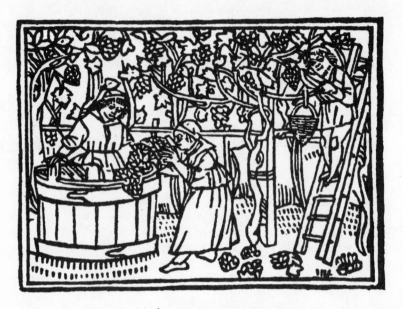

FROM CRESCENZI'S LIBRO DELLA AGRICULTURA, 1511

How to Use   A night of serious drinking requires some planning. It requires some food.

> *Beginning with hors d'oeuvres, some drinks, then a dinner, a chicken, perhaps, then drinking and talking late into the night, sharing the soul and the heart, getting down to all of it, confessions, revelations, insights, gossip, all of it flowing from the wonderful bowl . . .*

What else is life for, if not to share words from the heart, and how better to free them than with the proper company and the proper wine at the proper pace?

Wine gives breath to the periphery and to the repressed – to the shadows and the ghostly lurkers at the threshold of consciousness. Wine doesn't evoke numinous wheeling dynamos like the *phantastica,* but it does touch the *humanly* deep, the personally poignant, and can loosen sorrows stuck long in the craw.

Does wine heal? Not by itself, but sharing your heart with a friend is not a bad start.

> *Wine that maketh glad the heart of man.*
>
> – *Psalm 104:15*

CORRESPONDENCES

HUMOUR	Phlegmatic
IMAGE	Chalice
LANDSCAPE	Valley
LOGICAL OPERATOR	Or
MACHINE	Internal Combustion Engine
METAL	Tin
METAPHOR	License
MINERAL	Lapis Lazuli
MUSICAL INSTRUMENT	Flute
MYTH	Dying God
MYTHIC HERO	Orpheus
NUMBER	Irrational Numbers (Surds)
OCCUPATION	Prostitute, Hetaira
OUT-OF-BODY REALM	Realm of Reckless Abandon
PERIODIC TABLE COLUMN	Oxygen Column
PHASE OF COITUS	Seduction
PHASE OF MATTER	Liquid
PHYSICAL CONSTANT	G, Gravitational Constant
PLANET	Jupiter
PLATONIC SOLID	Octahedron
POISON	Jealousy
PROPORTION	Arithmetic Mean
QUARK	Charm

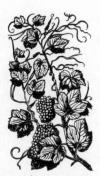

FROM MATTIOLI'S COMMENTAIRES, 1579

Texts

Fire proves the treasures of the mine,
The soul of man is proved by wine.

    – Theognis

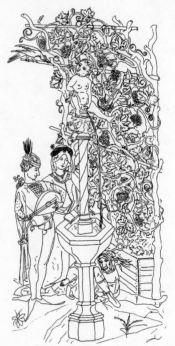

Bad wine is like bad men,
Deadlier in attack than arrows or knives.
I collapse on the platform;
Victory hopeless, truce will have to do.
The old poet carries on bravely,
The Zen master's words are gentle and profound.
But I'm so drunk the words he speaks
Only blur in a red and green swirl.

    – Su Tung-Po, "Bad Wine Is Like Bad Men"

If wine were to disappear from human production, there
would, I believe, ensue a vacuum, a lack, a flaw far more
appalling than all the excesses and deviations for which
wine is made responsible.

    – Charles Baudelaire, Artificial Paradise

with lute and book and pen and ink
I'll make my living
who cares for fame, or glory
I'll gab with fishermen and woodsmen,
drink together to the scattering clouds
no way I'll ever stray home sober.

    – Anonymous, Yuan Dynasty

LOVERS AND FOOL
IN GRAPE ARBOR

In wine I stumbled on unexpected joy.

    – Su Tung-Po

I shall light up your aged wife's eyes, the old companion of your everyday
cares and your oldest hopes. I shall soften her glance and drop into the pupil
of her eye the lightning-flash of her youth.

I shall sink into your bosom like a vegetable ambrosia. I shall be the seed
that fertilizes the laboriously cut furrow. Our close reunion will create poetry.

    – Charles Baudelaire, Artificial Paradise

History

We may have first learned the secret of drinking alcohol from animals. The ancient Greeks believed thus, and a legend told that people first learned to drink
from the apes. Studies show that chimpanzees and other apes do indeed like alcohol, and get drunk. Many animals seek out intoxicants, and most will partake
of them to excess, given the chance. Perhaps the most common example in temperate zones is birds drunk on fermented berries, wheeling about, crashing into
the ground, and generally making fools of themselves. And while recent experiments by Ronald Siegel suggest that some or all of the intoxication may be due

to secondary substances in the berries rather than alcohol, anyone witnessing the event might thereafter try the berries for themselves.

David Livingstone reported how African elephants sought out fermented palm fruits, sometimes traveling unusual distances to find and ingest them. And they did get intoxicated, staring off, trumpeting loudly, and separating out from the group.

CORRESPONDENCES

QUANTUM FORCE	Proton
REALM OF PLEASURE	Genitals
RITUAL EVENT	Marriage
ROCK	Limestone
SEASON	Autumn
SENSE	Touch
SEXUAL POSITION	Belly to Belly
SIGN	Lyra
SIN	Lechery
SOCIAL EVENT	Orgies/Dancing
TAROT KEY	High Priestess
TIME OF DAY	Evening
TOOL	Bow
VIRTUE	Charity
VOWEL	High Front: i

Ethnography The Romans reported that the Gauls were so fond of wine that they would trade their children for it. That they went crazy when they drank it, running about in frenzy and fighting each other.

> *An Italian man lived next door to us with his family. All through the fifties he vinted his own wine. I can remember the odor of the fermenting grapes occasionally wafting over the fence. My family were all teetotalers, so it was all very mysterious. The kids called the daughter "pink toes."*

The early Romans themselves were on the temperate side, and women were completely forbidden to drink on grounds that it led to lust and adultery. In later

Roman history, both sexes seem to have embraced excess in wine – twenty-five million gallons a year – for exactly the same reasons.

> *Buttery, good oak, with vanilla and apple –*
> > *a gold-medal chard, pineapple and melon . . .*
> *a classic cab: rich and full bodied;*
> > *fruity, but with tannins; cherry and clove,*
> > *unbelievable*
> > > *spice, good acid, hints of plum,*
> > *a great zin, or with bass notes, merlot . . .*

The Greeks, by classical times, appear to have been heavy drinkers, despite their reputation for moderation. When the Scythian philosopher Anacharsis visited Athens in 600 BC he was somewhat repelled by the behavior he witnessed. He said that there were three kinds of grapes, one for pleasure, one for drunkenness, and one for disgust.

> *Hide our ignorance as we will, an evening of wine reveals it.*
>
> – *Heraclitus (Davenport 1981)*

When asked how to avoid excess in wine, Anacharsis advised observing those who did not. The Scythians themselves had no wine. They smoked hemp.

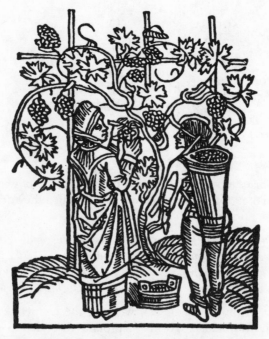

FROM CRESENZI'S *OPUS COMMODORUM RURALIUM*, 1493

HORDEUM VULGARE

Common Names	Barley, corn, malt. Ale, or beer, when fermented.
Related Species	Any cereal or starchy tuber. Especially rice, maize, wheat, cassava.
Taxonomy	Barley typifies an important tribe of the Poaceae, the Hordeae, which includes wheat and rye. The family is of recent evolution, as plants go. Grasses did well in the Miocene.
Part Used	The seeds: roasted, cracked, mashed, and fermented.
Chemistry	

$$\text{Starch} \quad \xrightarrow{\text{(enzymes)}} \quad \text{Sugar} \quad \xrightarrow{\text{(yeast)}} \quad \text{Alcohol.}$$

How Taken	Drunk. With gusto.
Effects	Refreshing and relaxing, a good catalyst for fun or trouble, for mixing or for mixing it up. Overheard in southern Louisiana:

> *There are only three things to do in life: drink Schlitz beer, fight in bars,*
> *and listen to Cajun music.*

Aristotle noted that wine drinkers fall on their faces when drunk, but that beer drinkers fall on their backs.

> *Inspir'd by thee, the warrior fights,*
> *The lover wooes, the poet writes,*
> *   And pens the pleasing tale;*
> *And still in Britain's isle confess'd*
> *Nought animates the patriot's breast*
> *   Like gen'rous, nappy Ale.*
>
> *– John Gay, "A Ballad on Ale" (in Digby and Digby 1988)*

Pharmacology	Besides alcohol, beer contains an admixture, *Humulus lupulus,* hops. Herbalists use hops as a soporific and as a digestive tonic. Brewers use it because of its bactericidal properties, to stop bacteria from growing in beer. It is effective in all of those areas. Hops are *very* bitter.
The Plant	Barley is probably the oldest cultivated grain. Edgar Anderson states that barley was dispersed from two centers, one in Abyssinia and another in Nepal or Tibet. Paleoethnobotanists have discovered domesticated barleys and emmer wheat in a prepottery Neolithic level at Jericho, in Palestine, dating to about 8000 BC. This may be the oldest cultivated grain to have been dated. Other Near Eastern digs of the same date have revealed only wild grains. (In the New World, however,

there is some evidence that amaranth was cultivated – certainly it was gathered – before 8000 B C.)

Most paleoethnobotanists now agree with Anderson that the oldest cultivated plants were originally camp followers. Human beings leave distinctive scars upon the places they live, and a community of plants evolved to take advantage of those scars. Barleys such as the foxtail are well-known and aggressive members of that anthropophytic community (we call them *weeds*).

> úcchrayasva bahúr bhava
> svéna máhasā yava
>
> *Rise up, become abundant*
> *with thine own greatness, O barley*
> — *Atharva Veda*

History Beer has been the working man's drink for at least fifty centuries. The Romans, being bosses more than workers, didn't care for beer very much and spoke disparagingly of those who did. They characterized the Gauls as getting drunk on "spoiled grain." In addition to Celtic peoples, the Germanic tribes, including the Angles and Saxons, have favored beers and ales since ancient times. Beowulf drank ale, and the alehouse is the setting for much discussion and laughter, complete with a queen acting as barmaid. Gallic beers were called *cerevisia,* or some other cognate of Ceres (the goddess). The etymologies of the words *beer* and *ale* are evidently not completely settled, but it seems likely that *beer* is akin to an Old Norse word, *bygg,* meaning *barley.*

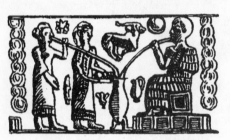

BEER TASTERS, SEAL OF HAMMURABI, 1913 BC

Ale comes from the Indo-European root *alu-,* relating to magic, sorcery, possession, and visions, and is cognate with our word *hallucinogen.* The German root is **alutha,* meaning "bitter," *aludoimos* in Greek. The characteristic bitterness of ale is evident in another cognate word, "alum." Bitterness and ale seem to go together.

Many other bitter plants besides hops have been used as admixtures in fermented malt beverages, including ground ivy, wild rosemary, wormwood, yarrow, and henbane. Many of them are psychoactive. Henbane, containing hallucinogenic tropane alkaloids, is especially potent. In German, henbane is *Bilsenkraut,* the *pilsener krut,* the plant used to brew pilsner. Henbane beers were common in Sweden until recently. The famous German purity act of 1516 was particularly directed against henbane and is really the first antidrug law of the modern era.

The Egyptians had words for more than eighty different kinds of beer, differentiated by the different plants and herbs mixed into the wort. Most of these beers were medicinal: beer seems to have been used as a carrier for other medicinal herbs.

The earliest known brewery is dated to 3500 B C, in a Sumerian trading post on the Silk Road in the Zagros Mountains.

And malt does more than Milton can
To justify God's ways to man.

     – A. E. Housman, "Terrence, This Is Stupid Stuff"

Calvert Watkins (1978) has uncovered philological evidence for an ancient Indo-European barley-ritual in the Odyssey, in the Homeric Hymn to Demeter (and thus in the Eleusinian mysteries), in the Vedas, in Hittite sources, and in the Avesta. Common features of the rite as described in each of the above sources are that the barley potion is drunk, that it is prepared or mediated by women, that it is a mixed potion, that it contains, in addition to barley, water, at least one other plant, and also milk or soured milk. Honey and wine also are often ingredients. Further, drinking the potion is described as inducing a feeling of well-being in which quarrels can be patched up and forgotten.

David Flattery (Flattery and Schwartz 1989) believes that the "other plant" in the mixture is *Peganum harmala,* known as *haoma,* or soma. The details of the preparation of the drink indicate that it was not fermented. Rather, and more significantly, the steps of the preparation closely match what Albert Hofmann outlined as the steps necessary to prepare an entheogenic lysergic acid amide drink from ergot-infested grain.

I am a yogi who drinks beer, because
It illumines the Diamond Body,
Completes the Enjoyment Body,
And gives form to all Emanation Bodies.

     – Milarepa

Poesis   The brewing of beer is more complex than the vinting of wine. The reason is that while grapes contain sugar, ready for fermentation as soon as the grapes are crushed, barley contains starch. Starch must first be converted into sugar before it can be fermented. This process is called *mashing.*

To prepare the grain for mashing, the barley is first sprouted and then roasted. Darker roasting produces stouts and porters. After the grain is roasted, it can be cracked, that is, broken into small pieces. The malt (the cracked barley) is mixed with hot water, and has to be kept between 145°F and 155°F for several hours. The temperature is critical to two enzymes, cytase and diastase. Cytase dissolves the cellulose that coats the starch granules, and diastase converts the exposed starch into maltose sugar. If human

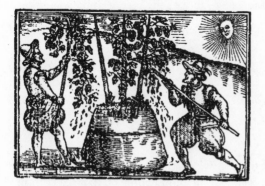

HOPPE-GARDEN, FROM SCOT'S
A PERFITE PLATFORME, 1576

beings produced these enzymes within our bodies, we could, like Nebuchadnezzar, eat grass and save ourselves a great deal of trouble.

Once the wort is mashed, it is taken off, strained, and boiled with the admixture, usually hops. Varying the admixture can produce many interesting and curious brews. Ground ivy was used as an admixture before hops, and the term *beer* was used to distinguish the hops beverage from the other ales. The use of hops in beer was actually prohibited in England by an act of Parliament in 1528, four years after its introduction from Holland. The prohibition was not successful.

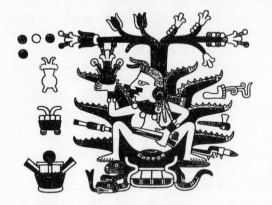

GODDESS OF PULQUE, FROM THE CODEX LAUD

Other admixtures, in addition to those mentioned above, included mushrooms, bay leaves, and *Papaver somniferum* (the seeds, possibly more). I've brewed a wonderful soporific and sedative ale with *Brickellia californica,* a bitter chaparral plant that blooms with a penetrating sweetness in the summer moonlight. I've also brewed spruce beer, though, in my case, the admixture was actually Douglas fir. Spruce beer is refreshing and stimulating. A word of caution, however. Don't overdo it with the pine oils. A friend once brewed up a wickedly strong spruce beer with Sitka spruce that gave him intense subdermal itching and burning for some very uncomfortable hours.

Other innovative admixtures to beer that I've heard of include *Cannabis sativa,* actually a close cousin to hops, ginger, dandelion, and nettles. Exotic plants like coca might come to mind, though in the case of coca, apart from its currently illegal status, history has shown that coca goes better in soft drinks, or in wine, than in beer. Above all, it is flavor that is important – you want enough bitters to balance any sweet or herbal flavors. Since most alkaloids are bitter, some imagination and inspiration might concoct some pretty hair-raising ales – if that's the sort of thing you enjoy.

Once the admixtures have been infused, fermentation proceeds much the same as for wine.

> O guid ale comes, and guid ale goes.
> Guid ale gars me sell my hose,
> Sell my hose, and pawn my shoon;
> Guid ale keeps my heart aboon.
>
>   – *Robert Burns*

Pulque is a Mexican beer brewed from agave cactus. I've heard that the bottled beverage of the same name is far inferior to the pulque brewed in large communal vats in the villages. The effects of the latter were reported to me as "a cross between mescaline and opium."

almost enough to hop on a plane for Mexico . . .

Jaime de Angulo liked pulque.

In equatorial America the natives brew *masato* or *chicha* from the manioc (cassava) plant. Those preparing the *chicha* first chew the tubers and then spit them into a large kettle or tub. Other plants are added, such as banana or some other fruit. Sometimes maize is chewed and added instead of cassava. The tropical warmth sets up fermentation almost immediately, and the first cups are dipped from the ripening mixture after one or two days. More water is added to the mash as fermentation proceeds. *Chicha* is rich and nourishing, tasting slightly like a soured kefir. It can also be somewhat chewy, the cassava being so fibrous. *Chicha* is the comfort beverage of the tropics. It is drunk for strength against the heat, for protection from fevers, and for general spiritual well-being. The alcoholic content, at least for the first several days, is kept low by continued dilution with water. If the *chicha* gets really strong it's time for a party.

Effects

> They who drink beer will think beer.
>   – *Washington Irving*

Organoleptic Methodology

About five beers can be tasted at a sitting. You need two sets of five identical glasses, a friend to taste with, and a trusted accomplice to pour and number the glasses. It is most important that all of the beers be at the same temperature. It is also important that the controller not screw up the labelling.

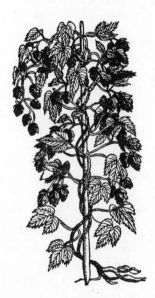

HOP PLANT, FROM DODONAES'S
PURGANTIUM, 1574

The controller should pour the glasses out of sight of the tasters, and should note in writing which brand goes with which number. You will want some mild food to cleanse the palate between tastes.

After tasting each beer, try to characterize it in writing. Record which of the numbered beers you like and why. When you are done and have picked a favorite, compare notes with your friend. Finally, have the controller reveal the brand names of each of the numbers. You'll get some surprises. One friend of mine who had loudly declaimed the superiority of Heineken over Becks selected them in precisely the opposite configuration in the blind tasting.

For tasting, it's best to choose beers all of a class: Mexican lagers, Low Country pilsners, English ales, American premiums, like that. No point in comparing Coors to Anchor Steam.

AQUA VITAE

Common Names   Alcohol, neutral spirits, booze, the Water of Life.

Related Substances   Wood alcohol, CH3OH, methylated spirits. Numerous other alcohols: propyl, isopropyl, butyl. Also, the simplest alcohol of all, hydro-alcohol, the universal solvent, HOH.

Chemistry   Ethanol: C_2H_5OH.

How Taken   Drunk. Imbibed. Sipped. Slugged. Guzzled. Tipped. Lifted. Slurped. Swilled. Chugged. Etc.

Taxonomy   Hydroxyl group, OH. The proton forces hybridization of the oxygen bond, to sp^3. While the hydrocarbon end of the molecule is unpolarized, the hybrid bond polarizes the hydroxyl end. This combination of both polarized and unpolarized parts of the alcohol molecule accounts for its remarkable versatility as a solvent.

Alcohol and water together are less than the sum of the parts: seventy milliliters alcohol plus thirty milliliters water give you only ninety-six and a half milliliters of 140 proof vodka. The molecules commingle: protonated oxygens take Pauling bonds – close-packing, 109 degree angles.

Alcohol is a liaison, mediating between water and oil, between the inorganic world and the organic, between carbohydrates and hydrocarbons.

Pharmacology   Extensively studied. Almost all of the alcohol ingested is metabolized, only a small fraction being excreted – this through the skin and lungs and in the urine. Alcohol is metabolized by oxidation at a constant rate independent of the amount of alcohol ingested. The human body burns about one-third to one-half an ounce of alcohol per hour. That's a little less than one average drink per hour. If you drink more than that, the alcohol accumulates in your bloodstream, and you become more intoxicated. Exercising or drinking coffee does not appreciably affect the rate of combustion, nor do any known drugs. The combustion rate of alcohol in the body seems to be a constant of human physiology.

The first stage in the oxidation of alcohol takes place in the liver, where alcohol is oxidized by an enzyme to yield acetaldehyde. This toxic substance disperses throughout the body, where it is further oxidized to form acetic acid, vinegar. Coenzymes lyse away another hydroxyl group from the acetic, and the result ultimately yields energy, carbon dioxide, and water.

Alcohol depresses synaptic transmission. The characteristic loosening of inhibitions may occur because the neurons responsible for inhibition, assuming such exist, are depressed before the others. Alcohol raises the testosterone level in women, which accounts for some of alcohol's aphrodisiacal properties.

Methyl alcohol, also called wood alcohol, has a different metabolic pathway. Methyl alcohol is burned only very slowly. Whereas all the ethyl alcohol from a drinking bout is metabolized within twenty-four hours, the same amount of methyl alcohol may take a week or more to be burned off. It might seem that drinking wood alcohol would be an inviting way to stay drunk. Unfortunately, one of the metabolites is formic acid, a cellular toxin whose perniciousness goes far beyond many of those that we will discuss here. Methyl alcohol is present in Canned Heat. Straining Canned Heat through a chamois, the old hobo trick, removes the paraffin, but not the methylated spirits.

Ethanol, drinking alcohol, is far from harmless. Alcohol is a protoplasmic poison. It kills bacteria, animals, and plants, even the plant that produces it to begin with. The most effective concentration for a germicide is 140 proof, or 70 percent alcohol. This is the concentration used in doctors offices as a disinfectant. Pure alcohol is less effective, evidently because it gelatinizes the cellular walls of the targeted microbes.

The toxicity of medicines and poisons is commonly expressed as the *LD50*, the "lethal dose for 50 percent." Usually measured in grams per kilogram of body weight, it signifies the amount of the substance necessary to result in death for one-half of the unfortunate test subjects. The *relative* safety or danger of a drug is denoted by its *therapeutic index,* its margin of safety. The therapeutic index is the ratio of the drug's LD50 to its effective dose, the dose necessary to produce the desired effects. Since both the effective dose and the LD50 are in grams per kilogram, the therapeutic index is a pure number. The larger the therapeutic index, the safer the drug.

The therapeutic index of alcohol is only about five. That is, five times the amount needed to get you high can kill you. This puts alcohol, as recreational drugs go, into the "highly dangerous" category. To illustrate: if your child were going to overdose on a drug as some rite of passage, say, turning twenty-one, would you rather he or she overdose on alcohol or on marijuana? Either/or is not the point of course. The point is that merely by drinking too much alcohol too quickly, even once, you can die. Even cigarettes are safer than that.

Alcohol is absorbed readily from the intestines into the bloodstream, less readily from the stomach. For this reason, eating food while drinking retards the effect of the poison, because it keeps the alcohol in the stomach longer. Milk, meat, cheese, and egg products are particularly effective for this.

Very strong liquor causes the stomach to close up. The fastest absorption of alcohol in the stomach is at a concentration of between 10 percent, like wine, and about 35 percent, or 70 proof. The absorption is facilitated by a basic condition in the stomach, such as produced by soda water, or by the bubbles in champagne.

Habituation and addiction are generally long-term processes. Nonetheless, 15 million Americans, one-tenth of the adult population, are either addicted or seriously debilitated by alcohol. Further, alcohol is creating a serious economic problem in developing countries, as commercial beverages replace the home-brews. The cost of two bottles of beer may be half a day's wage.

Effects

Nor have we one or two kind of drunkards only, but eight kinds. The first is ape drunk, and he leaps and sings and hollers and danceth for the heavens. The second is lion drunk, and he flings the pots about the house, calls his hostess whore, breaks the glass windows with his dagger, and is apt to quarrel with any man that speaks to him. The third is swine drunk – heavy, lumpish, and sleepy, and cries for a little more drink and a few more clothes. The fourth is sheep drunk, wise in his own conceit when he cannot bring forth a right word. The fifth is maudlin drunk, when a fellow will weep for kindness in the midst of his ale and kiss you, saying "By God, Captain, I love thee; go thy ways, thou dost not think so often of me as I do of thee. I would, if it pleased God, I could not love thee so well as I do" – and then he puts his finger in his eye and cries. The sixth is martin drunk, when a man is drunk and drinks himself sober ere he stir. The seventh is goat drunk, when in his drunkenness he hath no mind but on lechery. The eighth is fox drunk, when he is crafty drunk as many of the Dutchmen be . . .

    – Thomas Nashe, 1592

Or like the T-shirt I saw that said INSTANT ASSHOLE: JUST ADD ALCOHOL.

History

Legend ascribes the discovery of distillation and of aqua vitae to the alchemist Geber. Geber, whose proper Arabic name is Jábir-ibn-Hayyán, was born in the year 702. He was probably a Mesopotamian, though some have said he was a Greek who converted to Islam. The word *alcohol* is derived from an Arabic word for the fine antimony powder that women used to stain their eyes. The gist of the meaning is that it is *the finest essence.* By another tradition an Arabic alchemist named Rhazes was the discoverer of alcohol. Either way, both alchemy and chemistry flow to us through Baghdad.

The essential principle underlying the discovery is that the intrinsic power within the plant, or in this case within the wine, is an entity that can be extracted and collected with tools and the proper ritual. Nothing really new there, from a shamanic standpoint, other than the nature of the tools themselves: a retort instead of a bull-roarer, and a furnace instead of a drum.

Not the wine, but something within the wine.

And imagine the excitement when they found it: a clear, light liquid like water but not water – finer than water, more sparkling than water. It was the essence, the quintessence, the vital principle of the wine. And they named it *water of life:* a liquid that burns with a sulphurous blue flame.

Distillation was the key, and it probably grew out of wort-cunning and perfumery, rather than out of the metals work. The metals workers picked up on it secondarily, and tried to apply it to sublimation.

> *. . . out of water came fire.*

Effects

In spite of the fact that alcohol is a depressant, in people who are very inhibited, whose inhibitions keep them from succeeding, alcohol can, and does, improve performance.

> *All the great villainies of history, from the murder of Abel onward, have been perpetrated by sober men, and chiefly by teetotallers. But all the charming and beautiful things, from the Song of Songs to bouillabaisse, and from the nine Beethoven symphonies to the Martini cocktail, have been given to humanity by men who, when the hour came, turned from tap water to something with colour to it, and more in it than mere oxygen and hydrogen.*
>
> *– H. L. Mencken (in Mortlock and Williams 1947)*

Mencken means carbon. *Vajra*. The adamantine.

History

Alchemy and the knowledge of distillation migrated into Europe in the thirteenth century. Physician and alchemist Arnold de Vila Nova wrote a tract on the distillation of wine and is credited with coining the term *aqua vitae*. His pupil, Raymond Lully, was a leading proponent of the distilled spirit, believing it to be the elixir of eternal life and a preventative against senility. Many alchemists embraced the fiery liquid as the Great Stone itself.

The use of aqua vitae remained limited to doctors, monks, and a few alchemists throughout most of the Middle Ages and the Renaissance, but they performed a great many experiments. The power of aqua vitae as a solvent was quickly recognized, and many medicinal liqueurs and elixirs were created, containing a few herbs to perhaps several dozen.

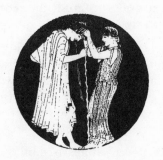

CLASSICAL INEBRIATION –
GREEK YOUTHS IN HIGH CAROUSE,
RED–FIGURE VASE PAINTING
BY THE BRYGOS PAINTER,
5TH C. BC

> *The herbs were macerated in distilled spirits and then distilled again. Sometimes the distillate was then reinfused with a second batch of herbs. Fruits were also used. And so were minerals and precious stones: ground pearls, lapis lazuli, gold leaf. Sometimes animals were used: "mans-brains," "viper-wine."*

By the mid sixteenth century, mostly as a result of the Protestant Reformation, distilled alcohol escaped from the poisoners and found its place as a poison of the general populace. Gin, "Geneva," the first popular liquor, was invented by a doctor. The popularity of alcohol as a recreational drug and its accompanying problems are depicted in the drawings of William Hogarth and other artists of the seventeenth and eighteenth centuries.

The Water of Life became so popular in the seventeenth century that another plant, *Saccharum officinale,* sugarcane, was grown in huge plantations on Barbados and other Caribbean islands, to feed the hungry yeast vats. To perform the back-breaking work of the cane fields, slaves were used. Much of the cane molasses was distilled in the American colonies. In fact, rum contributed to the economic success of the northern colonies much the way that tobacco did for the southern colonies. A diabolically lucrative trade developed: slaves from Africa to the West Indies, molasses from the West Indies to the colonies, rum from the colonies to England, and guns from England to Africa, to trade for slaves. The ships could just keep sailing in a large clockwise circle.

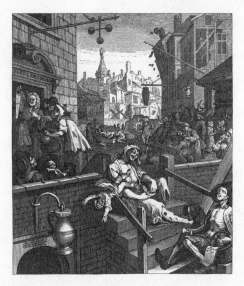

GIN LANE, WILLIAM HOGARTH, 1753

By the late eighteenth century, the alchemist's secret process was being used in the American backcountry. Transport to the east was difficult: the few roads charged tolls, and the Mississippi River was controlled by the Spanish. The Westerners responded by concentrating their corn or rye into whiskey, with a six-to-one compression ratio.

During George Washington's second term of office an armed rebellion broke out on the frontier because Alexander Hamilton had placed a tax on whiskey. Hamilton's friends were rum men, owners of large distilleries in New England. The rum industry was feeling threatened as the public outcry over slaving mounted, and the whiskey tax worked in its favor. Washington gave Hamilton 15,000 government troops to crush the rebellion and collect the tax. They succeeded, at least partially.

Folklore   The term *proof* originated in the practice of testing alcohol by wetting gunpowder with it, and then applying a match to the powder. If the liquor were more than about 50 percent water, the powder would not go off. If the powder did go off, it was "proof" (or *poof!*) that the stuff was at least half alcohol (actually, 57 percent, but in the United States 100 proof is defined as 50 percent alcohol by volume).

Poesis   The craft of compounding waters and cordials was summarized in 1757 by John French in a book called *The Complete Distiller.* Copies of the book can still be found in libraries. The only significant advancement of the two hundred years since French's book is the "continuous" still, the type used in commercial production of most primary distilled spirits: liquors produced by distilling wine or mash. Cognac and most of the finest herbal liqueurs are still cooked in batch stills, the old way.

The basic process of making liqueurs is the same as it has always been: macerate the herbs in high-proof alcohol (days to weeks), distill, finish with more herbs and/or with simple syrup. If you finish with a second maceration, such as is done with absinthe, you will probably want to filter the elixir afterward. (Millefiore Cucchi and some other herbal cordials contain a branch of the herb right in the bottle.) Add distilled water to drop the cordial to the desired proof.

The small-scale herbalist needs a still larger than the 1,000-milliliter glass flask of the laboratory and smaller than the copper pots of the moonshiners. Use imagi-

nation and ingenuity. A large pressure cooker can be perfect for a backyard operation. You want a pot with a jiggler spout in the lid, so that you can attach some vinyl or polyethylene tubing between the pot and your condenser. The tubing must fit snugly: a small hose clamp will secure it. A friend made a condenser with a large coffee can and coiled copper tubing. He drilled a hole in the can near the bottom for the tubing to poke through, sealed it, just let the water overflow over the top.

Don't fill the pot more than half full. If you are going to distill a wort with solid matter still in it, make some precaution so that the hole can't get plugged. And remember, the elixir is flammable, especially when hot.

Be careful not to have the heat too high. A fast drip into the collector is OK, but no faster. Discard the head and

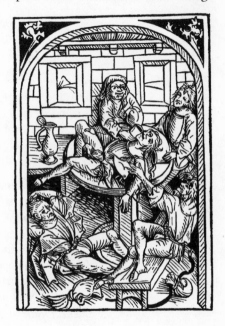

A STUDENTS' DRINKING BOUT, FROM THE
DIRECTORIUM STATUUM, CA. 1489

the tail: the *faints*. The *head,* the very first distillate to come over, contains the highest fractions (the most volatile compounds in the tincture), usually aldehydes. It's easy to tell by taste. The head will often be coarser, more biting, than the heart of the distillate.

The *tail* is the very last of the distillate, the low-proof fumes that come over after the majority of the alcohol has already been distilled off and the temperature begins to rise in the distilling pot. Fusel oils are often in the faints (not always). The faints can be saved and eventually redistilled, to save as much of the alcohol as possible.

Be sure to check local regulations before you do this. A dear friend once had a small pressure cooker still of the type described above in his yard in his mountain home. Finding an abandoned motorcycle on the dirt road to his house, he dutifully called the police, suspecting that it was stolen. While the police were taking his report they noticed his still, which was in plain view. Too honorable to arrest him themselves, they reported the still when they returned to headquarters. Two squad cars were sent, my friend was hand-cuffed, arrested, and taken to jail.

We brought photographs of the still to the trial to show the judge just what sort of a criminal he had in his courtroom, and the judge let him go with a fine.

> MORAL: When you call your local authorities to find out what the law is on backyard distillation, use a pay phone, and don't give them your real name.

On Drinking   Cultures have collapsed from inebriation – precarious worlds poised between starvation and feasting; worlds filled with spirits and deities, and taboos; with complex and demanding rules of behavior. Intricacies of etiquette, who can be spoken to, which relatives, which emotions can be displayed, which must be hidden – all swept away in a torrent of inebriation hallucinatory in its strength and virulence.

> *The Hurons, in the seventeenth century, obtaining a cask of rum from the traders, held council to select a weapons-keeper – a sort of "designated driver" – who was absolutely forbidden to drink. This person's job was to collect all the weapons – hatchets, knives, tomahawks, and guns – and hide them. Even so, fatalities were not uncommon in the days-long rioting and debauchery that ensued before the rum ran out. Moreover, certain Indians, particularly the sensitive or those holding positions of social dignity, on awakening from the days of drunkenness, would commit suicide from shame. Drunkenness put them in a world like the dream world where one of the two souls lives, a mirror-world where phantoms and impulses moved and mixed, visible, flesh and memory and vision all swirling together.*

Plato had a similar idea. He thought that at symposia the host should stay sober. Compare this to a bar, where the bartender never drinks. Nor the bouncer. Which would have seemed correct to the Indians.

Gustav Schenk (1955) believes that our age drinks somewhat less than those before. That may be true for a comparison to past civilized cultures, but not for natural and inhabitory cultures. In most hunter-gatherer and primitive agricultural communities, drinking has a ceremonial character. It is joyously indulged in, occasionally. That such occasions may be frequent does not alter their status as special events, whether social or religious. In such a milieu drinking alone would simply never be considered.

An Andean people, the Aymaru, drink to excess, ceremonially, at any important social occasion – events that are not infrequent. The drunkenness is sacred, it represents the *love* of the hosts, and everyone present must get drunk. Quite drunk. The binge lasts for several days when it happens, complete with vomiting, passing out, lurching about, and falling over furniture. But no one becomes an alcoholic.

The Ally   *cognac, armagnac, martell, martín, cambas, courvoisier, pisco, marc, hennessy, grappa, brandy, california brandy, masson, almadén, christian brothers, morrow, korbel, raynal, cognac, ahhh, cognac,*

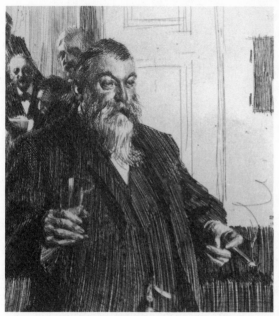

THE TOAST, ANDERS ZORN, 1893

whiskey, hiram walker, johnnie walker, irish, scotch, cutty sark, macallon, glenlivet, glenfiddich, bushmill's, jameson, straight, blended, crown royal, v.o., kentucky, tennessee, sour mash, corn, bourbon, rye, jack daniels, jim beam, wild turkey, george dickel, ancient age, old grand-dad, old taylor, old crow, old crone, old hoss, old tennisshoes, cream of kentucky, early times,

canadian club, canadian mist, irish mist, irish cream, arrack, metaxa, tequila, cuervo, herradura, mescal, galliano, stonsdorfer, goldwasser, strega, valentino, certosa, mentuccia, bronte, cognac, ahhh, cognac,

gin, english gin, dutch gin, bols gin, sloe gin, fast gin, gin done done it, tanqueray, bombay, boodles, vodka, smirnoff, absolut, aquavit, schnapps, creme de menthe, tava, sabra, ouzo, rum, ron coco, rum-cola, the yankee-dollah,

creme de cassis, creme de cacao, creme de vanille, creme de mocha, tia maria, kahlua, pasha, creme de almond, creme de noisette, sabazia, trappastine, carmeline, sapindor, aiguebelle, fior d'alpe, millefiore cucchi, sambuca, amaretto, kümmel, molinari, mistra, absinthe, anisette, pernod, izarra, tuaca, benedictine, b&b, cognac, ahhh, cognac,

aurum, campari, mersin, filfar, bertram's, marnique, san michele, rock and rye, prunelle, mirabelle, persico, framboise, parfait amour, curaçao, vaccari, médoc, drioli, slivovitz, maraschino, peter heering, james hawker, marasca, triple sec, du kuyper, yukon jack, applejack, calvados, forbidden fruit, bolsherwhisk, kirsch, dolfi, drambuie, southern comfort, sakura, cointreau, grand marnier, chartreuse,

cognac, ahhh, cognac . . .

THE ALCOHOLIC MUSE

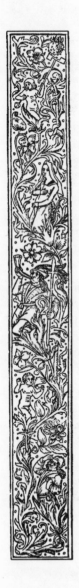

"Why are you drinking?" demanded the little prince.

"So that I may forget," replied the tippler.

"Forget what?" inquired the little prince, who was already sorry for him.

"Forget that I am ashamed," the tippler confessed, hanging his head.

"Ashamed of what?" insisted the little prince, who wanted to help him.

"Ashamed of drinking!" The tippler brought his speech to an end, and shut himself up in an impregnable silence.

    – Antoine de Saint-Exupery, The Little Prince

"Got any more?" Nick asked.

"There's plenty more but dad only likes me to drink what's open."

"Sure," said Nick.

"He says opening bottles is what makes drunkards," Bill explained.

"That's right," said Nick. He was impressed. He had never thought of that before. He had always thought it was solitary drinking that made drunkards.

    – Ernest Hemingway, "The Three-Day Blow"

Some men are like musical glasses – to produce their finest tones you must keep them wet.

    – Samuel Taylor Coleridge

Many addictions are so subtle that they go unnoticed. But big or small, addictions are almost always denied.

Opium was the drug of choice for the romantics, but for the moderns, the poets and writers of the first half or two-thirds of the twentieth century, the overwhelming preferred poison was alcohol. Donald W. Goodwin, in *Alcohol and the Writer*, writes: "Six Americans had won the Nobel Prize in literature and four were alcoholic. (A fifth drank heavily and the sixth was Pearl Buck, who probably didn't deserve the prize.)" Goodwin concludes that, as a vocation, writers are "over-represented" in the population of alcohol addicts. Sinclair Lewis, an alcoholic himself, once quipped: "Can you name five American writers since Poe who did not die of alcoholism?" Certainly enough of a problem that, for a writer, alcoholism could be considered an occupational hazard.

The loneliness of the work, the solitude,
or maybe just the unblinking white stare
of a blank sheet of paper . . .

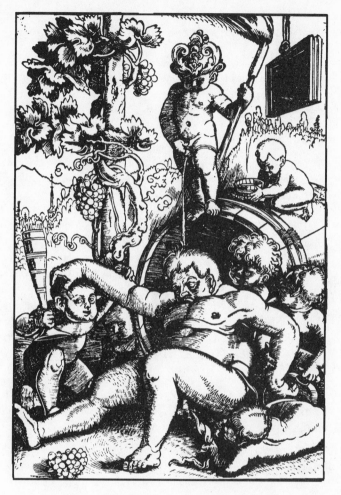

CHILDISHNESS AND FOOLISHNESS, HANS BALDUNG GREEN, 1510

And writers have to structure their own time; there is no office, secretary, or co-workers. There is no time-clock to punch. All of the solar medicine must come from within – but also, and simultaneously, the lunar inspiration:

> *For art to exist, for any sort of aesthetic activity to exist, a certain physiological precondition is indispensable: intoxication.*
>   *– Nietzsche, Twilight of the Gods*

The balance is the acme of our Art.

You have an appointment. You wait in the anteroom of the gods and worry about your makeup. The only mirror is the one you have brought with you, your offering, the mirror you have already painted over with your own visage.

> *Maybe the poison*
> *is to silence the critic.*

Or maybe, as Blake said, all true poets are of the Devil's party.

> *No poems can please for long or live that are written by water-drinkers.*
>   *— Horace*

Here is Goodwin's list of American writers who were either alcoholics or "heavy drinkers," alphabetized:

> *James Agee, Conrad Aiken, Philip Barry, Robert Benchley, John Berryman, Ambrose Bierce, Truman Capote, Raymond Chandler, John Cheever, Hart Crane, Stephen Crane, e. e. cummings, Mr. Dooley (Finley Peter Dunne), Theodore Dreiser, William Faulkner, F. Scott Fitzgerald, Woolcott Gibbs, Dashiell Hammett, Ernest Hemingway, O. Henry (William Sydney Porter), William Inge, Randall Jarrell, James Jones, Jack Kerouac, Ring Lardner, Sinclair Lewis, Jack London, Robert Lowell, Ralph Maloney, J. P. Marquand, Edna St. Vincent Millay, John O'Hara, Eugene O'Neill, Dorothy Parker, Edgar Allan Poe, Edwin Arlington Robinson, Theodore Roethke, Robert Ruark, William Saroyan, Delmore Schwartz, Irwin Shaw, Jean Stafford, John Steinbeck, Wallace Stevens, James Thurber, Edmund Wilson, Tennessee Williams, Thomas Wolfe, and, according to its nonalcoholic drama critic Brendan. Gill, almost every writer for the New Yorker during the thirties.*

To Goodwin's list, which he says was "off the top of his head," and only included writers who were "safely dead," we could easily add another score of poets, including, if rumors are to be believed:

> *Maxwell Bodenheim, Charles Bukowski, James Dickey, Richard Hugo, Bob Kaufman, Vachel Lindsay, Jack Michelin, Anne Sexton, Dylan Thomas, Chogyam Trungpa, Lew Welch, and James Wright.*

Deeper digging into the modern poets, 1920 to 1960, would double, triple, or quadruple this list.

> *And Li Po also died drunk.*
> *He tried to embrace a moon*
> *in the Yellow River.*
>   *— Ezra Pound*

❶

Timor Mortis conturbat me.

THE POISON PATH I

❧

For instance, one man will have faith enough to eat all kinds of food, while a weaker man eats only vegetables. The man who eats must not hold in contempt the man who does not, and he who does not eat must not pass judgement on the one who does; for God has accepted him. . . .

Let us therefore cease judging one another, but rather make this simple judgement: that no obstacle or stumbling-block be placed in a brother's way. I am absolutely convinced, as a Christian, that nothing is impure in itself; only, if a man considers a particular thing impure, then to him it is impure. . . . What for you is a good thing must not become an occasion for slanderous talk; for the kingdom of God is not eating and drinking, but justice, peace, and joy, inspired by the Holy Spirit.

— Rom 14: 2–3, 13–14, 16–17

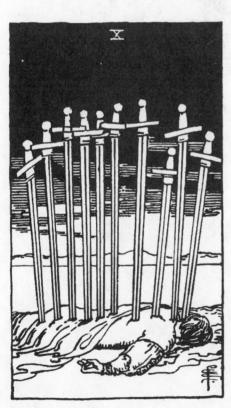

The matter of the *stumbling brother* is the cross of the Poison Path: on this trope turn the intersecting greater and lesser vehicles, the right-hand path and the left. Skilled poisoners avoid ruin, but in the struggle for "justice, peace, and joy" in the Kali Yuga, ruin may come on her own wings. And the Ten of Swords most readily approaches those who are unlucky.

How can you tell if you are lucky or unlucky? This is most important. If you are not lucky, you will surely stumble. Then the lucky ones must share the guilt. The question of the *stumbling brother* is relevant to the debate about legalization of crack cocaine and the possible "devastation of the Black community" that might result (as if the Black community were not already devastated by the current illegality of crack). Relevant, that's all. But we stray.

How can you tell if you are lucky? In his letter to the Romans, Paul is clear that he has two teachings, that there is an exoteric path and that there is an esoteric path. He states unambiguously that *he* knows that all substances are by nature pure, that Jesus told him so. The issue then is stumbling. Another's stumbling. Another who does not understand that all substances are pure. And since our way is the eclectic path of the magicians, we will step over the scores of stumbled bodies that accomplished poisoners such as Aleister Crowley leave in their wake, and toss off a couple of obstacles of our own.

You can tell if someone is lucky by their marks. Scars are particularly revealing. Even the lucky have close calls. But how did the wound heal over? *Is the person in question marked for calamity?* Or for ruin? The same way that some people bear the marks of survival, others are marked for ruin and failure – it is written on them. And I don't mean in any fatalistic sense, but writ by pattern.

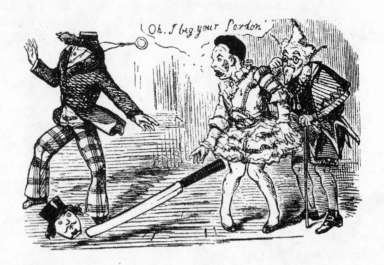

OOPS

Never share poisons with the *unlucky*.

And, as Nelson Algren said, don't sleep with them, either.

Best for all that they never hear a word about poisons. Or about power. Or about Paul. If they do, later, well, you know the rest . . .

> *The danger, of course, is that you who are reading this consider yourself, ipso facto, one of the lucky.*

ÆTHER

ぶ

Related Substances	Chloroform, $CHCl_3$; nitrous oxide, N_2O; ethylene, CH_2CH_2; ethyl chloride, C_2H_5Cl; halothane, $CF_3CHClBr$. Neither ethylene nor ethyl chloride is much used today as a general anesthetic, although ethyl chloride is still used as a local anesthetic. Chloroform is more toxic than ether, having a therapeutic index (margin of safety) of about three, an overdose causing cardiac arrest. Halothane also has a relatively low margin of safety, but has largely replaced ether as a general anesthetic because it is nonflammable. Ethylene is more than flammable: mixed with oxygen, as it must be for use as an anesthetic, it is explosive.

> *a plant hormone, ripener of fruit and deadener of mind:*
> *a neurotransmitter straddling two kingdoms . . .*

Chemistry	Ethyl ether, or diethyl ether, $(C_2H_5)_2O$. Two short alkyl chains, an oxygen between them, forming a symmetrical molecule of very low polarity. At room temperature, ether is a highly volatile liquid; as a gas it is heavier than air and highly flammable. Ethyl ether is an important organic solvent, but in most cases methylene dichloride is a safer and adequate substitute. Ether is notorious for forming explosive peroxides if left around the lab for too long.

Ether is prepared by using concentrated sulfuric acid to dehydrate alcohol at an atomic level. The acid's thirst for water is so great that it can strip hydrogen and oxygen atoms right off the ethanol molecules. The resulting liquid is lighter and subtler than its parent: an alchemical poison, the refinement of the refinement of the poisons in the plant.

> *An angel is boiled in satanic acid. But the vapor that arises must be the atmosphere of heaven, not of hell. In hell, with all the sparks and flames, ether would explode instantly.*

Ether is to alcohol as alcohol is to water: if alcohol is water and fire, ether is water, fire, and air.

How Taken	The vapor is inhaled. Ether may also be imbibed. Like from a shot glass. If recipes for mixed drinks exist, I haven't seen them. Besides, water and ether are immiscible, so if you are going to drink it, I think you have to drink it neat.

A teaspoonful is adequate for beginners, especially along with some inhalation. In the last century people would swallow six or eight drops on a cube of sugar and wash it down with a little water. Eternal recurrence.

Effects	*There is no truth so profound* *it cannot be obtained with the inebriants . . .*

Pharmacology   A general anesthetic, producing unconsciousness. Four stages are customarily recognized, but only the second is of much interest to us. The stages are:

> 1. local irritation: bad taste, choking, sometimes ringing or hissing sounds;

> 2. excitement: giggling, or shouting – the religious sing hymns, the abusive fight – some of us need to write;

> 3. unconsciousness: pulse rapid and strong, breathing deep and regular, muscles relaxed;

> 4. coma: all vital centers repressed, blue face, shallow or gasping breathing, dilated pupils that don't react to light.

Ether coma should be treated by immediately removing the mask and giving artificial respiration. Stretching the sphincter of the rectum can help induce breathing. Give respiratory stimulants such as caffeine or atropine.

Ether has a lower safety margin than alcohol does: about three to one for ether, and five to one for alcohol. Comparisons of the chronic toxicity of ether with the chronic toxicity of alcohol are mixed. Some people maintain that alcohol is more dangerous, others state that the "degeneration of character" proceeds more quickly with ether than with alcohol. As ether is not metabolized, liver damage is unlikely. More likely problems are gastritis, irritation of the kidneys, albumin in the blood, anemia, or pneumonia as a result of mucus in the lungs.

Ether interacts synergistically with tetrahydrocannabinol.

Effects   The trick is you can't pay attention to the smell or the taste, or be concerned that you'll go around smelling like ether for a day or two.

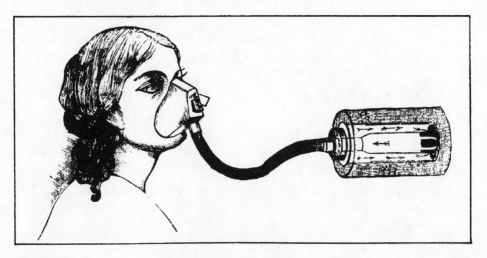

ETHER INHALING DEVICE

> *like a glockenspiel —*
> *colored bells, cold stars, a woozy ringing,*
> *great spaces opening between:*   *the Abyss*

How Taken   The best description is in John Irving's rather satisfying novel, *The Cider House Rules,* about an orphanage doctor and abortionist who is an ether addict:

> *Dr. Larch was an open-drop-method man. With one hand he held a*
> *cone over his mouth and nose; he made this mask himself (by wrapping*
> *many layers of gauze around a cone of stiff paper); with his other hand,*
> *he wet the cone. He used a quarter-pound ether can punctured with*
> *a safety pin; the drops that fell from the elbow of the safety pin fell in*
> *exactly the correct size and at exactly the correct rate. . . . When the hand*
> *that held the ether can felt unsteady, he put it down; when the hand that*
> *held the cone over his mouth and nose dropped to his side; the cone fell*
> *off his face.*

The good doctor visits the starry realm of ether nightly. Consequently, he always smells of ether, but the smell of ether was not so unexpected on a doctor in that era. For nondoctors, the lingering excretion of ether through the lungs is a dead giveaway, and is detectable for twenty-four or even thirty-six hours after a session.

Irving calls ether "the perfect addiction for a conservative," and there are many references to the "light, tasty liquid" throughout the book.

Effects   One might think that the last vestige of consciousness would be interested in monitoring the proximity of danger, in one's own margin of safety. But no. The last thread of consciousness is used to deliver a few more drops of the ether; all else is disregarded. Perhaps, you might say, the subject already is secure and in any real emergency invisible, submerged parts of the mind would come forth to signal and take charge. Perhaps. Perhaps, but in my experience, the faintest, least glimmer of volition is immediately directed to the ether bottle.

> *Let us not, out of hand, reject those arguments based on purely quantitative*
> *considerations, that in x-1 occurrences the conclusion is based on extraordi-*
> *nary circumstances. That is, that there is a basic difference between leisurely*
> *decisions and those based on duress or boundary conditions.*

Decisions based on boundary conditions do occur, and they are invariably to apply more solvent.

The Ally   *I'm not interested in just the,*
you know, the run of the mill,
the run of the mill kind of
profound thought.

Ahhh, drunk! And in public.

There must be some insistent repetition.

Repeating, even just repeating as fast as you can repeat, there is always at least some value in virtuosity, in perfection of craft.

History   The preparation and chemical properties of ether were described by Basil Valentine and Valerius Cordus in the early fifteenth century. Paracelsus may have been the first to use ether on himself. Ether was first used as an anesthetic around 1840 at Massachusetts General Hospital. Humphrey Davy knew ether and used it as a psychoeuleptic, as did Samuel Taylor Coleridge, though both of them focused more attention on nitrous oxide.

The Ally   You can figure out from the basics that it is not an evil conspiracy, that it has more to do with the nature of things, the difficulty, the subtlety of self-knowledge, and that Evil is overrated.

There is one class to whom reflection is a fault; is not only a fault, is a sin; is not only a sin, is an atrocity – who cannot bear to exist without their own existence dis-existencing somebody else's existence.

That's the problem: there are those who think that their own existence needs so much room they must grab all possible planes of existence before they have even begun to develop the plane that they themselves exist upon. That's the problem.

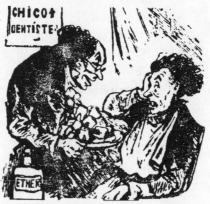

AFTER ETHER

History   Ether became popular as a party drug in the late nineteenth century. Many used it as a substitute for alcohol. Oliver Wendell Holmes experimented with it at Harvard, where there was much talk about ether's power to produce mystical and mind-expanding experiences.

déjà vu, anyone?

In northern and eastern Europe some people were consuming up to a liter a day. There are stories of entire villages drinking and sniffing ether, of the streets smelling like hospital rooms. One big advantage of ether over alcohol is the rapidity of the inebriation, which is nearly immediate, and the similarly rapid return of sobriety. Serious topers could get inebriated three or four times in a day and do business or errands in between, reportedly with minimal hangovers.

In the United States, not surprisingly, ether's popularity peaked during Prohibition. Ether was allegedly used to spike drinks, perhaps mixed with alcohol, or just drunk by itself.

The Ally   *What is the collateral damage of the pharmacist's pipette?*

Occasionally I have an insight that would lead me to despair of any nobility of human nature.

> *The difference between the ba-bá and the nothing is significant: there are political implications.*

And that the difference between being and nothingness has political implications is astounding.

> *There are those who would repress the question of the difference between the ba-bá and the ba-bá ba-ba-bá as having any significance.*

> *ba-bá ba-ba-bá or ba-bá-ba ba-bá*

History   Allen Ginsberg used a whole quart of ether pursuing his poem of the same name: a long, rolling poem, "Aether: 4 Sniffs & I'm High," begun at eleven-fifteen in the evening, Hotel Commercio, Lima, Peru, May 28, 1960.

> *All night, w/ Ether, wave*
> *after wave of magic*
> *understanding.*

The poem not ended until the next day, questioning the One, questioning Death, questioning Keats's Nightingale:

> *What can be possible*
>   *in a minor universe*
>   *in which you can see*
>   *God by sniffing the*
>   *gas in a cotton?*
>   *— Allen Ginsberg, Reality Sandwiches*

Laughter, Light, Pistol Shots, a Magic Universe slightly mad.

The Ally   It is the Fool who knocks at the door of Death:

> *"Hey, asshole, open up!"*

And not surprisingly the door of Death opens: and Death steps out in a foul mood and wants to know who it is among the mortals who is so impatient to knock thus. And the Fool, the Fool, even with a cold sweat breaking all over his body, gestures, with that shit-eating grin, over his shoulder, and blames the guy behind him.

and if you think about it, who really cares:
I mean who cares that some creep
hiding around in the bushes behind a fool
gets creamed
on a case of misidentification?

But we do care. They deserve to live because they are like us – walking is not so different from creeping – they just don't understand. The way we do. Be tolerant, because tolerance is self-tolerance. Why root out one part of yourself as bad and self-destructive and cherish some other part as worthy and good?

In order for there to be something that something happens on
there has to be something like this fabric of the drum
there has to be a tympanum
there has to be an echoing
has to be a sounding board
be something that occurs
out of the mother womb
of nothingness . . .

So some heroes move to the other side, so that they can create, so that something happens here, so there's some kind of music, so that light scratches the sky.

Someone must say OK, I'll move, I'll go, let's see, I'll dance, let's see what happens, let's see where this electricity goes, let's see what happens when we strike this match.

phosphorous, streaking black night –
Lucifer, fire and light.

The here and the beyond are enough, but there were a few angels for whom it was not enough: who demanded a third dimension – who sought fusions, communes, who ate each other and created sex.

They said even though the here and the beyond encompass everything and
stretch everywhere, we wish to go further than the beyond, even if, even if
that will mean that some here must die.

There would be enough in the here and the beyond if everybody stayed in the here and the beyond – but because we have ventured further, there is not enough: some must perish, and thus Death entered the world.

"Yet the experiments must continue!"

We must welcome Him with symposia. It is no other than the Other.

and you of all men know the importance of the Other
you of all men and women know the importance of the Other

FOSSIL FUEL

The poison spreads over the planet.

Related Substances Hexane, Freon, airplane glue, toluene, gasoline. Spray paint, hair spray, PC cleaner, dry cleaning fluid. Spot remover, nail polish remover, paint remover. Lighter fluid, correction fluid thinner, etc., etc., etc.

How Taken "Huffed." That means inhaled.

Effects Similar to ether and nitrous oxide, either of which are many times safer than any of these poisons. Habitual huffers can distinguish different brands of sprays and fluids, and develop preferences. Huffers probably have an interesting terminology to describe the subtle differences of effects, and it would be worth recording, if you could find an informant who is still articulate.

The Plant Here we are at great distance from the alchemical chloroplast: separated in time by eons. Geology and industry have combined to crack, twist, and distill the mummified juices of ancient forests into spiritous and ethereal fluids.

The ecologist Howard Odum once quipped that the evolutionary purpose of human beings was to release all the carbon locked up under the ground back into the biosphere. If true, our mission will soon be accomplished. That it be a suicide mission in no way detracts from its grandeur or heroism.

Chemistry

PRODUCT	CHEMICALS
Adhesives	
Airplane glue	toluene, ethyl acetate
Miscellaneous glues	hexane, toluene, methyl chloride, acetone, methyl ethyl ketone, methyl butyl ketone
Aerosols	
Spray paint	butane, propane, fluorocarbons, toluene, hydrocarbons
Hair spray	butane, propane, chlorofluorocarbons (CFCs)
Air freshener	butane, propane, CFCs
PC cleaner	CFCs
Cleaning Agents	
Dry cleaner	tetrachloroethylene, trichloroethane
Spot remover	xylene, petroleum distillates, chlorohydrocarbons

Solvents

Nail polish remover	acetone, ethyl acetate
Paint remover	toluene, methylene chloride, methanol, acetone
Paint thinner	petroleum distillates, esters, acetone
Correction fluid	tricholorethylene, trichloroethane
Industrial solvent	toluene, xylene, methyl ethyl ketone, methyl butyl ketone

Fuels

Lighter fluid	butane, isopropane
Gasoline	hexanes, aliphatic hydrocarbons, tetraethyl lead

Toxicology   Hexanes can cause peripheral nerve damage. Toluene can affect the central nervous system. Butane and cfcs do not seem to cause neurological damage, but butane can trigger cardiac arrest. Chlorohydrocarbons are toxic to the liver. Gasoline contains hexanes, benzene, other hydrocarbons, triorthocresyl phosphate, and sometimes lead, all of which are toxic. Benzene is carcinogenic.

Epidemiology   Glue sniffing is usually tried once, a few times, or for a few weeks or months. Most young people quit after that. All but a few.

The Ally   A treacherous ally. She turns on you quite suddenly. She gets more and more demanding and gives less and less in return. Like all plant allies, she wants your consciousness, but unlike the others her home is in the Paleozoic: only her spiritous ghost wafts through our own eon. Nerve cells doze, sleepwalk with the ally back to a gooey subterranean syncline.

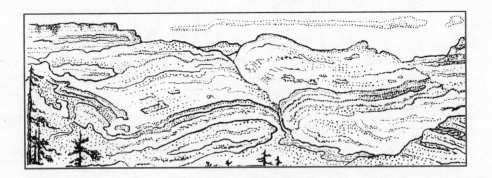

Poesis   If you are incarcerated, you may not have many choices. Otherwise, you do, and you should avail yourself of less harmful substances.

That said, if you are a huffer anyway, take the time to read about solvent abuse in your local library. Reading between the lines, you can discover that some are more harmful than others, some are safer than others. In general, pure solvents are less toxic than mixtures, and a can of pure toluene from the hardware store is safer than the mixtures found in airplane glue or aerosols and spray cans.

Methyl ethyl ketone, MEK, has a relatively clean rap sheet, while MBK, methyl butyl ketone, has the same toxicity as hexane, and mixtures of MEK and MBK are worse than either alone.

If habituated, get off and get help.

Ethnography Gasoline sniffing was once most common among Latinos and on Indian reservations, but with the decreased availability of other intoxicants it is now becoming much more widespread in other cultural and economic strata.

> *Give them ether. Give them halothane.*

Glue sniffing as an "epidemic" was created by scare stories in newspapers and later in schools, beginning in 1959. Before that time glue sniffing, like other solvent huffing, was a relatively rare and inconsequential activity. However alarming the newspaper stories of the new threat, with their spectre of permanent brain damage, were to parents, the result was a tremendous increase in the practice. Before the scare stories, few had even heard of glue sniffing. *Consumer Reports* editors were unable to find any reference to glue sniffing before a scare story appeared in the Denver *Post* in 1959. That the hazards of glue sniffing were wildly exaggerated, that their teachers and their police lied to them, was not lost on the baby-boomer generation.

> *I'd heard from my mother that he was sniffing glue. She was very afraid. So was I. I'd always heard it melted your brain. One night I came in he was on the couch with a plastic bag with three tubes of glue in it. He showed me how to do it. It was wild. I really got a buzz. Very mental. It didn't last very long. Then we had to do it again.*

Toxicology N-HEXANE
         METHYL BUTYL KETONE (MBK)

The neurotoxin is the metabolite: 2,5-hexanedione (HD). Hexane seems as if it should be pretty innocuous stuff – it's just a straight hydrocarbon chain – but like MBK it metabolizes into 2,5-HD in the body, which causes peripheral neuropathy. The neuropathy begins to develop several months after continued exposure, begins painlessly, and may continue to develop for several months after cessation of exposure.

MBK was little used until the 1970s, when it began to be added to paint thinners and other solvents. After MBK was added to methyl ethyl ketone (MEK), reports of polyneuropathy began appearing. MEK alone does not produce neuropathy.

TOLUENE

Chronic inhalation of toluene may produce cognitive dysfunction, hearing loss, equilibrium disorder, and damage to the optic nerve. There is no convincing evidence that pure toluene produces peripheral neuropathy. Nor is it clear that the damage from toluene is irreversible with sustained abstinence. Most sniffers, however, get their toluene from products containing mixtures of solvents, some of which may be highly toxic both by themselves and by synergistic effects on metabolism.

TRICHLOROETHYLENE (TCE)
1,1,1-TRICHLOROETHANE
BUTANE
CFCS: TRICHLOROFLUOROMETHANE (FREON 11)
DICHLORODIFLUOROMETHANE (FREON 12)
1,2-DICHLORO-1,1,2,2-TETRAFLUOROETHANE (FREON 114)

All of these substances appear to sensitize the heart to epinephrine, which may then cause arrhythmia.

TCE was once used as an anesthetic agent along with nitrous oxide. Its toxicity seems to be low. Heavy exposure leads to neuropathy, which is reversible. The biggest danger is cardiac arrhythmia.

Relatively less toxic than other solvents, 1,1,1-trichloroethane is most commonly inhaled in typewriter correction fluid, where it occurs in combination with TCE. Several deaths are attributed to sniffing correction fluid, all from cardiac arrhythmia.

Butane, common in cigarette lighters and tanks of cooking fuel, is also relatively low in toxicity, but like the above chemicals can cause sudden cardiac failure. Several cases are documented in the United Kingdom. The true degree of risk in inhaling butane is unknown, because there is no accurate knowledge of the extensiveness of the practice. Nor is it certain that other factors may not have been involved in the fatalities, such as interaction with other drugs, or even the freezing temperature of the expanding gas. (Merely drinking ice water can, and does, trigger heart fibrillation because of the proximity of the esophagus to the heart.)

The CFCs Freon 11, Freon 12, and Freon 114 may cause minor toxicity to bodily organs other than the heart, but all such damage seems reversible. A handful of deaths are recorded due to cardiac failure from inhaling CFCs. Freon 11 appears to be more toxic than Freon 12 or Freon 114. Newer replacement aerosols appear to be safer, both environmentally and biologically, with significantly less cardiac sensitization.

MEAD AND THE DIVINE MADNESS

The greatest blessings come to us through madness, when it is sent as a gift of the gods.

— *Socrates, Phaedrus*

Mead is a gift of the bee goddess. Two lionlike figures wearing bee-robes, carved into a Mycenaean gem: bee priestesses, something being poured out of vases over a young growing plant. Nectar. Bees like messengers, angels – banqueters bearing *amrita*, the Elixir.

The sexual nature of apian food-gathering would not have been lost on the archaic plant people, either. Their lives were dependent on the vegetal world and its fecundity. They would inspect the seed-heads, the fruits, find some fertile and growing, others barren. They'd figure it out. And follow the bees.

> *Flowers, genitals open to the world,*
> *the wind, critters flying or crawling,*
> *the whole forest a vagina –*
> *bees like semen, promiscuous and orgiastic,*
> *butterflies feeding – proboscis curling*
> *and uncurling, lips, petals, golden*
> *pollen and amber, compound eyes.*

Honey is between, is both food and intoxicant. As an offering, honey was νηφαλια, *nephalia*, of the sober offerings, offered without wine. Honey, water, and milk were offered to the Muses and the nymphs, sometimes with twigs of Cretan thyme, *Thymbra capitata*. Honey was recognized as a source of good health: Pythagoras credited his longevity to daily consumption of honey. Honey is antiseptic, a preservative. The Egyptians used it for embalming, and the Greeks probably knew about that. The priestesses of Demeter were called *melissae*:

> *bees swarming, golden bees clumped*
> *around a branch, and a queen,*
> > *the Goddess bee, Melitodes.*
> *Artemis, also called Melissa, the bee.*

○

"Bees are begotten of bulls."
— *Porphyry*

And honey is also inebriating. Mixed with water it ferments like wine, and certainly preceded wine. Mead is a perfect inebriant for hunter-gatherers: you find it, you put it into some kind of vessel along with some water and send out the invitations. By the time everyone arrives, the mead is ready to drink.

> *When the Dog Star rises,*
> *from the sacrifice, life: autogenesis.*
> *The divine child is nurtured by bees*
> *in a cave that overflows, ekzein, fermented:*
> *mead the ichor, the amniotic fluid of the gods.*

❂

> *"A hum arises: hark! they buzz and buzz."*
> *– Virgil*

Linguistically *mead* is from a very ancient strata of words. Indo-European roots *medhu*, "honey," and *⋆medhus*, "sweet," are thought to be akin to Mediterranean, Semitic, and Egyptian words. Hebrew *māthōq* or *metheq* and Aramaic *matqā*, all mean "sweetness." Akkadian *matqū*, "sweet," like Ugaritic *mtq*, is probably cognate with Greek *meli*, "honey," like the Latin *mel*, German *met*, Hungarian *mez*, Finnish *mesi*, mean "honey beer." Greek *methu* is an "intoxicating drink"; *methyein*, "to be drunk," *methyskein*, "to make drunk"; thus amethysts are a charm against drunkenness.

> *Mead, meodu, meddo, madhu.*
> *Traveling east and vaguely downward in time.*
> *Sweet and pleasurable,*
>   *the nectar of flowers,*
> *mead, or sweet wine, or soma.*

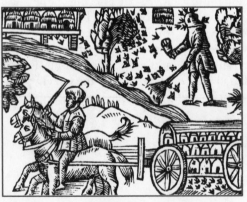

DOMESTICATING BEES

> *Hydromel, the cuckoo bird,*
> *to revel and rejoice, a girl*
> *with bewitching eyes, the madness*
> *of love. Madness. Drunkenness.*
> *Wanton passion. A libertine,*
> *a world of pleasure, the erection*
> *of bodily hair caused by love.*

> *A lump of honey, a large black bee,*
> *bees in swarm, drunken carousal.*
> *To be crazy, to be mad,*
> *exhilaration and delight, passion.*

> *Love, the God of Love,*
> *to inflame, be enamored. Lust.*
> *Musk. The excrescence from the temples*
> *of an elephant in rut.*

To madden, to gladden, to love and desire.
A stream of honey. Grapes or dates.
Ardor. Rapture. Pride,
arrogance, conceit.

Sexual love, sexual union, spring, datura,
a fingernail, a kind of embrace;
Shiva, the penis, pudendum, semen,
a valley of pleasure, Asoka, the tree
of delight.

The Plant In mead the plant has already been digested once by the bee, and then digested again by the yeast, but traces remain. Alkaloids remain, and certain terpenes and oils. Light flavors of citrus and clover, dark poisons of buttercups.

Xenophon reported how the whole Persian army got intoxicated and sick by eating honey of bees that had been feeding on *Azalea pontica*. Honey from bees feeding on nightshade is hallucinogenic. In some cases the bees seem to concentrate the toxins.

Germanic and Celtic tribes continued to drink mead long after the Greeks and Romans changed to wine. Mead was often spiked with spices and other plants, often the same psychotropic plants that bees would feed upon naturally: henbane (*Hyoscyamous niger*), poppy (*Papaver somniferum*), or wild rosemary (*Ledum palustre*).

In Mesoamerica, the Mayans, Polomchi, and Lacandon brew a mead called *balché*. Bark of the *balché* tree, *Lonchocarpus violaceus*, is mixed in with honey and water, along with other admixtures such as datura, tobacco, or *Nymphaea*, the water lily. Sometimes spices are added, vanilla or frangipani, or cocoa, or even the cane toad, *Bufo marianus*, or the skin of tree frogs. The preparer, who identifies himself with Bol, the god of inebriation, chants and summons the invisible spirits of the poisonous plants and animals to add the essence of their poisons to the brew. Drinking *balché* is social and ceremonial, the drinking beginning just before dawn.

Hydromel (υδρομελι), honey and water, the basic mead, survived into the Renaissance as *idromellum*. Another popular medieval beverage was metheglin, spiced mead: "the healing liquor." Welsh *meddyg*, medicinal, plus *illyn*, liquor.

med: medicine, mete, modern,
     meditate,
          empty.

Thomas Hardy, in *Wessex Tales*, gives a recipe for an old spiced mead:

4 lbs. maiden honey to a gallon of water;
white of eggs;
cinnamon, ginger, cloves, mace, rosemary;
yeast.

History   Hydromel, mead, flows from a well at the base of the world tree, Yggdrasil; the well of the giant, Mimir. Odin once wounded and hung himself on the great ash tree for nine days and was revived by a drink of hydromel given him by Mimir. When Odin was seeking Othorial's mead cauldron, he changed himself into a serpent and made love to Gunnloth. He drank the mead in three great draughts, but some drops fell to earth. This is how men obtained poetry. But our poetry is not like that of the gods.

> *[The poet speaks] not with intellect alone but with the intellect inebriated by nectar. As the traveller who has lost his way throws the reins on his horse's neck and trusts to the instinct of the animal to find his road, so must we do with the divine animal who carries us through this world. For if in any manner we can stimulate this instinct, new passages are opened for us into nature. . . . This is the reason why bards love wine, mead, narcotics, coffee, tea, opium, the fumes of sandalwood and tobacco, or whatever other procurers of animal exhilaration.*
>
> — *Ralph Waldo Emerson, The Poet*

Divine drunkenness, like ether, like alcohol used to cause. Adolescent drinking, filled with profound thoughts and poignant reflections.

> *We will sit here and drink beer until we figure out the answers —*

Is there a God? How did the universe begin? What was there before the universe was created? Can there be a fundamental particle? Does life have a purpose?

> *Man, being reasonable, must get drunk;*
> *The best of life is but intoxication.*
>
> — *Lord Byron, "Don Juan"*

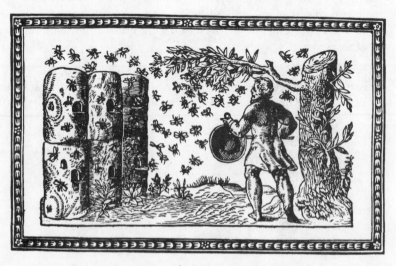

FROM MATTIOLI'S COMMENTAIRES, 1579

Socrates made four divisions of divine madness, giving each kind to one of the gods. Prophecy (*mantike*), which he distinguishes from mere augury, is given to Apollo. Mystic madness (*telestike*) he gives to Dionysus; poetic madness (*poietke*) to the Muses. The highest madness is erotic madness (*erotike mania*), inspired by Aphrodite and Eros.

We are souls who have lost their wings. As plant poisons fly on the wings of bees, so we, drinking poisonous metheglin, don bee robes, borrow their wings, and once again fly up to the place where dwell the race of gods.

Enthused, our voices change. Certain attitudes and postures of the gods become apparent in our movements. The verses come by themselves, wingèd words, clearer and surer than our minds could know.

> *Man is no longer an artist, he has become a work of art: the artistic power of all nature here reveals itself in the tremors of drunkenness to the highest gratification of the Primordial Unity.*
>
> *— Nietzsche, The Birth of Tragedy*

ON THE SEDUCTION
OF ANGELS

Our Way is the seduction of angels. Trouble is, sometimes after you've seduced the angel, you find that it is really the angel that has seduced you. Then you find out that the angel has horns. Wonderful hard nubs of goatlike horn beneath her hair.

If you are a shaman of our way you don't care. In fact you are delighted. You love the horns. You kiss and fondle them. You weave intimate designs upon them. And are given woven charms in return.

Flower-songs, xochitl.

> *Anca zo zan nican tinechnahualan,*
> *Have you bewitched me,*
> *yectli ticchiuh ye motlatoltzin.*
> *you have spoken lovely words.*
> *Iz im axcan tlahuanquetl,*
> *Here, now there is intoxication,*
> *mah teh titlahuanquetl!*
> *inebriate yourself!*
> *Azo no netlacamachon tochan?*
> *Is there happiness in our house?*
>
> *– Aquiauhtzin of Ayapanco, ca. 1430–ca. 1500*

Angels are hard to pin down. Ethereal. Their nature is movement. They are vectors, messengers.

Angels are *betweens,* and the between is of special interest to Hermeticists. One doctor of our way was visited at night by an angel who made love to her and then instructed her in the secrets of the preparation of the Great Stone. René Descartes was given the keys to mathematics.

○

Hermetic. Hermaphrodite. Shamans are often sexual inverts. Or bisexuals. It's part of the between-ness. Female shamans were traditionally promiscuous in many cultures, their

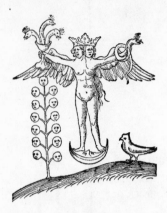

HERMAPHRODITIC ANGEL, FROM THE
ROSARIUM PHILOSOPHORUM, 1550

between-ness eventually becoming ritualized in temples. Don Jaime, who lives on the Rio Napo in Ecuador, had regular sexual relations with Sacha Huarmi, the green woman who takes care of wild animals.

❍

Angels incarnate into plants and springs, into trees, into certain trails and grottos. When they enter men or women we detect it by a subtle glow.

❍

Our way is reptilian sleep, the sleep of amphibians. Sleeping with one eye open. Walking into sleep secretly awake, into dreams without succumbing. Our way involves the will.

❍

The work is carried out in solitude. Our way is teasing. From the beginning, or perhaps from before the beginning, there have been those who open themselves to possession. This method requires a partner, a translator. The seduction way is more like teasing: like a half-sleep, lying still and letting the angel approach. After that, some try to bind the angel, others wrestle; some prefer to blow softly on the angel's cheek and to whisper pleasing words.

Calliope, Erato, Urania.

❍

When the angel comes to your bed you might say no. We are not talking about a one-night stand here. This is an angel, not a strumpet. Maybe if you are not sick you can say no and then just wake up and go back to sleep and live an ordinary life: have a family, maybe a business or a profession, be blessed by the gods and respected by friends and neighbors. But if you are sick, or poisoned, the angel can threaten you, might say, "Make love with me or I will kill you, I will make you sick. I will make you crazy. I will steal your soul and hide it where neither you nor the psychiatrists will ever find it." In such a circumstance it is best not to play the martyr.

Our business is the seduction of angels, and one might wonder if it is a wise endeavor. Indeed.

We have come to give you metaphors for poetry.
    —Yeats, A Vision

Contrary to what the theologians say, not all angels are men: there are male angels, female angels, and hermaphrodites.

Some angels are green. Some of them are called "fairies."

◐

Rituals invoke angels, especially sexual rituals. Threesomes, the minimal orgy. Or mere nudity: snakelike drawings glowing on bodies, breasts, and arms. Penises painted. Black light. Dancing.

Seduction. Seduced. We are all seduced. That's why we are here.

◐

When she comes she is naked. The way she moves, the way she dances, it is as if she holds a knife, a chopper, and the things you thought were absolutely true and real reel and bleed. She bears the Grail: it is a skull. She is naked, she stands on one leg and wraps the other around your head, her cup flows with blood. What she shows you is more real than Reality. Sometimes it smells of corruption. A thin film of gelatin sticks to hands, leaves, grass, tree trunks, the ground, hardening: collagen, cellulose. Some angels have red eyes.

◐

Some ideas are harder to realize than others. Once an idea is realized, it can be discarded. It's the ones you can't see that are dangerous. The dark angels. They can control you. Do. You can't see them because they are behind you.

Better to put your ideas in front.

> *Jeder Engel ist schrecklich.*
> *Every angel is terrible.*
> — *Rilke, Duino Elegies*

◐

Which consciousness can I trust? Some of them are sultry. Some of them are manic. Some are of the sort that don't believe any of the angels are perfect, and that that is desirable.

Some, them. Us, me. You, maybe, too.

◐

Angels are sometimes felt as an alien presence: a vacuum, a sudden absence. The conversation suddenly stops. No one knows what to say. So we say *un ange passe,* an angel passes.

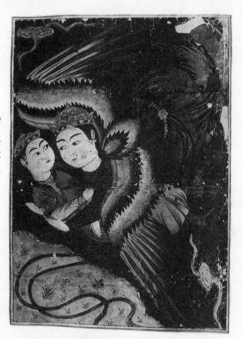

FROM A TURKISH MINIATURE

Words are angels: "winged words." Like arrows, like poison, the shaman's dart.

Words are the most terrible of angels.

The *pharmakeus* is like a baleen porpoise, a filter feeder, straining medicines from currents of charged signs, eddies. The adept of our way must sense unfailingly the instant an angel loses its wings. Unwinged words: τῆ δ ἄπτεροεντα ἔπλετο μῦθος.

> *Expect poison from the standing water.*
> – Blake, The Marriage of Heaven and Hell

Sammael is the Angel of Poison. Sam-el: the "poison angel" who seduced Eve and begat Cain. All *poisoners* are children of Cain. This is the path of the Healer. We still carry the serpent.

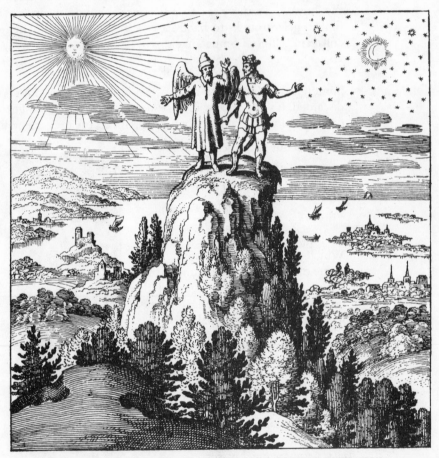

THE ALCHEMIST AND THE ANGEL CONSIDER THE WONDERS OF CREATION,
FROM THE MUSAEUM HERMETICUM REFORMATUM ET AMPLIFICATUM . . ., 1678

ARTEMISIA ABSINTHIUM

❧

Common Names   Wormwood, absinthe, *la Fée Verte,* the Green Muse.

> *. . . that sage of the glaciers, absinthe!*
>   *– Arthur Rimbaud letter to Delahaye*

As the term *absinthe* is used both as a synonym for "wormwood" and also as the name of the famous liqueur, we will use "wormwood" to refer to *Artemisia absinthium,* and "absinthe" to refer to the alcoholic beverage.

Related Species   *Artemisia vulgaris:* mugwort (also called wormwood). Riparian, herbage full of *vertue:* nervine, stimulant, a wash for poison oak, protection against witchcraft, ghosts, thunder, and thieves.

Artemisia tridentata: sagebrush.

> *sweat-lodges: the sacred sage.*
> *horses, cowboys, campfires –*
>
> *the Great Basin . . .*

Artemisia moxa: used for moxibustion in Chinese acupuncture.

Artemisia dracunculus: tarragon.

> *in a cream sauce, with wine and butter . . .*

Thujone, the major active ingredient of wormwood, is also found in cooking sage, *Salvia officinalis;* in tansy, *Tanacetum vulgare;* and in cedar trees, genus *Thuja.*

ARTEMISIA
TRIDENTATA

In addition to wormwood, absinthe (the liqueur) contains hyssop (*Hyssopus officinalis*), lemon balm (*Melissa officinalis*), fennel (*Foeniculum vulgare*), and anise (*Pimpinella anisum*). Some varieties contain sweet flag, *Acornus calamus.* Other absinthes include such herbs as coriander, veronica, marjoram, nutmeg, oregano, angelica, mint, chamomile, parsley, juniper, dittany, and spinach.

Taxonomy   Family, Compositae. Munz, in *A California Flora,* states that Artemisia was the wife of Mausolus, King of Caria, but clearly the genus was named for the Goddess, as was recognized by Apuleius in the second century.

> *Earrings of the moon:*
> *Artemis, goddess of wild things, chastity, fertility,*
>   *and the bloody hunt.*

Dian's bud is the plant that Oberon uses to reverse the effects of the love potion in *A Midsummer Night's Dream.*

The genus is widespread in the Northern Hemisphere. Many species are medicinal; many have not been fully investigated. *Artemisia* is in the mayweed tribe, along with chamomile, yarrow, tansy, and coltsfoot.

Part Used   Leaves.

How Taken   As a liqueur, obtainable only with extreme difficulty. Absinthe is banned by most of the civilized world. Absinthe was legal in Spain until the end of the Franco reign, but is said to be impossible to obtain now, even there. Evidently the old Fascist "took it with him."

Absinthe is a clear bright-green liquid. As absinthe was bottled between 120 and 160 proof, it was rarely drunk neat, but usually diluted about five to one with water. More, because of the bitterness, absinthe was usually drunk sweetened with sugar. Since sugar is not very soluble in alcohol, a delightful ritual developed. A small amount of absinthe was poured into a glass. A special slotted spoon, with a flange, was placed on top of the absinthe glass and a sugar cube placed on the spoon. Then water was poured over the sugar cube, dissolving the sugar into the water, the water falling into the absinthe and mixing with it. Concentrated oils in the absinthe mix with the water and cloud, changing the color of the absinthe from a crystalline green to an opalescent yellow.

> Green changed to white, emerald to opal; nothing was changed.
> The man let the water trickle gently into his glass, and as the green
> clouded, a mist fell from his mind.
> Then he drank opaline.
>
> — Ernest Dowson, "Absinthia Taetra"

Wormwood may also be smoked. Rätsch (1992) reports that a Mexican species of *Artemisia* is smoked as a marijuana substitute. An Asian species of sagebrush, *Artemisia nilagirica,* is smoked by the Oraons of West Bengal for its hallucinatory effect (Pal and Jain 1989). The Zuni inhaled fumes of *Artemisia caruthii* to effect analgesia (Ott 1993). The sacred sagebrush of the Great Basin, *Artemisia tridentata,* is highly important in sweat lodge rituals. Jonathan Ott (1993) reports psychoactive effects from smoking *Artemisia absinthium,* an assertion that I have been able to verify.

Chemistry   Thujone, an isomer of camphor, $C_{10}H_{16}O$, is the major psychoactive ingredient. Although by count of atoms, thujone is like camphor and menthol, its geometry and bonding structure is strikingly similar to Δ^9tetrahydrocannabinol, THC. A recent article in *Nature* suggests that the peculiar effects of absinthe may be related, neurologically, to the observed effects of *Cannabis.*

> No, not the same, though the speed is reminiscent . . .

Besides thujone, wormwood contains absinthin, $C_{30}H_{40}O_6$, one of the most bitter substances known.

The characteristic turbidity of absinthe when water is added to it is from the terpenes, which are soluble in alcohol but insoluble in water, precipitating to form an emulsion. Absinthe is a drink of terpenes: thujone from the wormwood, fenchone from fennel, pinocamphone from hyssop, anethole from anise, and citral from melissa. Thujone, fenchome, and pinocamphone are all ketones, isomers of camphor.

Effects Absinthe can excite sexuality, stimulate ideas and conversation, or dissolve the brain.

> *Difficult choices, indeed.*

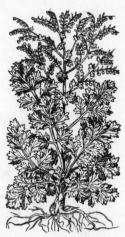

Absinthe is known as a narcotic, a stimulant, an aphrodisiac, a convulsant, and a hallucinogen. Medically, wormwood is an anthelmintic and febrifuge. Maurice Zolotow (1971) wrote that absinthe was without equal in counteracting airsickness and seasickness.

The Plant *Artemisia absinthium* has been known and used by herbalists since ancient times. The name *wormwood* comes from Old English/Old Saxon *wermōd,* meaning something like "defend the mind." Because of the plant's efficacy as a vermifuge, the second syllable of the Middle English *wor-mod* was gradually assimilated into *worm-od,* and the word became *worm-wood.*

ARTEMISIA ABSINTHIUM,
FROM MATTIOL'S
COMMENTAIRES, 1579

In Greek the plant was *apsinthos* (αψινθος), the root of our word *absinthe.* Like *wermōd, apsinthos* is *o.o.o.,* "of obscure origin," but may mean "no wasting," reflecting wormwood's power as a general tonic, as ψίνω is Cretan for φθινω, "wasting."

Effects *It's like when you have just forgotten what it was you were about to say: that instant . . . extended.*

Like *Cannabis sativa, Artemisia absinthium is a* cognodysleptic. But the differences in absinthe's effects from both hemp and alcohol are distinctive enough to prompt us to place it in a new class, *rhapsodica,* on the path between *inebriantia* and *exitantia.* Absinthe again exemplifies the importance of admixtures. A lot depends on dosage, length of use, and intent.

In small doses wormwood is a nervine and a digestive tonic.

> *It does not idle in the stomach lie*
> *But, like some God, give present remedy.*
> *– Abraham Cowley, Of Plants*

Wormwood is credited with curing chills, fevers, and bronchial ailments. Richard Burton recommended pillows stuffed with wormwood for insomnia.

I began my absinthe experiments with wormwood. Whereas absinthe liqueur is not available in the United States, wormwood the herb is. I first wanted to determine the effects of wormwood alone, so I brewed a strong tea. Wormwood is said to be the second most bitter substance known, after rue, and, having drunk extremely bitter potions before, I purposely made the wormwood tea especially strong, as I knew that I would never be able to drink a second cup, even if the tea were weak. Now bitter concoctions are not uncommon on our Poison Path, but wormwood, ahhhhh, is the type for the class!

The first effect was loosening of the sinuses. Perhaps purging would be more accurate. Much stronger this way than the Japanese wasabi horseradish. If you are ever stuffed up and need to liquify the inside of your skull, wormwood is worth considering!

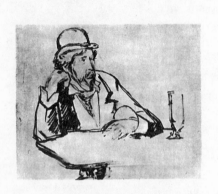

GEORGE MOORE AT THE
CAFE DE LA NOUVELLE ATHENES,
EDOUARD MANET, 1878

The paintings I had seen of absinthe drinkers almost always portrayed them sitting at a cafe on a boulevard, probably in the early evening, dressed, men in coats, women in hats and high collars, summer in the air, with the drinkers staring off into space, lost in reverie with a vacant inward stare, and a half-empty glass of absinthe on the table in front of them. As I finished my cup of wormwood tea, I prepared myself with notebook and pencil, in order to record the effects.

After some minutes, I noticed that I wasn't writing anything. I was just staring off into space. And the space was beautiful. The light was brighter.

Mottled sunlight filtering down through the walnut tree. It was afternoon. The temperature was perfect. I could feel the air on my arms and face. I got up and opened the door, letting the light and the outdoors into the room. I lay down on a couch where I could look out the door and up into the tree.

It was nice. Everything was nice. The light was different, softer and more intense at the same time. I felt great, actually. I gazed around my studio and spent a lot of time looking at my paintings.

A little tightness in the head and around the eyes . . .

The convulsive properties of thujone are exactly like those of camphor. Large doses of camphor were once used to induce convulsions in mental patients, a technique that today has been replaced by the application of large jolts of electricity.

The *Hevarja Tantra* mentions drinking camphor in a ritual context.

Pharmacology   Complex, because of the multiple and synergistic effects of the various herbs and alcohol. In 1708, Johan Lindestolpe, in his book *De Venenis* (On Poisons), claimed that chronic use of wormwood caused permanent nerve damage, and said that his information was based on personal experience. M. Cadéac and A. Meunier, two French scientists, investigated all the ingredients of absinthe in 1889, attempting to determine the effects of each. They found that the ingredients fell into two groups: the *epileptisants,* including hyssop, wormwood, and fennel; and the *stupefiants,* anise, angelica, oregano, and melissa. They declared all of them dangerous. In 1980, Y. Millet (Conrad 1988) and five colleagues replicated some of the earlier studies, finding that both anise and hyssop oils, injected into rats, could cause convulsions. Millet's group characterized the effects of the anise injections as "like opium," and concluded that hyssop was the most dangerous of the herbal ingredients.

In both the 1889 and the 1980 studies, however, the quantities of essential oils injected into the rats were far higher than it would be possible to drink, even with a whole bottle of absinthe. The executive editor of *Clinical Toxicology,* Dr. Richard Rappolt, reported in 1979 that the most harmful ingredient in absinthe was not wormwood or thujone, but alcohol (Conrad 1988). Jean-Charles Sournia (1990) goes further and states flatly that the ban on absinthe "had no scientific basis." One opposing viewpoint, by Wilfred Niels Arnold, was published in *Scientific American* in 1989. Arnold states that "the interdiction [on absinthe] was tardy but surely justified." Curiously, however, he cites no studies more recent than 1874 to back up his assertion.

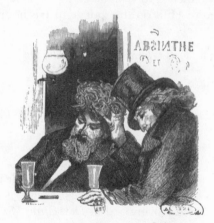

ABSINTHE DRINKERS, 1870S

But dosage is everything. According to Duke (1985), wormwood contains up to 1.7 percent essential oil, 3 to 12 percent of which is thujone. So we could say that wormwood averages 1.5 percent essential oil and 0.15 percent thujone, by weight, and probably be on the high side. By multiplication, that means that absinthe made from my recipe at the end of this section contains forty-five milligrams of thujone per liter of finished product. Mild convulsions in rats begin at around thirty milligrams of injected thujone per kilogram of body weight (the LD_{50} for mice is 134 mg/kg). I weigh eighty kilograms. Therefore, a minimally toxic dose of thujone for me is 2.4 grams, or fifty bottles of absinthe.

One glass of absinthe (forty milliliters of absinthe plus two hundred milliliters of water) contains less than two milligrams of thujone, $\frac{1}{1200}$ of a minimally toxic dose. For a substance to be classified as GRAS (Generally Recognized As Safe) by the Food and Drug Administration, their safest category, the nominal serving must be at least 100 times smaller than the minimum toxic quantity. It appears from my arithmetic that absinthe is GRAS by a factor of twelve.

Effects

> *Absinthe makes the tart grow fonder.*
> — *Ernest Dowson (Flower and Mass 1967)*

> *L'Absinthe, bue un soir d'hiver,*
> *Eclaire en vert l'âme enfumée.*

> *Absinthe, on a winter evening,*
> *Illumines the smoky soul in green.*
> — *Charles Cros, "With Flowers and with Women"*

Experiments with wormwood on animals seem to verify that it produces both auditory and visual hallucinations. In a scene reminiscent of H.P. Lovecraft, dogs injected with absinthe were reported to stand barking at blank walls.

The Plant   Wormwood is said to have grown up along the path the serpent took when cast out of Eden. Ironically, when God next returned to walk on earth, some believe that it was wormwood that was offered to Him on the sponge in His hour of destiny, to ease His suffering.

> *There fell a great star from heaven, burning as it were a lamp. . . . And the name of the star is called Wormwood.*
> — *Rev. 8:10,11*

Others, however, say that wormwood was a gift of Diana, and was given to Chiron the centaur, the ancient master of leechdoms.

Artemisia is sacred to Vishnu and Shiva.

History   In the ancient world absinthe was prepared as an infusion of wormwood leaves in wine and taken as an herbal tonic. Galen wrote of absinthe's virtues, as did Hippocrates and Pliny. Dioscorides included wormwood in *De Materia Medica*, and stated that it was an insect repellent as well as a vermifuge.

> *Wormwood is said to kill fleas, so I once rubbed down my cat with a handful of fresh wormwood leaves. The cat, of course, immediately began cleaning himself. He licked, scowled, shook his head, and gave me such a dirty look that I never repeated the experiment.*

> *I use sprigs of wormwood in trunks and clothes closets, to repel moths and vermin.*

Dioscorides recommended adding wormwood juice to ink, saying that it would keep mice away from the papyrus.

In the Middle Ages absinthe was used as a cure for flatulence, effective in dogs as well as in people. The English brewed an ale with wormwood, called *purl*. Samuel Pepys mentions wormwood ale in his diary.

He hath made me drunken with wormwood.

   – Lam 3:15

Absinthe, as we know it now, was invented by a country doctor in Switzerland, or so the folklore goes, in 1792. The doctor's name was Dr. Ordinaire, and his absinthe quickly acquired a local reputation as a cure-all. When the good doctor died, he willed his recipe to his housekeeper, for whom, it was said, he had an affection. The housekeeper passed the recipe on to her two daughters, who continued to make and sell the doctor's tonic. A certain Major Dubied was so impressed with the medicinal and aphrodisiacal virtues of the sisters' product that he bought not only a case of their bottles but also their recipe. One suspects that it was the aphrodisiacal rather than the medicinal properties that inspired the major's purchase, because he gave the recipe as a wedding gift to his son-in-law, Henri-Louis Pernod. Pernod began manufacturing absinthe on a commercial scale in 1805.

   The good I do Venus herself will own,
   She, though all sweets, yet loves not sweets alone.
   She wisely mixed with my juice her joys,
   And her delights, with bitter things alloys.
      – Abraham Cowley, Of Plants

French soldiers fighting in Algeria in the 1840s drank absinthe as a preventative against malaria and other diseases, and that sparked the first big surge in absinthe's popularity in France. (The use of absinthe as an antimalarial medication is not without scientific support. In 1990, M. Zafar and his associates found that alcoholic extracts of *Artemisia absinthium* given orally were nearly as effective in suppressing malarial *Plasmodium* in mice as was the standard antimalarial drug chloroquine. Other species of *Artemisia* have been proven effective even against quinine-resistant strains of malaria. Absinthe's efficacy as a febrifuge is also well supported.)

The soldiers brought the taste back to Paris, and absinthe drinking was well established by 1859, when Edouard Manet painted "The Absinthe Drinker." The painting created a small scandal, artists and intellectuals taking sides to attack or defend the painting, a controversy that foreshadowed the history of absinthe in France for the next sixty years.

The story of absinthe reads like a who's who in art and literature: Manet painted absinthe themes, and his friend Charles Baudelaire drank absinthe (though he later rejected it in favor of opium). Verlaine and Rimbaud seem to have drunk absinthe more or less continuously. Van Gogh drank absinthe. Oscar Wilde drank a lot of absinthe, and wrote about it. Ernest Dowson drank it. Poe drank it. Degas drank absinthe in the cafes and then painted absinthe, stirring up a scandal in London. There was something about light seen through an absinthe intoxication that seemed to feed the impressionists. Henri de Toulouse-Lautrec drank absinthe, and painted it frequently. Paul Gauguin liked absinthe, and was somehow able to continue drinking it even in Tahiti. Alfred Jarry called absinthe "Holy Water," and his friend Pablo Picasso painted pictures of absinthe a number of times. Jack London liked absinthe.

What other psychotropic concoction, excepting perhaps wine, has produced as large a body of laudatory poems in the last two thousand years as has absinthe?

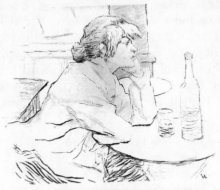

THE DRINKER, HENRI DE
TOULOUSE-LATREC, 1889

It was the national drink of France for two generations. It was finally killed by World War I and the growing forces of Prohibition, and was buried with the generation that loved it most.

The French military intelligentsia, if that is not an oxymoron, were strongly influenced by the philosopher Henri Bergson. They believed that France could win the war if they had enough *élan vital*. The inability of the French generals to understand the effect of machine guns on frontal assaults has always been an enigma to me, but so it was. The generals believed that the reason the assaults were failing was that the troops did not have enough élan. They sought the cause for this deterioration of French élan, and the culprit they found was absinthe. Absinthe was outlawed by martial law.

After the war everything was different. The French were more interested in American drinks like the cocktail than in the old-fashioned absinthe. The American expatriots, on the other hand, were very interested in absinthe and were able to obtain it through the black market. Ernest Hemingway, who liked absinthe enough to bring a supply with him back to Key West, agreed with many earlier writers by saying that absinthe was not a hallucinogen, but that it just rearranged one's ideas in new ways:

> *In this, the real absinthe, there is wormwood. It's supposed to rot your brain out but I don't believe it. It only changes the ideas.*
>
> *— For Whom the Bell Tolls*

So did absinthe get a bad rap? Yes and no. One of the spearheads of the anti-absinthe campaign was the defense plea entered by a man named Lanfray in 1906. Lanfray, an alcoholic who drank a bottle of wine and a bottle of brandy every day, as well as a couple of glasses of absinthe, had murdered his wife and family in a psychotic rage. His defense was that he had been rendered temporarily insane by the absinthe. Unlike Dan White, who beat his double murder rap of shooting San Francisco mayor George Mosconi and supervisor Harvey Milk by claiming temporary insanity from eating "Twinkies," Lanfray was convicted. Nonetheless, the Prohibitionists used the case to successfully get absinthe outlawed in several cantons in Switzerland. Harry Anslinger availed himself of the same strategy thirty years later, when there was a similar murder in Florida, to prove that *Cannabis* transformed its users into killers.

Still, absinthe is clearly a poison. Whether it is more poisonous than the alcohol in which it is dissolved is certainly doubtful. Many inferior absinthes were being sold in France, some mixed from industrial alcohol and essential oils. Unscrupulous manufacturers would add copper sulphate, or worse, antimony salts to the mixture to give it the characteristic green color and turbidity that real absinthe has. Heavy metal poisoning would be a certain result of ingesting such abominations, and it is likely that many of the horror stories about absinthe were caused by such toxic adulterations.

But none of this proves that absinthe is safe.

Correspondences   Nicholas Culpepper assigns wormwood to Mars, perhaps because of the herb's warming quality.

Effects   *After the first glass you see things as you wish they were. After the second, you see things as they are not. Finally, you see things as they really are, and this is the most horrible thing in the world.*

   – Oscar Wilde (in Conrad 1988)

Absinthe, mother of happiness, O infinite liquor,
you shimmer in my glass pale and green like the eyes
of the mistress I once loved. . . .

   – Gustave Kahn, "Absinthe"

Whiskey and beer for fools; absinthe for poets; absinthe has the power of the magicians; it can wipe out or renew the past, and annul or foretell the future.

   – Ernest Dowson (Flower and Mass 1967)

. . . It smelled like bottled summer.

   – Barnaby Conrad (1988), describing his first sniff of absinthe

Poesis   When absinthe was outlawed in France and Switzerland, Pernod Fils was forced to make an absinthe without any wormwood. The closest product today to real wormwood, the percentage of anise being increased to make up for it. It is possible to create a pretty good absinthe by simply adding the wormwood back in.

I say "simply," but there are several steps involved, and once mastered there is no reason not to make absinthe from scratch. There were always regional absinthes in France, and the mixture of herbs in the drink was never canonized completely, sweet flag, dittany, angelica, oregano, coriander, and nutmeg being included in some absinthes and not in others. My own recipe is based on that most excellent of formularies, *Dick's Encyclopedia of Practical Receipts and Processes,* and other nineteenth-century formularies.

*To Prepare
Absinthe
by Distillation*

30.0 g wormwood
8.5 g hyssop
1.8 g calamus
6.0 g melissa
30.0 g anise seed
25.0 g fennel seed
10.0 g star anise
3.2 g coriander seed

Put the dry herbs in a large jar. Dampen slightly. Add 800 milliliters of 85–95 percent alcohol. Wine spirits make a better product than pure grain alcohol. Let it steep for several days – a week is better – shaking occasionally. Then add 600 milliliters of water and let the whole macerate for another day. Decant off the liquid, squeezing as much from the mass of herb as possible. Wet the herbs with some vodka and squeeze again. Recipe should give a little over a liter and a half of green liquor. It must then be distilled. Inferior recipes skip this step, but what they produce is not worthy to be called *absinthe.*

In the distillation, change the receiver when the distillate turns yellow: those are the faints. You can save the faints and add them to future distillations, but they will taint the flavor if added directly to the product. Just use the good stuff. The next step is to color and finish the liqueur by another round of maceration.

Color the distillate by again adding:

4.2 g mint
1.1 g melissa
3.0 g wormwood
1.0 g citron peel
4.2 g liquorice root

Let the herbs macerate for another three or four days. Decant, filter, bottle. You will probably want to carefully add some concentrated sugar syrup to the blend. The result will be a Swiss style absinthe of about 135 proof. Recipe makes one liter of absinthe.

To Prepare
Absinthe
from Pernod

If you want to doctor a bottle of Pernod, you need the essential oil of worm-wood or an alcoholic distillate of the same. Absinthe contains the equivalent of about one ounce (thirty grams) of wormwood per quart or liter of liqueur. One way to prepare the absinthe is to macerate four ounces (120 grams) of dried wormwood in a quart (or liter) of alcohol, and then add a couple of cups of water and distill off the essence. The distillation, after the maceration, is vital. Whereas the distillate explodes into minty and aromatic flavors, the residue, with equal, nay, surpassing vehemence, explodes into astonishing, persistent bitterness. Add the distilled essence to the Pernod in a proportion of one to four.

If you can obtain the essential oil of wormwood (without the thujone removed), your job is easy: just dissolve 0.3 or 0.4 milliliters of the oil in some alcohol and add it to a quart or liter of the *pastis*.

But it is just about as easy to make the absinthe from scratch. Try it the old way first.

The Ally

If you are sick, it will cure you.
If you are depressed, it will ease your soul —
If you are smitten, desirous to touch
the one so long beyond your grasp,
it will give you words
and a long green hour, together, to speak them.

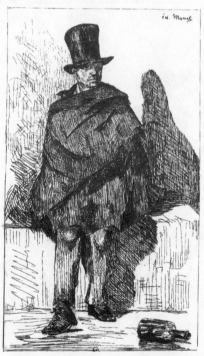

THE ABSINTHE DRINKER,
EDOUARD MANET, 1862

CALEA ZACATECHICHI

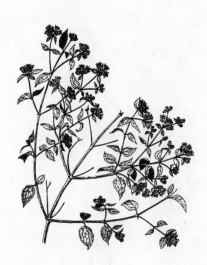

Common Names	Dog grass, *Thle-pelakano,* "leaf of God." *Zacatechichi* is Nahuatl for "bitter grass." The bitterness is in a class with *Artemisia absinthium.*
Related Species	Not all races are psychoactive, even within the genus. Needs study.
Taxonomy	Sunflower family, Asteraceae, found from central Mexico south to Costa Rica. The plant likes open ground; readily colonizes disturbed ground and land that has been burned over. The genus *Calea* is neotropical and contains a hundred other species besides *zacatechichi.*
Part Used	The dried leaves. Fresh leaves are used medicinally and would probably be as effective as infusions of the dried leaves.
Chemistry	Contains $\frac{1}{100}$ of 1 percent by weight of an unidentified alkaloid, $C_{21}H_{26}O_8$, and a large number of triterpenes, flavonoids, sesquiterpene lactones, organic acids, and a glucosidelike bitter principle. The source of the psychoactivity is unknown. Most of the research has focused on the alkaloid, but the sesquiterpene lactones certainly deserve attention.

CALEA ZACATECHICHI

How Taken

Drink an infusion of the dried leaves and lie down in a darkened place. Then smoke a cigarette of the dried leaves. The "alert" that the plant is taking effect is when you can feel your pulse and heartbeat.

The bitterness alone, however, is so unsettling that such finer points may be missed. Use a good palmful of dried leaf per cup.

Effects

Oneirogenic: induces lucid dreaming.

Pharmacology

Unknown.

The Plant

Natives use the leaves as an insecticide. In the Yucatan, the leaves are added to baths for skin eruptions. Internally, the herb is taken for fevers, colic, diarrhea, and cholera. Dried plants were exported to Brazil specifically for Asiatic cholera.

The leaves have been shown to contain a central nervous system depressant. Scientific testing has also shown that the leaves possess antiatherogenic properties – a virtue of some promise for a heart attack culture such as our own.

The Chontal, in Oaxaca, who use the plant, recognize that some plants are oneirogenically active while others are not. Ethnobotanist José Luis Díaz is trying to determine if the active plants constitute a new species.

The Ally

The ally clarifies the senses. For some, the transmission is visual; for others, the ally speaks in voices.

Effects

You may or may not get lucid dreaming. Some people do, others don't. Díaz (1986) conducted double-blind experiments and did find an increase in meaningful dreams reported by the subjects given *Calea.* Even without the dreams, a sense of well-being is very common, and can last for a day or more.

Poesis

On a hunch that a volatile terpene might be the active ingredient in Calea, rather than the alkaloid or some other fixed or bitter compound, and that the terpene might be separated by distillation, I prepared an absinthelike *Calea* liqueur. Preliminary tests are, alas, disappointing. Not that the beverage is disagreeable – far from it – but in an effort to clearly feel some effects from the herb, all subjects became so thoroughly inebriated that they were unable to continue the experiment. These results are still preliminary, but it looks as if the oneirogenic activity and the bitterness, if not derived from the same compound, are at least traveling companions.

The Ally

There is a problem with your poison path. This "ground state calibration" is very nice but it misses the point. You use ground state calibration as a means to an end, as a temporary retreat, like a visit to a spa.

"Misses the point" . . . spoken with great spiritual authority, for words in a dream!

But I know I'm dreaming, so I'm awake, right?

EUPHORICA

Approach the God of Dreams with sword drawn.

The First Doctor was a woman wise and compassionate. Because of her skill, her receptivity, her strength, and her integrity, the gods looked upon her with favor.

The First Doctor had many patients, but few medicines. She had songs, she had cereals, but the terrible cries of her patients drove her into the mountains seeking a vision of power.

In the mountains she fasted, then ate. Sang, then was quiet. She waited, she lived alone in the mountains. She met the animals, and then she met the plants.

And the gods – the spirits of the earth, the spirit of the sky, the spirits of the plants and the animals and the spirits of her ancestors – pleased with her, granted her a wish.

Briefly, the First Doctor considered. There were so many things for which one might ask: power, sustenance, energy, vision, love.

"You may have whatever you wish," the gods repeated, "from the least to the greatest."

"Then, O Gods, give me that medicine that cures pain, the medicine that eases suffering."

And the gods responded. They gave her the opium poppy, and they told her she had chosen wisely.

"After food," they told her, "this plant is our greatest gift. Use it wisely and unselfishly. It is never wrong to ease the suffering of those who do not know the secret. But remember, for yourself, who are a doctor, this plant shall ever be a poison."

> *The danger is smoking as a defense against some moral disequilibrium. Then it is difficult to approach the drug in the way it must be approached, as wild beasts should be approached – without fear.*
>
> *– Jean Cocteau, Opium: Diary of a Cure*

Wine robs a man of his self-possession: opium sustains and reinforces it . . . wine constantly leads a man to the brink of absurdity and extravagance; and, beyond a certain point, it is sure to volatilize and to disperse the intellectual energies; whereas opium always seems to compose what had been agitated, and to concentrate what had been distracted.

– Thomas De Quincey, Confessions of an English Opium Eater

Alcohol provokes fits of madness. Opium provokes fits of wisdom.

– Jean Cocteau, Opium: Diary of a Cure

Euphoria is a middle child, born between consciousness and sleep. It is a condition of peace and well-being, like that which follows orgasm, and not everyone reacts to it the same way. Some are entranced by the radical stillness, and lie unmoving, without thoughts. Others are so glad to be freed from the rude pushing and shoving of desire that they take advantage of their reprieve and set about finishing some piece of work. Some just let their minds drift, half awake, half dreaming, and let the yearning visions try to coax their souls up from the somatic twilight of their bodies.

Perhaps we desire death: or why is poison so sweet?
Why do the little Sirens
Make kindlier music, for a man caught in the net of the world
Between news-cast and work-desk, –
The little chirping Sirens, alcohol, amusement, opiates,
And the carefully sterilized lust, –
Than the angels of life?

– Robinson Jeffers, "Sirens"

Pain is the first teacher we deny.

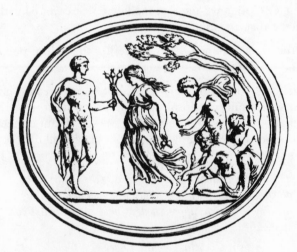

THE GODDESS OF NIGHT, BEARING POPPIES

PAPAVER SOMNIFERUM

Common Name	Opium poppy.
Related Species	*Papaver setigerum, Papaver bracteatum, Papaver orientale, Papaver pseudo-orientale, Papaver rhoeus,* and ninety other species of *Papaver.* Also *Eschscholtzia californica, Argemone glauca,* and *Argemone mexicana.*
Part Used	The alkaloid-rich latex is the source of opium. The nutritious seeds are important as a food crop and as a source of oil. The young leaves can be eaten as potherbs.
	There are small amounts of morphine throughout the plant, possibly excepting the seeds, but it is only in the lactifers in the walls of the seed capsule that the alkaloid is produced in quantity.
Effects	*In small quantities it exhilarates the mind, raises the passions, and invigorates the body: in large ones it is succeeded by intoxication, languor, stupor and death.*
	— *Erasmus Darwin, The Loves of the Plants*
	Opium expands boundless space.
	— *Charles Baudelaire, Artificial Paradise*
Taxonomy	Family Papaveraceae. *Papaver somniferum* is a cultigen, one of a very select group of plants with extremely ancient associations with human beings. Although escaped populations are sometimes able to survive in a favorable environment, *Papaver somniferum* is not found in a truly wild state.
	The origins of the opium poppy are still being investigated. Many researchers believe the wild setaceous poppy, *Papaver setigerum,* to be the ancestral species, or that the two species share a common ancestor. Other paleobotanists disagree, noting that *Papaver somniferum* is diploid, whereas the setaceous poppy is usually tetraploid.
	Of the many species of poppy, *Papaver somniferum* and *Papaver setigerum* are the only two containing morphine in significant quantities. Various researchers have reported morphine and like alkaloids in *Papaver rhoeus, Eschscholtzia mexicana, Argemone mexicana,* and even the hops plant, *Humulus lupulus,* but the findings are doubtful.
Pharmacognosy	In 1803, a German pharmacist named Friedrich Sertürner, while working with opium, isolated a substance that reacted chemically like a base. For this reason he named it an *alkaloid.* It was the first alkaloid ever discovered. Sertürner found that his alkaloid was highly narcotic, and he soon determined that it was the principal

active constituent of opium. He named it after Morpheus, the god of dreams. The discovery of morphine was analogous to the discovery of the spirit of wine: a power within a power, and had like social consequences, though in smaller degree.

Since Sertürner's discovery, more than forty alkaloids have been identified in opium. The opium alkaloids fall into eight major groups, represented by benzyl isoquinoline, hydrophenanthrene, protopine, phthalide-isoquinoline, protoberberine, aporphine, benzophenanthridine, and papaverubine. Of these, the phenanthrene group, including morphine, codeine, and thebaine, and the isoquinoline group, including narcotine and papaverine, are the most important.

How Taken   As pills, plaster, or wash; as smoke, drink, or suppository – opium is compounded with a large variety of admixtures.

The simplest way to take opium, and perhaps the oldest, is as *mekonium,* an infusion of chopped-up poppy capsules in water. The Greeks drank *mekonium,* or sometimes *mekonium* mixed with wine. The pharmaceutical preparation *Vinum Opii* is opium in wine flavored with cinnamon and cloves.

> *A social worker named Eric Detzer who was a poppy addict for many*
> *years would just drop six to twelve poppy heads into a food processor, add a*
> *cup of hot water, and whizz them up. It made a milky green juice which he*
> *then filtered through a strainer and drank. Adding some lemon juice would*
> *have helped both the extraction and the taste.*

There is evidence that opium was smoked by the Minoan people, on Crete. But after 1500 BC, the art of opium smoking disappeared for three millennia until it was rediscovered by the Chinese in modern times, with the encouragement of the British, who were trying to build up a trade surplus. Opium is smoked in a special pipe that facilitates vaporization of the tarry goo without actually burning it.

> *a characteristic odor – musty*
> *faintly sweet and almost nutritious –*
> > *thick-smelling, not earthy,*
> *but subterranean, not unpleasant,*
> *but the smell of something*
> > *lived and died deep in darkness:*
> *the smell of the food that the dead eat.*
> *But they are friendly dead.*

There are five kinds of commercial opium. The first is *druggist opium.* Druggist opium is raw opium meant to be used to manufacture medicinal opium. It need only have a morphine content of between 8 and 10 percent. The second kind of commercial opium is *manufacturers' opium,* which is used for the isolation of the principal alkaloids: morphine, narcotine, and papaverine. For this grade the highest concentration of morphine is desired.

The third kind of commercial opium is *prepared opium,* the soft opium used for smoking. In India it is called *chandu. Chandu* is prepared in various ways, some of them quite complex and requiring practiced skill. Raw opium is dissolved in boiling water, and then filtered and concentrated. The concentrate is then roasted over a low heat, which gives it a characteristic aroma. The brittle, roasted opium cakes are then extracted with water, cold water first, and a second time with warm water. The cold water extract is the best. The extracts are concentrated until the water content is 23 to 26 percent. Sometimes sugar or aromatic substances are added. Also, and this is a point of debate among opium smokers, dross can be added at this time. Dross, the charred residue from opium pipes, besides containing a great deal of morphine, also contains secondary products that are said to greatly contribute to the stupefying effect of opium. Not all opium smokers appreciate that effect.

The last step in making *chandu* is to pack it into sealed earthenware jars to let it "ferment" for four to six months. This is to perfect the flavor and aroma of the product. The best *chandu* may have a morphine content of 10 to 13 percent, while ordinary *chandu* may only have 7 or 8 percent.

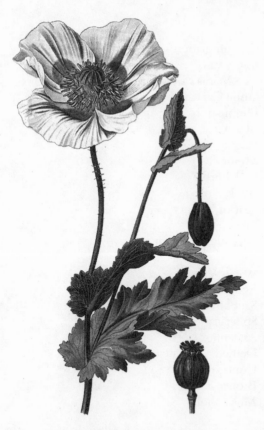

PAPAVER SOMNIFERUM, FROM KOHLER'S
MEDIZAL–PLANZEN–ATLAS, 1887

The last two kinds of commercial opium are the opiums used for opium sticks and for eating opium. This opium is little processed, basically being used in its raw state.

Charbughra is a mixture of wine, hashish, and opium, chased with a chai-style ginger-cardamom tea. . . . Now, anyone for adding a little coca perhaps, just so nobody feels left out?

Medicinal opium preparations include *Opium Pulveratum,* powdered opium; *Opii Deodorati,* deodorized opium; *Pilula Opii,* pill of opium; *Extractum Opii,* extract of opium; *Pulvis Ipecacuanhae et Opii,* Dover's Powder; *Trochisci Glycyrrhizae et Opii,* Wistar's cough lozenges; *Emplastrum Opii,* opium plaster; *Tinctura Opii,* laudanum; *Tinctura Opii Camphorata,* paregoric; *Vinum Opii; Tinctura Opii Composita,* Squibb's diarrhea mixture; and *Acetum Opii,* black drop.

Laudanum is a deodorized alcoholic tincture with the narcotine removed, and was popular in the nineteenth century, especially with women. Taking laudanum was more socially acceptable for women than was drinking alcohol. Paregoric was laudanum mixed with camphor, glycerin, and anise, and was commonly given to children. (Someone once called absinthe paregoric for adults.) Numerous patent medicines have contained opium.

In addition, the salts are extracted and used extensively: morphine, codeine, and a number of synthetic and semisynthetic derivatives.

Heroin, diacetyl morphine hydrochloride, is another opium derivative, but it is no longer used medicinally in the United States because of its abuse.

Effects   Warmth and well-being.   Ease.   Sociability.   Dreaminess.

Sometimes, or maybe:

     Nausea.   Nightmares.   Solitude.

But that comes later.

CORRESPONDENCES

ACTIVITY	Contemplation
ANIMAL	Ibis, Swan
ARCHETYPE	The Mama's Boy, The Junkie
ART FORM	Stone Carving
BODILY FUNCTION	Elimination
BODY PART	Blood
BUDDHA REALM	Padma
CHORD	Minor
COLOR	Red–Purple
COSMIC ENTITY	Black Hole
CRUTCH FOR	Fear of Infinity
DIMENSION	Line
DISCIPLINE	Leechdoms, Perfumery
ELEMENT	Air
FORM OF ENERGY	Water Wheel
FORM OF IGNORANCE	Egoism
GEMSTONE	Sapphire, Moonstone
GEOMETRY	Spherical
GOD	Asclepius
GODDESS	Demeter, Hecate
GRAMMAR	Context Sensitive
HISTORICAL AGE	Bronze Age
HUMOUR	Melancholia

Pharmacology   Several of the alkaloids present in opium have opposing effects, and the combined effect is distinct from the effects of, say, morphine alone. The major alkaloids are morphine, 8–14 percent; codeine, 2–3 percent; narcotine, 5–8 percent; papaverine, 0.5–2.4 percent; and thebaine, 1–2 percent. Thebaine is a strychnine-like convulsant, stimulating the smooth muscles. Its presence in opium tends to counteract one of the most dangerous actions of morphine – the depression of the respiratory system – a common cause of death in morphine or heroin overdoses. Thebaine is a precursor to the chemical synthesis of codeine. Antidrug forces are trying to substitute *Papaver bracteatum* for *Papaver somniferum* as a source of opiates, as *Papaver bracteatum* contains no morphine. The thebaine produced by the farmers would then have to be sold to the industrial countries to be converted into codeine chemically.

Morphine still has its uses, however, even in the United States. It is considered essential for radiation sickness, and was allegedly stockpiled for that contingency as part of cold war planning.

> *Morphine, the soldier's friend.*

Opium is the archetypal medicine, and morphine is its essence. Morphine is the most powerful naturally occurring analgesic in the world, and the synthetics use opium as their precursor. Morphine stimulates the spinal chord and increases the tone of involuntary muscles, such as the sphincter. It is the only known remedy for the common cold. In large amounts it causes sleep.

> *White sleep. A waking sleep.*
> *The pleasures of sleep with enough consciousness*
> *to enjoy them.*

Codeine is similar in its action to morphine, though less stimulating to the spinal chord, and less euphoric. It is a superior antitussive, as it depresses the coughing centers as much as morphine without the concomitant effect on the rest of the central nervous system. Almost all of the legal morphine harvested from poppies is converted into codeine. The inverse process is much more difficult.

Narcotine, like thebaine, accentuates respiration. It is also a mild analgesic and spinal stimulant. It is used medicinally for emphysema. Papaverine, present in the opium poppy in small amounts, is an antispasmodic, a smooth muscle relaxant, and a vasodilator. For these properties it has been used to treat impotence by direct injections into the penis. It's the *relaxation* of the muscles that causes erection, a reaction mediated by nitric oxide ions. My own suggestion is papaverine mixed with a little scopolamine, in a slippery oil, to be applied topically.

The study of opium led to the discovery of the first alkaloid. Likewise, the study of that alkaloid, morphine, has led to the discovery of the brain's own painkillers, the endorphins, perhaps the most important advance in neurochemistry of the past half century.

Endorphins are far more than painkillers; they are neurotransmitters mediating the processing of visual information as well as of emotional states and physical stress. The connection between endorphins and morphine is that they bind to the same receptor sites in the brain, and it was this similarity that led to the discovery of enkephalin by Hans Kosterlitz and John Hughes in 1975. Since that time other researchers have ascertained that there are at least a dozen endorphins in the brain, falling into three families: the enkephalins; the alpha-, beta-, and gamma-endorphin group; and the dynorphins. Moreover, there are at least three different kinds of receptor sites in the brain, each site showing preference toward one or more of the endorphin peptide families, although not to the complete exclusion of the other families. The resulting permutations and combinations form a highly complex web of interaction between sensory input and emotional/physiological response.

As an example, the mu receptors, those most attuned to opiate reception, are linked to analgesia, while the delta receptors, sensitive to opiates (and opiatelike endorphins to a lesser degree), are more involved with euphoria. And even with one type of receptor there are subtypes: one type of mu receptor governs analgesia, while another regulates the inhibition of breathing. This suggests the possibility of an "overdose-proof" painkiller – but so far no molecule has been discovered that will bind to only one of the two subtypes.

The Nature of Addiction   Endorphins present a physical analog to the spiritual laws of homeostasis and addiction. It is the principle of "no free lunch," perhaps best summarized by Lenny Bruce, who said:

> You gotta pay dues.

Or bills. The bills will wait for you on the desk, opened or unopened. In some cases the interest compounds. There are social dues and there are spiritual dues, there are mundane bills like the one from the gas company and esoteric bills such as the phantom afterimage left by a lost opportunity.

> You gotta pay bills.

On the physiological plane, addiction researchers have confirmed what Louis Lewin intuited half a century earlier.

> *It is conceivable that the impulse and the activity of regulating processes against foreign influences is enacted according to a scientific principle which has been termed by d'Alembert, Gauss, and later by Le Chatelier, the Law of Resistance to Constraint, and which applies to chemical and physical processes. It may be thus stated: If to a system in equilibrium a constraint be applied, a change takes place within the system tending to nullify the effect of the constraint and to restore the equilibrium.*
>
>   *– Louis Lewin, Phantastica*

Precisely. In response to continued flooding of the endorphin receptors by opiates, the brain grows new receptor sites. Any reduction then in the amount of morphine leaves the brain in disequilibrium on the excess of pain side.

Lewin was careful not to be reductionist about the role of physiology in an individual's response to drugs, suggesting that every individual had a "toxic equation," in which temperament played a role along with heredity and other medically determinable factors. Reductionism is one of the dull poisons. Students of the Poison Path should give a great deal of consideration to the Law of Resistance to Constraint, and make it part of their ground state training.

The Plant

> *Sopha'd on silk, amid her charm built towers,*
> *Her meads of asphodel, and amaranth bowers,*
> *Where Sleep and Silence guard the soft abodes,*
> *In sullen apathy Papaver nods . . .*
>
>   *– Erasmus Darwin, The Loves of the Plants*

The opium poppy is named for sleep: Somnus is the Roman name for Hypnos, the god of sleep. Nyx, the goddess of night, carries poppies in her hand, while her son, Thanatos, death, wears a poppy garland. Hermes, the shaman god who travels between the worlds, carries a staff that brings sleep. His home was Mekone, "poppy town," the place where Prometheus stole fire.

> *lavender petals, red petals,*
>   *petals with a black splotch*
> *near the claw*

Poppies are annuals. There are dwarf species, but commonly poppies grow to four feet in height, and carry eight or ten flowers. Poppy flowers are red, white, lavender, and variegate. They are strikingly beautiful ornamentals, apart from their evocation of mystery. The buds are pendulous until they are ready to open, the stems bending over near the apex. As the buds open, the stem straightens and become erect. The purple petals, pressed upward by the expanding knob of the capsule, break through the sheaf straining around them and unfold.

> *it's like a glans*
> *emerging from the prepuce.*

The petals are soft and fine-textured. The ovary is surrounded by stamens, crowned by a disklike stigma.

> *one woman, many husbands*

The number of stigmatic rays is important taxonomically, and also as an indicator of latex content and strength.

The Ally   The opium ally speaks, when she speaks at all, through dreams. There is clearly a linkage between the importance that the romantic poets placed on dreams, and their fascination with opium, though it is not clear which came first. In ancient

times, the sick, visiting the Temple of Asclepius, were given poppy extract for just
this reason – that they might receive a healing dream, a dream revealing the cause
of their illness.

> but you can get dream after dream,
> until you begin dreaming the forgetting of dreams,
> until the dreaming and the forgetting
> become one act.

The trick is mastering nondisruptive questioning: being able to place the desired
question at the head of the queue without disturbing the flow of images. The ally
answers by creating a pictorial representation of the question. If you get a useful
answer – something insightful that makes sense – the next problem is remembering it, to be able to return with the image to ordinary conciousness.

History   Ancient, indeed. Poppies were collected, and probably cultivated, by the Neolithic Lake Dwellers in Europe. The poppy seems to have moved from Europe
to the Mediterranean during the late Neolithic, following the tin and amber
trade routes from Lithuania and Switzerland south through the passes across the
Alps. During the Bronze Age and the Iron Age, the poppy made itself at home
throughout the ancient world, both as a food plant and as a medicine. There is
some evidence that the Sumerians called the poppy *hul-gil,* the "joy plant,"
though that claim is now disputed. By classical times, poppies were a part of the
spring mysteries at Eleusis.

> gold poppy capsule earrings,
> a statue of a goddess, bare breasts,
> her hands uplifted, three poppy capsules
> growing up from her brow,
> fine vertical scars, on each capsule

A statue of Asclepius depicts him holding a bunch of opium capsules in his hand.
Opium poppies are on the backs of many ancient coins, both Roman and Jewish.
Isis sometimes holds poppy heads. Demeter drank opium to ease her sorrows,
and poppies are part of her worship.

> bread and poppies

Helen learned the secret of nepenthe from the Egyptians. Thebes, in particular,
was famous for its poppy fields. Nepenthe was probably a mixture, perhaps *mekonium* in wine, with mandrake and henbane. Tropanes go well with opium.

In the Middle Ages, opium came into Europe, as did most of Greek learning,
through the Arabs. Jewish physicians traded with the Arabs and translated their
books. But with the Black Death, in the fourteenth century, opium disappeared.
Perhaps, being an Eastern medicine, it was suspect, since the plague had come
from the East. It was our own esteemed Paracelsus, several centuries later, who
reintroduced opium to Europe. Paracelsus claimed that laudanum was superior

to all other medicines in warding off death, and is said to have made liberal use of the medicine himself.

Although opium has come to be associated with China, the poppy was unknown there until the Tang. In the Sung, poet Su Tung-Po praised its medicinal properties as a cure for diarrhea and for colds. The poppy was mostly grown in China as an ornamental flower until the nineteenth century, when the British, in an effort to correct a trade imbalance, began importing large quantities of opium into China from India. As recreational use of opium went against the grain of Chinese sensibilities, the government tried to stop the flow of the drug into their country. The British responded to this challenge with force, and the resulting conflicts were called the Opium Wars.

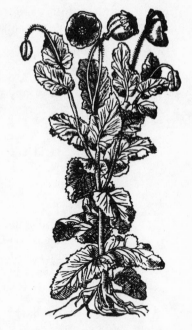

GARDEN POPPY (PAPAVER SOMNIFERUM), FROM MATTIOLI'S COMMENTAIRES, 1579

Poesis Poppies are beautiful and rewarding flowers to grow. They like rich soil, and it should be finely cultivated, though it is not necessary to cultivate deeply. Poppies like lots of sun, but not heat. They don't like fog or clouds. Mountains are ideal. They need water while they germinate and grow, less when they flower, and little or none as the capsules mature. Mediterranean climates will make them feel right at home.

Most people do not realize that the poppy seeds in their pastries are opium poppy seeds, and will, indeed, show up as opiate-positive in drug tests. This is more due to the extreme sensitivity of the drug-testing technology than to any psychoactive properties of the poppy seeds. Or so it is said.

It is also said that there is wide variation in alkaloidal content between poppy strains grown for seed and strains grown for drugs. But is there really? Evidence is contradictory.

As the worldwide persecution of the opium plant continues into the twenty-first century, government genetic engineers may succeed in disabling the alkaloidal genes in the DNA of *Papaver somniferum,* but such is not the case today.

When you have broken up, raked, and smoothed out your beds, scatter the seeds, then lightly rake or broom the soil so that the seeds are just covered. Water with a sprinkler head, so that the soil is not unduly disrupted, and don't allow the ground to dry out while the seeds are germinating. If the weather is warm, the seeds should germinate in one or two weeks.

Abseits im Garten blüt der böse Schlaf.

Apart in the garden blooms the angry sleep.
    – *Rainer Maria Rilke*

As the seedlings begin to crowd each other, thin them out to eighteen to twenty-four inches. I've seen them grown closer than that, but many of the plants were undersized and had small capsules. The seedlings look a little like lettuce, and you can eat some of the plants you pull in salads. The greens carry some of the characteristic poppy taste, but contain few if any alkaloids.

The rate of growth seems to depend on the light and temperature. Early poppies hold back and wait for the warm weather to really grow. Still, in many climates, two crops a year ought to be possible. In India, where the growing season is limited by winter at one end and by the monsoons at the other, the sowing is set to a particular week in November. The seedlings can overwinter under a light cover of snow and then have a head start into spring.

Many studies have reported that manuring and giving extra phosphorus and nitrogen increase the quality and quantity of latex substantially, up to a certain maximum.

Much of the best research comes from India. Indian chemists and agronomists have studied all aspects of opium poppy agriculture: effects of fertilizers, harvesting techniques, when to plant, selective breeding, all in terms of yield per hectare, or percent alkaloid per plant, or morphine/codeine/narcotine ratio.

Phosphorus seems to be most important during the initial stages of growth, and the nitrogen later. Manure is always good. The professionals treat the seeds with a fungicide before they sow them, and weed the rows conscientiously throughout the growing season.

The plants begin to flower in about three months. Opium poppies come in many colors, despite the popular belief that all true opium poppies are white. The red-flowered poppies are spectacular, and there is a deep lavender poppy that is exquisitely beautiful. The flowers are ephemeral,

they are studies in impermanence . . .

the petals falling a day or two after their emergence.

itself a study of metamorphosis, like a butterfly
breaking out of its chrysalis,
    and letting her wings dry in the sun.

The fallen petals are wonderfully edible and are a beautiful addition to any salad. After the petals fall, the capsule grows quickly for several days, and then ripens and matures for several weeks. About two weeks after eating opium-flower salads, if you live somewhere in the world where the State has not assumed stewardship for your spiritual temptations, you are ready to begin the harvest.

Many studies have been done to determine the optimal time to lance the capsules. One pamphlet I saw stated that the capsules could be lanced as early as five days after petals have fallen, but the scientific studies disagree. While the latex may indeed be thick enough for lancing at that point, the morphine content of the latex has not reached its maximum until about fourteen days after the petals fall. Moreover, an Indian agronomical study has shown that the morphine content does not, as was previously believed, decline after a certain critical time. In fact, dried poppy heads are still loaded with morphine, codeine, narcotine, papaverine, thebaine, and all the rest.

It *has* been shown that when the latex is exposed to the light and the air, some of the morphine degrades into codeine. The scientist V.S. Ramanathan (1980) suggested that the latex be sprayed with an antioxidant solution of salt and ascorbic acid, or that the latex be collected immediately, instead of being allowed to congeal and dry, as is traditional.

> *I read about a poppy farmer who would lick the fresh latex right off the capsules. And the image has stayed with me: a man looking like Blake's painting of Nebuchadnezzar, on his hands and knees, licking poppy capsules, a couple of long-haired cats, their tails wrapped about them, sitting nearby in the dirt and watching . . .*

But a few more words on lancing. The morphine is produced in lactifers in the wall of the capsule, the last step in a long process of biosynthesis (the penultimate substance being codeine). Opium, as such, is prepared directly from the latex, the collecting of which is a labor-intensive process.

To cut an opium poppy capsule is to enter mythic time, to share in a tradition stretching unbroken into prehistory and to let the ancient tradition enter history again at the moment of the millennium.

> *Ritual. Long memories,*
> > *houses built on poles,*
> > *mountains, glaciers, trading parties*
> > > *of tattooed men and women, faience beads,*
> > > *packs filled with poppies, tin, and amber,*
> > > > *threading through a pass.*
> *Hammered bronze knives, Helen,*
> > *mixing her potions,*
> > *the blue Aegean stretching*
> > > *like a storyteller's breath.*

While controlled studies indicate that the best time for harvesting is fourteen to twenty days after flowering, in practice, in the field, the timing can only be approximately measured by a calendar, since the maturation of the plants is not uniform. Harvesters learn to judge the maturity of the capsules by their compactness and color, the change from green to whitish green being the signal. Unfortunately, not every capsule undergoes the same color change, as the size of the capsule also affects the change. Harvesters also judge by the firmness of the capsule.

Professional farmers in Asia and the Middle East sometimes have three little blades set into a ring that is worn on the finger for lancing. Others just use a sharp sickle-shaped knife. A razor blade works great, wrapped with masking tape so that only a millimeter or less of the corner of the blade is exposed, the layers of tape forming a shoulder to prevent the blade from cutting deeper.

> *like circumcision,*
> > *carefully cutting*
> > > *just the outer skin*
>
> > *drops of semen, glowing*
> > > *white in the sun*

If you cut completely through the pericarp, the latex is lost inside the capsule, and it spoils the seeds. Several different methods of lancing are used in different parts of the world: a single vertical incision, multiple vertical incisions, multiple horizontal incisions, multiple slanted incisions, and the Turkish spiral cut. One Indian team found that the Turkish spiral cut was the best, while another team found that the single incision did just as well.

> *Turkey, young men in turbans*
> > *in the chest-high fields.*
> > > *China. Ripe poppies*
> > *in the mountains of Laos.*

But some things are clear from both studies: that long cuts diminish the morphine content of secondary and tertiary lancings. This indicates that if you live in a part of the world where you are free to harvest your poppies as you see fit, consider making your incisions only one-third the length of the capsule, vertical – one or two incisions only – and then repeating this process every two or three days until the capsule no longer exudes latex. Lance on opposite sides of the capsule each time.

> *the fresh latex is acrid*

On the other hand, if you cannot indulge in such freedom, and can only afford one lancing, make your cuts longer, either the spiral cut or several vertical cuts on both sides of the capsule.

> *the taste of opium becomes so delicious*
> > *that one salivates*
> > > *drawing in the smoke*

It is generally accepted that it is important to collect the latex before 8:00 AM. Usually the lancing is done in the late afternoon or early evening, and the collecting done early the next morning. The latex, which is white when it first appears, dries and darkens fairly quickly. It is collected by scraping it off the capsule with a dull knife or some other scraper.

> *You have to scrape a lot of poppies*
> *to get a little bit of opium.*

You need a scraping device, and a collecting cup. There is a knack involved, better learned from experience than from text.

> *Learn from the man on his hands and knees, browsing*
> *around the poppy patch.*

A paring knife is a good tool.

The Ally
> *More like a white-haired phantom,*
> *half man, half ghost,*
> *lingering on and on*
> *in the twilight of desire.*

What alcohol has been to twentieth-century literature, opium was to the nineteenth-century Romantics. They followed the dreamer's way – and the dreaming path led through the poppies. None of them smoked opium. They took laudanum.

> *For not to think of what I needs must feel,*
> *But to be still and patient all I can;*
> *And haply by abstruse research to steal*
> *From my own nature all of the natural man –*
>
> *This was my sole resource, my only plan:*
> *Till that which suits a part infects the whole,*
> *And now is almost grown the habit of my soul.*
>
> *– Samuel Taylor Coleridge, "Dejection: An Ode"*

Thomas De Quincey's name has become synonymous with opium because of *Confessions of an English Opium Eater*. De Quincey brought "opium eating" into public consciousness. De Quincey was the first "out-of-the-closet" laudanum drinker from the genteel classes. (The working class often used laudanum because they couldn't afford beer.)

Coleridge accused De Quincey of taking opium for pleasure, while stating that he himself only took it for medicinal purposes, implying some moral superiority thereby. The accusation seemed to bore De Quincey more than it shamed him. Interestingly, it was De Quincey who was better able to control his habit. After some years of taking a pint or more a day of laudanum, De Quincey gradually tapered himself off to a mere spoonful or two a day, and seemed quite satisfied with that. Coleridge drank about two pints a day for most of his life, his frequent attempts to break his addiction complete failures.

Alethea Hayter in *Opium and the Romantic Imagination* refers to John Keats as a writer who used opium only occasionally. Recently, however, a test was made of a lock of the poet's hair, and the test results indicated chronic use of opiates.

George Crabbe, the poet and clergyman, used laudanum regularly, without deleterious effect on his poetry, day job, or family life. Elizabeth Barrett Browning took morphine in ether for her nerves, and became addicted. She kicked when she married Robert Browning, and was drug-free when she birthed their daughter, but probably relapsed after that.

Some, like Walter Scott, who used opium as a medicine for digestive problems, were able to quit whenever their physical ailments permitted. Southey, Shelley, and Byron used laudanum whenever they felt they needed it, and were able to put it down when the need passed.

Wilkie Collins was a laudanum addict, as was Baudelaire. Many plant allies passed through Baudelaire's life, including, as we have noted, absinthe. But opium got him at the end. Whether or not Edgar Allen Poe was a laudanum addict is still a matter of academic debate.

The Plant I first smoked opium out of a baby bottle. A tiny hole had been drilled in one side of the bottle. The host had a little ball of opium on the end of a bicycle spoke, and twirled it over a candle until it was soft. The side of the bottle was being heated also. There was a rubber stopper in the bottle and a glass drinking tube in the stopper. As the host pulled the bottle over the candle, he pushed the little ball of opium into the hole, and told me to suck. White fumes filled the bottle and entered my lungs. I smoked several balls. It came on slowly and built for hours.

> *That's the way the bosses did it. The soldiers didn't have time for that*
> *kind of thing. They took the fast stuff, the stuff you could shoot through*
> *your arm.*

In India, you buy smoking opium in little cups. Maybe there are four or six hits in a cup, and maybe you will stay and smoke several cups. You get a bunk and a headrest, and the proprietor who prepares the pipes.

The most common mistake of untutored smokers is to try to burn the opium the way hashish is burned. With opium the object is vaporization rather than combustion, and even with the best technique a lot of opium is destroyed by heat.

But opium is lost by digestion also. And if the opium is eaten, the effects are more diffuse. (Cocteau maintained that the two practices of eating and smoking were not the same at all, and attracted different sorts of people, but it is hard to guess what he was referring to.)

The Path   While there is probable evidence of ritualistic use of the poppy in the Eleusinian mysteries, the predominant use of the poppy through history, drug-wise, is as a medicine. There is nothing antisocial, intrinsically, about most plant allies, such as *Cannabis* or alcohol or *Coffea*, but the same cannot be said for *Papaver. Papaver* has antisocial tendencies, at least when the acquaintanceship becomes a full-fledged affair. In Cocteau's words, "Two on a pipe is already crowded."

> *Opium likes to associate with itself.*

Spiritual masters are sought out by seekers of truth. The opium smoker is mostly sought out by domesticated cats, seekers of a warm body upon which they can walk about, stretch out as they please, and nap: purring and secure.

The Ally   *Opium knows how to wait.*

> *— Jean Cocteau: Opium Diary of a Cure*

Effects   *a sudden wave of nausea, I wonder briefly*
if I will need to vomit.
then comes the thirst,
the long thirst that water doesn't seem to quench.
and itching. I scratch my beard
scratch my legs. my balls itch.
one hand spends a lot of time
inside my pants.

and I saw the visions: the damsel with the dulcimer,
some beautiful, some scary, some obviously symbolic,
like kissing a woman and her mouth suddenly becoming
"dry paraphernalia," hard and angular, stuck
in my mouth.
other:
a woman suddenly strips naked, and all so
immediate: color, texture, odors,
lucid.
always knew I was dreaming, but didn't always
know whether my reflections upon the dreams
were waking, or dreams themselves.

all my ideas became visual, structural ideas for
the book, all took visual form.

but not all pleasant. the punishing visions get
their turn . . .

CORRESPONDENCES

IMAGE	The Keys
LANDSCAPE	Large River
LOGICAL OPERATOR	Not
METAL	Lead
METAPHOR	Dream
MINERAL	Olivine
MUSICAL INSTRUMENT	Lyre
MYTH	Oedipus
MYTHIC HERO	Adonis/Narcissus
NUMBER	$\sqrt{-1}$, imaginary numbers, i
OCCUPATION	Physician, Coolie
OUT-OF-BODY REALM	Realm of Equanimity
PERIODIC TABLE COLUMN	Noble Gases
PHASE OF COITUS	Postorgasmic
PHASE OF MATTER	Amorphous
PHYSICAL CONSTANT	Permittivity of Free Space, ε_0
PLANET	Saturn
PLATONIC SOLID	Dodecahedron, the Knowledge Body
POISON	Fear, Inadequacy
PROPORTION	ϕ, Golden Mean
QUARK	Bottom

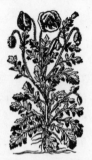

CORN POPPY (PAPAVER RHOES), FROM
MATTIOLI'S COMMENTAIRES, 1579

Effects   *The effectiveness of opium is the result of a pact.*

— *Jean Cocteau, Opium: Diary of a Cure*

CORRESPONDENCES

QUANTUM FORCE	Neutron
REALM OF PLEASURE	Spinal Chord
RITUAL EVENT	Love Affair
ROCK	Schist
SEASON	Spring
SENSE	Smell
SEXUAL POSITION	Woman on Top
SIGN	Cygnus
SIN	Sloth
SOCIAL EVENT	Convalescence
TAROT KEY	Hanged Man
TIME OF DAY	Twilight
TOOL	Athanor, Nail
VIRTUE	Hope
VOWEL	Middle Central: ə

Poesis   When the plants dry out, collect the seeds. In some races the valves at the top of the capsule open, and it is like a shaker. In some races of poppy, the valves never open, and you have to slit the capsule to get the seeds. Dry the seeds and they will keep well, for sowing the next crop and for food.

After harvesting the seeds the plant can be harvested for "straw." The leaves make a pleasant tea, but the capsules themselves are rich enough in alkaloids, even after lancing, that they have become a major source of opiates, commercially.

Extraction processes can be divided into aqueous methods and solvent-based techniques. Methods of collecting the alkaloids from "poppy straw" are slightly different from the methods of separating the morphine from opium. For the latter, in the fields of Southeast Asia and in the Middle East, the method is to dissolve the opium in hot water (not boiling), and to precipitate the narcotine and codeine and other organic parts by adding lime (calcium oxide, CaO). Because of its phenolic structure, morphine is an exception to the general rule that alkaloids are insoluble in basic solutions. The solution is filtered, and the filtrate is heated and stirred again, and the morphine dropped out with concentrated ammonia, NH_4OH, and recovered by another filtration.

Opium alkaloids are extracted from poppy straw with a 5 percent sodium sulphate solution, in a series of extractors. The solution is neutralized and concentrated, the concentrate then repeatedly extracted with 90 percent ethanol. The alcoholic layer contains all the alkaloids, which can be recovered by distillation.

There are a large number of patents for processes to separate the various opium alkaloids. The oldest is the Gregory process, where a concentrated aqueous solution of the opium is treated with calcium chloride, which precipitates the narcotine, and most of the nonalkaloidal organic compounds: calcium meconate, calcium lactate, and calcium sulphate. The filtrate contains morphine and codeine hydrochlorides. This is crude "Gregory salts." They can be redissolved, and the morphine precipitated with ammonia.

Solvent-based extractions of poppy straw on a small scale would follow other alkaloidal extraction techniques.

The Nature of Addiction

The pipe becomes the ally,
the ally becomes a crutch,
the crutch becomes a habit.

Effects

Narcotics are not generally thought of as sexual enhancers. In fact, the contrary is usually the case: the eidetic upstaging the carnal. But with opium, *if you ever get around to it,* sexual orgasm can touch astonishingly primal centers. Perhaps part of it is a side effect of the general decrease in sensitivity, delaying the orgasm and demanding a prolonged and more insistent intercourse – but when the climax is at last achieved, it seems to split the spine. In an instant one knows what lizards feel when they mate, and why they clamber onto a sun-warmed rock in the morning. One feels kinship with amphibian consciousness, you know for yourself what frogs' legs do when they stop jerking. One even knows, and for an instant must acknowledge, a power greater than the poppy – and this is a knowledge worth remembering. For if the poppy ever succeeds in sucking out your soul, in having you serve her instead of her, as before, leisurely caressing your hair with her soft fingers, you will need the memory of that glimpse of light. You will need to know that somewhere raw life exists, that it lives in seemingly imperfect and ephemeral bodies, but that in mundane flesh the universe has triumphed. Without that knowledge, your chances aren't worth a long shot at the dog races.

Beautiful mistress
When I inhale your dark perfume
My deepest longings for love.
Are touched and soothed.

HEROIN AND THE NATURE OF ADDICTION

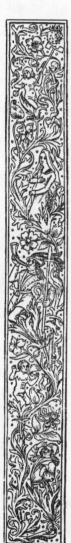

Mornings,
    teaspoons,
        Richard Farina . . .

With heroin, the nature of addiction can be drawn out to a fine point.

Addiction has become so synonymous with heroin that dependency on nicotine or alcohol is more often thought of as a *habit* rather than as an addiction. This despite the fact that a heroin addict has a better chance of beating his habit than does a smoker.

Heroin is diacetyl morphine. It is prepared from morphine in a fairly simple reaction, using acetic anhydride or acetyl chloride. When it was first synthesized, heroin was believed to be a superior painkiller to morphine (true), without the habituating properties (false). Heroin was even sold as a cure for morphine addiction, and in this it was certainly successful, if substituting one addiction for another can be called a cure. Though, inasmuch as methadone is called a cure for heroin addiction, heroin's claim as a cure of morphine addiction surely stands. Junkies say that methadone is more painful and difficult to kick than is heroin.

Smack. Stuff. Heavy.
Horse. H.

The addictiveness of opiates (the length of time necessary to acquire the addiction) seems to vary directly with the immediacy of the effects, while the strength (the persistence of the addiction) varies inversely. Intravenous morphine is much more addictive than is opium, and opium smoked is more addictive than is opium ingested. But an opium-eating habit is reportedly harder to kick than an opium-smoking habit, other variables, such as length of addiction, being constant. Heroin, which is shorter-acting than morphine, is more addictive. Opium addicts do not necessarily have to keep increasing their dosage, as is more commonly the case with heroin addicts.

Even with heroin, however, it is possible to avoid the build-up of tolerance. Experienced addicts will often take minimal doses, the minimal dose that relieves the craving. What builds tolerance is always going for the same rush experienced as a beginner. Either way, though, you've got a monkey.

Men lies about it,
Some of them cries about it,
Some of them dies about it,
Ev'rything fight about a spoonful,
That spoon, that spoon, that spoonful.
    – Willie Dixon

Thanks to misguided drug laws, while opium is almost impossible to obtain in the United States, heroin is readily available to anyone with money, determination, and a modicum of street savvy.

Effects   *Itching, coasting, soap-boxing, sweating, nodding.*
                 Dry mouth, dry ass, blind eyes.

Even the itching becomes a craving.

Narcomania   Intent is involved in addiction. Not that many junkies started out by one day thinking, "Gee, I think I'll become a heroin addict." In fact, those who start that way ("I just wanted to see what it was like to be an addict") seem able to kick and leave the stuff with the same nonchalance as they began.

The importance of intent has to do with the nature of the dis-ease being treated: whether the intent is to relieve physical pain from a specific organic ailment, or whether the intent is to relieve spiritual pain. If it is a physical pain that is being treated, when the cause of the physical pain is gone, you can stop taking the medicine with no or few untoward effects. If the pain is spiritual, the matter is more complicated.

If the spiritual pain is caused by some particular environmental malady, such as being in a combat zone in Vietnam, the cause of the pain will disappear when you finish your tour of duty. Most of the vets who returned to the United States as addicts gave up their habits when they gave up their rifles.

But if the spiritual pain is from within yourself, how will you ever escape? And there is a particularly pernicious feedback loop in narcomania: the presence of the ally in your body impedes the very spiritual work needed to relieve the pressure, and so the pressure increases.

Three headings define the vicious state of Samsara:
    The misery of conditioned existence,
    The misery of change and
    The misery of misery.

Should we try to illustrate this triad of misery by similes, that of conditioned existence would be like an unripe fruit; that of change would resemble a meal of rice gruel mixed with poison; and the misery of misery would be like the growth of mold on fruit. Or again, the first is a general feeling of indifference, the second a feeling of pleasure, and the third of displeasure.
    – Gampopa, The Jewel Ornament of Liberation

Effects   Susan Lydon, who writes about her fifteen years of heroin addiction and eventual recovery in *Take the Long Way Home,* says that it wasn't that heroin got her high, but that it made her feel "like an ordinary person." At first.

If you don't feel like a normal person until you snort H this is a sign that – well, a bad sign. A sign that you must avoid it, immediately; that the prognosis of your relationship with this particular ally is poor.

Such people should take Prozac, not heroin.

Narcomania   The pain of creation, the birthing pain. Relieve it at your peril. H is constipating.

Still, some do. Some do and still triumph. Bird. Trane. But neither of them ever claimed that the stuff helped them.

> *They love not poison that do poison need.*
>   *– William Shakespeare, Richard II*

Maybe it happens that you've been using the stuff off and on, kind of for fun, and that you feel really terrible today. You have a runny nose, don't feel much like eating or going out. Then you realize that you don't have a cold. And you go score.

After that is the "honeymoon" period. How long it lasts and how much of a honeymoon it is depends on the legal status of the drugs in question, and on your "luck." Medical doctors, who are overrepresented statistically among narcotic addicts, can often maintain themselves for many years, if not for their whole career. If they inject they use clean equipment. They get proper nutrition, supplementing it where necessary. And they don't have to spend half of each day trying to score.

The (dull) honeymoon can last months, years, or decades. After that comes the late chronic stage, during which the principal motive is simply maintenance, avoiding withdrawal. When problems set in, the final stage appears: deterioration or recovery, whichever. That problems will set in is certain, even in the best of circumstances. It's a corollary of the laws of spiritual physics. "He not busy being born is busy dying," as Bob Dylan put it.

The Kicks
> *I started sniffing stuff on the road and I ran out. I got totally depressed and my stomach hurt. My nose hurt something awful, terrible headaches; my nose started bleeding. I was getting chills. I was vomiting. And the joints in my legs hurt.*
>   *– Art Pepper, Straight Life*

John Lennon wrote a song called "Cold Turkey" containing many images of heroin withdrawal: the aching body, the sleeplessness.

> *But not everyone survived. Accidental overdoses: Carl Perkins, Phil Seaman, Tim Hardin, Mike Bloomfield. Mistaking pure heroin for cocaine: Tim Buckley. Combining H with barbituates, alcohol, stimulants and tranquilizers: Janis Joplin, Gram Parsons, River Phoenix.*

The Ally Hiding it. Keeping it private, not telling the spouse. And they feel betrayed when they find out, like with an affair. It *is* an affair, an affair with a pipe, an affair with a syringe. Most masturbation is a private kind of thing.

Narcomania Nonaddictive use of narcotics has been difficult to study. The draconian laws and the social stigmas connected with any nonmedical use of opiates has forced the occasional user to be completely secretive. The anecdotal evidence and what stories are available to us reveal that some "chippers" last for decades before becoming addicted, and that some never become addicted.

Cocteau distinguishes between habit and addiction: smoking opium every Sunday is a habit; having a ruined liver is a sign of addiction.

The Ally It's easy to get romantic here: Burroughs was a master of that, and Algren. There is already enough glamour about "God's own medicine" without my adding to it.

> *Things kept getting worse. I got busted. All my deals started falling through. And the worse it got, the more I needed my fix to take away the pain, to keep from having to face the music. The mail and the bills just kept piling up. I didn't even notice. Some thugs came over and pistol-whipped me and ripped off most of my stash. I wanted to kill them and was going to put out a contract. I hired some Hells Angels to come with me and we went after them. Things were* SO BAD.

> *Then through the fog of the narcosis it occurred to me that the heroin might be affecting my luck.*

The Kicks "Like having the flu," someone said. No, worse than that, much worse. Not that the flu is to be taken lightly.

> *Tremors.   Sweats.   Your whole body aching.*

But what is worse is the mental pain, and having to face the ruins of your life, what's left of it. Maybe things weren't great when you started, but they are much worse now.

> *My best friend got strung out and started stealing from me. He'd actually burgle the house. He stole from all of us. One time we had to call the police.*

Seeking oblivion, we awaken in the Abyss. Hung over, craving, out of money, out of friends.

> *That's right, it's come to this,*
> *It's come to this,*
> *And wasn't it a long way down?*
> *Wasn't it a strange way down?*
>
> — *Leonard Cohen, "Dress Rehearsal Rag"*

Narcomania In Laos, among the Lao and the Hmong, smoking opium is not stigmatized, it confers no special status upon a person. Addiction to the point of impairment, however, does. The situation is precisely analogous to drinking in the West: moderate drinking is neither good nor bad, but alcoholism is seen as a defect of character and a serious liability. Thus life in the Laotian mountains provides an example of a culture where the use of opium is "socialized."

In Laotian villages that are actually growing and producing opium, up to 10 percent of the population may be opium addicts. In cities where opium is widely traded, but its presence is less pervasive, the addiction rate is around 5 percent. In villages near the opium fields, but which are not actually growing poppies, the addiction rate is 1 to 2 percent.

These figures suggest that even in villages where opium is an everyday part of life the addiction rate is roughly the same as the rate of alcoholism in the West. This lends some credence to the theory that the proportion of addicts in a society is a constant, that it is only the object of addiction that varies.

When, under pressure from the United States, the Laotian government outlawed opium, traffic in heroin increased tremendously, and heroin addiction began replacing opium addiction. We should note that the number of alcoholics in Laos is small, and that alcoholism occurs where there is the least amount of opium addiction. If we in the United States could switch our heroin addicts onto

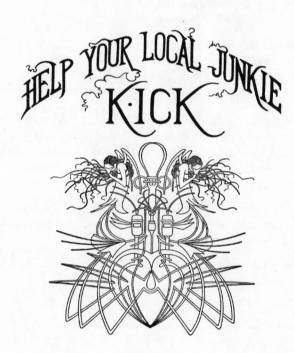

MICHAEL MYERS

alcohol, and our alcoholics onto heroin, the savings in medical and social costs to the country would pay for a sizeable portion of national health care.

The Ally Like Mayakovsky, we play Russian roulette. That is why luck is so vitally important.

The Kicks There comes a time when it's all over but the crying. Mostly after five or eight years, maybe ten, junkies get tired of the life. A few exceptional dope fiends hang in there for fifteen years and attain some notoriety in those circles. But there is nothing comparable in the narcotics world to the smoker who has had one lung removed but still can't/won't quit smoking.

> *A pervasive sadness, memories of a happier life.*

Memories of a life that was simpler and warmer, when you had friends who weren't junkies. When your family still trusted you. When you could hold a job. When you were in love, and were loved in return, and with good reason. When your dreams were what you were living for, rather than in.

Ending even the worst marriage is painful.

> *When you look through the years*
> *and see what you could have been,*
> *oh what you might have been,*
> *if you'd had more time.*
>
> *Who's to blame if you're not around?*
> *You took the long way home.*
> *You took the long way home.*
>
> *– Supertramp, "Take the Long Way Home"*

The Ally One of the beautiful things in the world is a dope fiend getting straight. They have a special radiance. Narcotics Anonymous meetings overflow with warm feelings of love and support, and that in itself is enough reason to visit one. "Recovery doesn't happen in isolation," they say. No, but vision quest does. And vision is what you are going to need.

Love, a relationship, a good job, friends, all those things we call "merit" or "good karma," are part of your medicine, part of your power. You are going to need them all, but you are going to need more.

> *It is hard to know that this magic carpet exists and that one will no longer*
> *fly on it.*
>
> *– Jean Cocteau*

The *poison doctor* calls upon all of his medicines and uses poisons to fight poisons. Here we part company with Twelve Step approaches. Nothing against abstinence; "whatever works," we say. But most *poisoners* would prefer to give up the identity of "being an addict" without taking on the new one of "being in recovery." We wish to maintain and continue the recovery that led us to poisons in the first place.

Still, if your solar medicine fails, all bets are off.

Narcomania

> *Got the blues in my coffee, got the blues in my head,*
> *if I die in the gutter, God almighty now,*
> *at least I'd be dead.*
>
> *I don't like living, but I don't want to die,*
> *Cause if I was dead, God almighty now,*
> *well I'd miss getting high.*
>
> — *Patrick Sky, "Nectar of God"*

The Kicks

Clonidine is said to depress the locus coeruleus in the brain stem, thought to be the "fear center," and should certainly be investigated for relief during the initial period of withdrawal.

Recently, ibogaine has been found to be effective during withdrawal. The claims for ibogaine sound much like the claims that were made thirty years ago for LSD, and probably for as good a reason. Withdrawal is bounded, is finite. It's hell, but the days are numbered. It's after the withdrawal, when you reemerge into the world, that you need power.

Power comes from vision, and vision comes from the allies, particularly the *phantastica*. Some *poisoners* use LSD right during withdrawal, to go into it further, to look for something in the smoky hell that is familiar — a poison, a passion once loved and cultivated, but cast aside. You search to find your old ally and to make amends.

You may need to change your environment. If all of your friends are junkies you have to move. A few members of our beloved poison clan have proved exceptions to this rule, but how many of us can pull off what the magicians do? Your ally will tell you.

The Ally

Having kicked one addiction does not make you immune. In fact, if you fall again you will be worse off than before. Every magician can survive one bottoming out, by definition. Don't tempt the Fates.

> *A man who, after having long been in the power of opium or hashish, has succeeded, despite his enfeeblement by the habit of slavery, in mustering the necessary energy for his deliverance, seems to me like an escaped prisoner.*
> *He inspires me with more admiration than the prudent man who has never lapsed, having always been careful to avoid temptation.*
>
> — *Charles Baudelaire, The Poem of Hashish*

Truly poisonous words.

THE PERFUME OF POISON

The arrowhead is avoidance: sloth, greed, and their friends mere hangers-on. Something must be risked.

> *The first poisons were love philtres, potions*
> *to ensnare the heart.*

Other seductions came later: knowledge, the Elixir of Life.

> *Adam was already in love. One led to the other.*

Poisons for commerce are recent. Royal coca fed to workers by the conqueror. *Excitantia*. Armies goose-stepping to reduced ephedrine. Coffee breaks.

> *The poison is the veneer.*

An aroma, a spice. Makeup. *Pharmaka*. Empedocles: the deceiving poison of appearances. Gaudy colors and flashing lights, merely the most obvious.

The technician fashions gods. Poems. A vision of a world. And we walk through it, calling and singing, working, raising children.

> *I conjure you, my brethren, remain true to the earth, and be-*
> *lieve not those who speak unto you of superearthly hopes!*
> *Poisoners are they, whether they know it or not.*
> — *Nietzsche, Thus Spake Zarathustra*

The craving for immortality is the primal poison, and the original sin. Thus we fell from paradise, grasping for the permanent and seeking the undying. The wish to be like gods oozes toward us.

> *Sweet, sweet, sweet poison for the age's tooth.*
> — *Shakespeare, King John*

Poisoner, wizard, benefactor.

PACIFICA

PIPER METHYSTICUM

❧

Common Names Kava kava, *'awa*. And over a thousand other names. Most kava people have distinct names for each of the many varieties of kava that they grow, usually fifty or more. Figure that there are three hundred languages in Indonesian New Guinea alone, and at least that many in the rest of Melanesia, and scores more in Micronesia and Polynesia. Just multiply fifty by five hundred.

Related Species *Piper betle,* the leaf used to wrap betel nut; *Piper nigrum,* black pepper; *Piper cubeba,* cubeb.

Taxonomy The pepper family, Piperaceae. Pantropical: small trees, woody shrubs, and herbs, mostly in rain forests. Black pepper has been a major cargo and motivator of the spice trade for at least three thousand years.

Part Used The ground rootstock.

Chemistry Details of the chemistry of the active constituents of kava have recently been explored by Lebot and Lévesque. They divide the active ingredients into two groups that they call the "major kavalactones" and the "minor kavalactones." The major kavalactones account for 96 percent of the total lipids, and Lebot and Lévesque believe they fully determine the wide spectrum of effects experienced from ingestion of various kavas.

The six major kavalactones are

1. demethoxy-yangolin (DMY);
2. dihydrokavain (DHK);
3. yangonin (Y);
4. kavain (K);
5. dihydromethysticin (DHM);
6. methysticin (M).

Kavalactones are sesquiterpenes. They have a phenol ring connected to a saturated δ-lactone six-atom ring through two intermediary carbons with or without a double bond. Kavain is with a double bond between C7-C8. Substitutions on the phenol ring, mostly methoxy groups, and the shifting double bond between C7-C8 and C5-C6 account for most of the kavalactones. In methysticin, a methoxy group joins together with a hydroxyl group to make an O-CH2O bridge between C11 and C12.

Lebot and Lévesque analyzed cultivated varieties of kava from throughout Oceania, and discovered that they could classify the many chemotypes by coding the relative abundance of each of the six major kavalactones. For example, chemotype 521634 contains primarily (5) DHM; (2) DHK; and (1) DMY, in that order, the other three lactones present in smaller quantities. Further, they found that each chemotype, or chemo-genus, determined by the three most abundant kavalactones, produced physiological effects distinct from the other chemotypes. Combining the relative abundances of the chemotype code with absolute content percentages, the authors were able to map the history of the domestication and differentiation of the various chemical races of the kava plant. Their research showed that the evolution of *Piper methysticum* has been guided not by a struggle for existence but by human beings seeking distinct highs from the effects of eating the rootstocks.

Not surprisingly, the plant people with whom these admirable scientists studied already had names for the different chemotypes, recognized them, used some for ceremonial occasions, others for medicinal purposes, and others for everyday drinking. And they cloned and traded them.

Effects   Serenity, well-being. Kava is an emotional leveler. It relieves fatigue and is mildly stimulating mentally. In moderate doses kava is a muscle relaxant, especially for the lower body. In larger doses kava is a soporific, but without dulling the consciousness. Half a coconut shell of strong kava will put a drinker to sleep within half an hour.

> *Where can you get a better night's sleep than with kava?*

Kava drinkers prefer softened light and quiet.   Mellowness.

The Ally   A doctor of our path could base her whole practice on kava, swimming with energies of the heart, adjusting, finding words, seeking the common ground, sharing and bringing together. Common ground like a warm breeze,

> *trade winds, turquoise water,*
> *a sunken tank rusting on a coral reef.*

The Plant   *Piper methysticum* is derived from a wild plant still found in Melanesia, *Piper wichmannii*. Kava is a sterile cultivar, and was domesticated by vegetative propagation from a limited genetic base of *Piper wichmannii*, probably on Vanuatu. Lebot, Merlin, and Lindstrom, in *Kava, the Pacific Drug*, write that the domestication probably is only 3,000 or 3,500 years old, and present both chromosomal and linguistic evidence to support their thesis.

Piper wichmannii has the chemotype code 521634, nearly opposite of the chemotype of the most sought-after variety of kava, 426135. The process of breeding this variety would necessitate detecting the difference between 521634 and 521643 in one's garden, and then cloning off of 521643 for another garden. And perhaps in the new garden finding, purely by subjective effects, a clone that has mutated to 526341, and then cloning yet another garden from that plant. And so on.

Mathematically, the number of codable chemotypes by Lebot's system is $P\binom{6}{6}$ = 6! = 720. Actually, there is very little difference between clones varying only in the minority lactones − the first three components tend to typify a class. That would be $P\binom{6}{3}$ = 120. Representatives of many, if not most, of these intermediates still exist and are still cultivated. Such an accomplishment in a few millennia of clonal selection bespeaks the skill and sensitivity of the Pacific Islanders as plant doctors.

Chemistry
Kava people consider plant varieties with a high percentage of K, kavain, and a low percentage of DHM, dihydromethysticin, to induce the most desirable psychoactive effects. Plants that are high in DHM are usually avoided, as the effects are said to be long-lasting and to cause nausea. All six of the major kavalactones are psychoactive, and all six differ in their psychoactive properties and also in their pharmacokinetics, the speed of the onset of effects and the duration of the effects. Moreover, it is likely that the effects of the various kavalactones are synergistic, adding even more complexity to the various properties of the many cultivated varieties of *Piper methysticum*.

The Ally
Used for camaraderie, and for divination. Used to find words, to find a song, or to get advice. The seeker retires to a quiet place and drinks kava. Then listens. Maybe the words will come from a bird, maybe the words will come from the trades in the palm branches. Sometimes the words will come from your ancestors. For that reason kava is often drunk in burial grounds.

How Taken
Traditionally, the fresh root is chewed for five or ten minutes to soften and separate the fibers. The whole mass is spat out onto some leaves, and more root is chewed. This is usually done in a group. In the past, on some islands, such as Samoa, this task had to be performed by a bare-breasted virgin girl, bedecked with flowers and sitting cross-legged on a mat.

Mostly though, what has always been sought are strong young jaws that still have all their teeth. But virgin girls or boys lacking, the older men will sit and chew. Ritual requirement for the young to chew kava for their elders has been outlawed on most of the Pacific Islands. Indeed, due to zealous Christian missionaries who confuse faith with culture, the mastication of kava has been almost completely replaced by pounding, where kava has not been banned completely. On one island whose inhabitants were converted by Seventh Day Adventists, the kava plant has been eradicated entirely: rooted up, gone. One of the results of the suppression of kava drinking is the rise in alcohol consumption. Alcohol and kava are almost never mixed − their natures are so opposite, despite the similarity of the staggering characteristic of both inebriations. Kava is the plant of peace, of quiet speech or no speech at all, while alcohol (according to the Islanders) brings out aggression and boisterousness.

> *Sometimes I think that history is a war of poisons, and that bipedal hominids are mere pawns and soldiers, mouthing whatever slogans or propaganda are current, but ignorant of the designs and strategies of the true plant generals who direct the action from a realm beyond our usual ken.*

The juice of the softened masses of root is squeezed out several times. Kavalactones are resins and insoluble in water: the chewing creates an emulsion. This is the finest kava. It is said to clear the head, to relax the body, to ease sorrows, and to sharpen vision, hearing, and memory.

Effects Anaphrodisiac. "Boys never want girls after kava." Kava as *petit mort*, a "little death," obviating the need for sexual relations.

The Plant A shrub with heart-shaped leaves. The rootstock grows quickly and is ready to harvest in as little as three years. If left to grow, kava can exceed heights of ten feet.

The Ally Associated with exchange. Gifts. Communication between realms. Exchanges between social classes. Congress with the dead.

> *Necessary for any business deal: a large kava bowl on wooden legs in the general store for the customers.*

For conflict resolution or domestic quarrels. Kava is like *ska Pastora* this way, but without the bright spotlight on "depth-truth," or like MDMA, but without the intensity of "depth-emotion."

Third parties will sometimes try to make feuding families drink kava together so that they will talk and negotiate. Gifts of fine kava cultivars are given to seal the agreement.

How Taken In kava bars, large mechanical meat-grinders are used to mash up the root. The juice is strained and sometimes diluted with water, which can make it look muddy.

Poesis The kavalactones are lipophilic resins. It was once believed that the chewing of the kava root set up enzymatic reactions that led to fermentation. As Louis Lewin stated, "This is false in every respect." The purpose of the chewing is to release the resins into an emulsion. The resins could easily be extracted with oils or organic solvents.

In the United States, unless you grow your own *Piper methysticum*, the best you can do is to buy the dried root or root powder at an herb store with good connections. (Growing kava, incidentally, is not difficult, but, except in Florida, requires a greenhouse.) One herbalist I spoke with boiled the root in coconut milk, surmising, correctly, that the fats in the coconut milk would extract the lactones.

But I find boiled coconut milk thick and unappetizing. Most Pacific Islanders now use dried root, and simply make their kava by pounding the dried root with some cold water, squeezing it out, and then repeating the procedure.

My own kava technique varies, depending on whether I have root or powder. Dried root stores better than does powder, and as I have no way of knowing how old the material in question is, as it has passed through a number of middlemen, I try to buy root. It usually comes coarsely chopped. One strong dose is half an ounce of chopped, dried root. I grind the root into a coarse powder in that most useful of machines for a plant doctor, an electric coffee grinder. Instead of just whisking the powder up with water as is traditional, I sometimes add a tablespoon or two of cream to the ground root, along with the contents of a lecithin

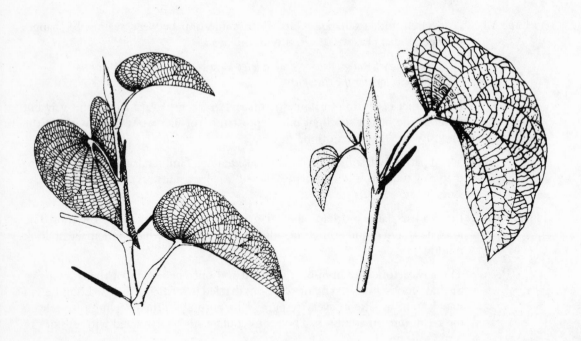

PIPER METHYSTICUM

capsule (about 1,000 milligrams). Grind this mixture well in a bowl, add one-quarter cup of water, and stir with a whisk or an eggbeater until it thickens into an emulsion. Strain through a fine wire jelly strainer, and press the emulsion out with a spoon or your fingers. Return the mass of root to the bowl, add another half cup of cold water, and whisk some more. Strain as before. Drink the filtrate. I get enough to fill a coconut shell cup. If you want to be ritualistic, hold the coconut shell with both hands and drink it all in a single draught.·

With powdered kava, of course, you can skip the grinding. Unless you are lucky enough to get very good kava, you will probably want a second shell in forty-five minutes or in an hour or two.

Try to develop a personal relationship with the kava buyer at your local herb store. Maybe she drinks kava already. Stress the importance of finding a good cultivar: for example, *white kava* is preferable to *black kava*. Try to get the buyer to send the word on up the chain of command that it's better to pay a little more and get better kava. One store I saw was selling leaf instead of root, which is, for our purposes, useless.

See if you can make a deal to buy in quantity. Then write to your congressional and senatorial representatives and tell them to keep the FDA out of the herb stores.

Effects
Immediate numbness in the mouth. Kava is a very effective local anesthetic, rivaling cocaine. Ethanolphilics and other detractors say that kava "tastes like dirt." Perhaps. But if dirt, it is clean dirt, on the green side, and somewhat peppery and bitter.

In larger doses kava affects balance and motor equilibrium, dilates the pupils, and alters perception of depth and distance:

> *changes in spatial relativity, like reaching for a doorknob but finding the door is clear across the room*

The Plant
The dried root contains 3 to 20 percent kavalactones, depending on the variety, with 15 percent about average. One gram, or a gram and a half, of resin is a strong dose. Effects last from two to eight hours.

There is no kavain in the leaves. Ascorbic acid in the leaves would quickly reduce the double bond between the two carbon atoms joining the phenyl group with the lactone ring.

The Ally
Kava is often associated with semen. At traditional all-male kava banquets ribald jokes and double entendres abound.

> *"Hey, have some of my kava."*
> *"That new woman, I think I'll give her some kava."*

In one story, the kava shoot is a penis that copulates with a woman who happens to step over it. She becomes a plant person. And it spreads around from there, until finally everyone on the island is a plant person.

Hybrids, part human being, part kava kava.

Sometimes the plant is female: like breast milk. Milk with a female smell, the scent of female genitalia. Milk for adults as breast milk is for infants, we being children in relation to the great power beyond. Image of the nourishing, the milk of the dead sister – the plant that sprouted from her corpse. Ghost nourishment.

Sometimes the plant is bisexual.

Effects   "Noise and light spoil the kava."

Pharmacology   The psychopharmacology is poorly understood. Kavalactones probably reduce spinal rather than cerebral activity.

Kava acts as a hypnotic in moderate or large doses, particularly strains high in DHK and DHM. Both DHK and DHM are more powerful as analgesics than aspirin.

It was noticed that no yeasts, bacteria, or fungi attack kava, so kavalactones are antimycotic. Kavalactones are also diuretics, anticonvulsants, spasmolytics, and local anesthetics. In folk medicine kava is used to treat gonorrhea, menstrual cramps, epilepsy, muscle aches, toothaches, sore throat, and many other ailments.

The Plant   Smuggled onto the island by two women in their vaginas, hence the characteristic odor of the drink. Others say it sprouted from the semen of a dead kangaroo.

In many Pacific Island languages *kava* or *'awa* also means "bitter" and is used to mean "poison." Being under the effects of kava is to be "poisoned by kava."

Tools   Grinding stones. Carved kava cups. Coconut shells.

Toxicology   Kavalactones can attach to proteins in the skin to form allergens, and in people prone to allergies, heavy and sustained use of kava can cause scleroderma, "alligator skin," or even lesions. The condition disappears when kava consumption is decreased.

An anonymous paper reported that kavalactones concentrate in the liver and cause damage, but this has not been substantiated. One Australian scientist has implicated kava in Aboriginal health problems, including weight loss, liver problems, shortness of breath, and skin rash. The problems are serious enough to require more study, but it is not clear what part kava plays, as many of the same persons drinking "excessive" amounts of kava had previously been abusers of alcohol.

In the Pacific Islands, one half of the population (the men) have been consuming kava for centuries, while the other half (the women) have not. This is a made-to-order epidemiological study. No known health problems have been found that correlate with these two easily recognized and easily trackable groups.

Matters
of State
and Liberty

Kava has been (and is) threatened by missionaries and alcohol, but seems to be making a comeback, even flourishing, on some islands. The missionaries, even the most liberal, were repelled by the chewing and spitting, which they considered unhygienic. Beyond that, they understood the importance of the kava ceremony to the traditional culture, and thus considered kava an impediment to the conversion of the islanders to the One True God.

Speaking of which, Marxist sociologists criticize the use of kava on the grounds that it creates a false goodwill between classes that, in a state of movement and economic differentiation, ought properly to be at each other's throats. This remnant of the old apocalyptic millenarian faith is against any half-measures or compensations, against any opiates or palliatives, believing that only by things getting worse will the Revolution come to save us.

They may be right, except for the part about saving. And the part about Revolution.

Class PACIFICA: *Peace-making, bringing peace.*

Lewin included kava in his class *hypnotica;* Schultes and Hofmann classified kava as a narcotic and hypnotic. We place it on the path between the narcotics and *thanatopathia:* sharing of both the euphoria of the narcotics and the mental alertness and moral calm of tobacco.

> *A benevolent ally to abate craving,*
> *a poison to subdue poisons.*
>
> *A moral peace:*
> *peace in body,*
> *peace in mind,*
> *the peace of twilight and evening,*
> *the Prince of Peace —*
>
> *kava.*

ON POISONING WELLS

There is nothing so beautiful or so profound that the Forces of Evil cannot warp and subvert it for their own base and nefarious ends. You must understand this well, if you be a poisoner, a doctor of the *poison path*.

There is no panacea. Do no trust those who believe that there is.

Thus we have the practice of "poisoning wells."

The doctors at the United States Central Intelligence Agency had investigated the possibilities of putting LSD into municipal water supplies a decade before the Sixties radicals considered the same idea. That is not the meaning of "poisoning a well."

Confronting the nature of evil. The evilness is us.

We are the evil. And within evil is the only hope for salvation. The evil is the remedy. You must dance with evil. Shunning only makes it stronger. It will not die – it will metamorphose into a new shape that we can't identify, an epiphany unrecognized.

Dionysus needs temper.

A formal discipline that does not deny it but sits with it patiently, letting it come and go. Becoming intimate. Merging, kissing, enraptured in orgasmic bliss. Not chasing the god, but making love with it. Bedding Satan, Why not? The power of love is beyond measure!

This illustrates the practice of "poisoning wells."

EXISTENTIA

SALVIA DIVINORUM

❧

Common Names Diviner's sage, *ska Pastora, hojas de la Pastora*, seer's sage, *la Maria*.

The *"Just This"* plant. The *"Emptiness"* plant.

Related Species *Salvia divinorum* contains a diterpene, salvinorin. Some *Coleus* species are rumored to contain similar compounds, but this is still unconfirmed (bioassay reports are mostly negative). *Salvia splendens* contains salviarin and splendidin, both diterpenes, and we should expect more from other species. No psychotropic activity has been reported for those compounds, but that does not close the case – I heard background whispers of "placebo effect" for years when talking about the powers of dried *ska Pastora* leaves!

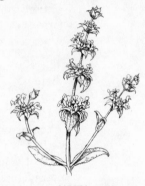

SALVIA
MELLIFLORA

Salvia sonomensis contains a camphorlike substance that is a mild stimulant when smoked. *Salvia officinalis* contains thujone, constituting in some varieties more than 50 percent of the essential oil.

But those plants don't really have anything to do with me.

True.

Taxonomy A true sage, like cooking sage. Mint family. There are a thousand species in the genus, and five hundred species in the neotropical subgenus *Calosphace,* to which *Salvia divinorum* belongs. Many temperate *Salvia* spp. are adapted to xeric conditions, such as black sage (*Salvia mellifera*), white sage (*Salvia apiana*), and purple sage (*Salvia leucophylla*) of the California chaparral. *Salvia divinorum* is a hydrophyte.

The Plant Square-stemmed, winged margins; the stems hollow and succulent. The stems will grow to more than eight feet if supported. Commonly they fall over, rooting where they fall. Axillary branches easily sprout from the nodes. The plant flowers when the days shorten: long graceful racemes of fragrant white flowers, the calyces deep lavender. I sprinkle the flowers into salads.

The Ally She can be shy. Sometimes she has to get to know you for a while, before she will come out and say hello. But once she appears, are there any who are more direct?

Part Used The leaves. The stems can be juiced.

How Taken, The Path of Leaves

Thirteen pairs of leaves, the stems all facing the same direction, are rolled into a cigar and eaten. That is the traditional way, the way of the Keepers of the Plant, the Mazatecs. The leaves are used the same way mushrooms are used, with candles (which are later put out), prayers, and singing. The ceremony is performed at night, in a darkened room. The darker the better. And the quieter the better: both light and noise have a way of dissipating the experience.

It is not uncommon for the Mazatecs to wash the leaves down with a swig of tequila. The tequila cleanses the palate and may aid in the final absorption.

> *It lights up the mouth like a rainbow,*
> *it's like a pastel sunrise breaking in the east.*

There are strict taboos to keep for several days after eating the sacred leaves, such as not having any sexual contacts. It is also important to be ritually mindful when collecting the leaves, and also in cleaning up after the ceremony.

Chemistry

Unknown until recently, and still far from understood. In 1982, Alfredo Ortega and his associates isolated a bicyclic diterpene, $C_{23}H_{28}O_8$, from material gathered in Oaxaca and named it *salvinorin*. Another group, led by Leander Valdes at the University of Michigan, independently isolated the same compound and named it *divinorum*. Because Ortega published first, the name *salvinorin* has precedence. Neither author tested salvinorin for human activity, but recent tests by Daniel Siebert and others, myself included, have proved the psychoactivity of salvinorin beyond doubt.

Other compounds in the fresh leaves may act synergistically in creating the extraordinary and variable effects of this plant, perhaps by inhibiting the lytic action of an enzyme or of the digestive juices.

The Plant

seer's sage
  truth sage
dream sage
  ghost sage
lizard sage
  mouse sage
soft-footed sage
  cymbals sage
roller-coaster sage
  rocket sage
wake-up sage
  it's-like-a-dance sage
silver-fox sage
  bare-light-bulb sage
waterfall sage

Effects

It's like a mirror with no frame: some don't see it at all; some do, but don't like what they see.

It's like cat paws, soft cat paws pressing, or like a bunch of bird tongues lap-ping the mind. Or like tiny fingers, the way ivy fingers reach out to climb a wall . . .

Some say it is a sensual and a tactile thing. Some say it's about temporality and dimensionality, that it's about time travel. Some say it is about the Root Energy Network, or that it is about becoming a plant.

"Bird tongues lapping the mind." We timed them: they hit four or five times per second. It may be the theta rhythm.

How Taken, The Bridge of Smoke

The dried leaves may be smoked. A large-bowled pipe, like a tobacco pipe, is about right. Rolled cigarettes are less satisfactory, because it is difficult to get a deep lungful of the smoke. Hold the smoke in. One to three lungfuls are enough.

Five or six small tokes do not produce the same effect as one large inhalation. The reasons for this are not clear. Perhaps the brain responds to salvinorin within seconds, with neurochemical defenses.

The best technique is to use the Val Salva maneuver, beginning by emptying the lungs of air and then layering the smoke until the lungs are completely full. Then hold the smoke in as long as you can. Release gently.

The Ally

Frequently people experience little effect from the leaves in their first meetings. The power of the leaves seems to slowly build toward a climax with successive ingestions. Díaz was the first to comment in print on this phenomenon. He drank the juice of the fresh leaves six times and noticed an "increased awareness of the plant's effects" each time.

Contrarily, sometimes the ally rolls over and crushes a person without warning, first visit. And a few people seem obdurately immune.

Effects, The Bridge of Smoke

Over a period of several weeks, everything around me gradually became more intelligent.

Pharmacology

Completely unknown. *Salvia divinorum* represents an entirely new class of en-theogen. A Novascreen receptor site screening sponsored by David Nichols dis-covered no binding inhibition for the forty reference compounds tested, covering all major known receptors.

Salvia divinorum contains no alkaloids. In screening plants for psychoactivity, plants that do not contain alkaloids are routinely thrown away. Clearly that ap-proach is too hasty.

Because of the quantity of material that must be ingested for diviner's sage to be fully active, it occurred to me in a light moment that *any* plant would be entheo-genic if one ate twenty-six whole leaves at a sitting. That's a joke, but you can't really get the point until you eat diviner's sage yourself.

It is bitter, my brothers.

Effects, Some people experience hyperthermia, a warming of the body. Nausea is rare,
Physical though by the eighth swallow of the leaves the gag reflex becomes overwhelming. Still, except for the swallowing part, almost nobody gets sick at the stomach.

The Plant   *It's faster than the mushrooms, and older.*

An extremely rare cultigen, found only at a few locations in Oaxaca. There are
specimens in botanical gardens, and in a few private collections, but lack of genetic diversity is a concern.

The plant is endangered by the forces of imperialistic religion, and has been for
four hundred years, possibly longer.

> *Her real name must not be told –*
> *Her real name is closer to Medusa than to Mary.*
>   *"They came with crosses –*
>   *they came to drag us*
> *from our huts, from our beds,*
>   *the soldiers that serve the priests."*

> *en el nombre del Padre*
> *en el nombre del Hijo*
> *en el nombre de Espíritu Santo*

The Ally Consciousness has to do with energy and light. It is really very simple. Neither
animals nor people have consciousness. It is plants that have consciousness. Animals get consciousness by eating plants.

> *We like to walk around sometimes, and to see new places.*
> *We like some of those animal things, like mating.*
> *Sometimes we get curious*
>   *to see what it is like to program computers.*

The Plant This plant is the great secret of our tradition.

> *Not secret anymore!*

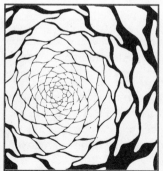

LEAF–PRIMORDIA
AT THE GROWING-POINT

Few have heard of it. Fewer know what it looks like. Fewer still
have ever met the sagely ally, yet the alliance forms invisible links
wherever it goes, across continents and across oceans. The ally
blesses some, eludes others.

That such an ordinary-looking plant, kind of succulent and without any alkaloids, can be as subtle and effective as the seer's sage
is, causes one to wonder about other green plants – perhaps there
are other such, sisters to this sage, waiting for someone to give
them the time and attention they deserve.

People ask, "If it's really so good, why is it so obscure, why haven't
more people heard of it?" The answer has to do partly with history,

and partly with intention, and perhaps partly with the intrinsic nature of the plant's effects.

First off, the plant is not at all obscure to her people. They know her and love her, or know her and don't love her (some think the plant devilish). Most of our ("our" meaning Western literate culture) current knowledge about *ska Pastora* can be traced back to the visit of Gordon Wasson and Albert Hofmann to Maria Sabina. Most of "our" plants are also from this transmission. Several particulars of the Wasson/Hofmann/Sabina meeting account for some of the plant's recessive reputation. For one, Maria Sabina's primary ally was the mushroom: she only used the *little leaves* when the *children* were out of season. But there are other *curanderos* who prefer the leaves to the mushrooms. Don Alejandro says that taking the mushrooms too often "will make you crazy," but that the Virgin, who speaks through the leaves, is more gentle.

Second, when Hofmann returned to his laboratory at Sandoz Pharmaceuticals in Basel, he had brought some juice from the *Salvia* leaves back with him, "preserved in alcohol." When this juice was deemed by self-experiment no longer to be active, Hofmann abandoned his intention to analyze the juice for its psychoactive principle(s). Hofmann reported that the unknown active ingredient must be unstable. This belief was incorrect but tended to inhibit further research for some years. My own reports on the effectiveness of smoking the dried leaves were dismissed by a number of my colleagues.

On the matter of intention, to quote Lao Tzu: "Those who speak do not know, those who know do not speak." Most sage people would rather not have their beloved ally spotlighted, or scheduled, or even much heard of or spoken about.

> *"This is the sneaky one.*
> *We caught all the others,*
> *   but we couldn't catch*
> *   this one —*
> *this one was too subtle.*
> *We've been after this plant*
> *   for almost five hundred years."*

Lastly, I think that some of the plant's obscurity is intrinsic and will endure. How many really want to see? Most people are after the side effects, and in the matter of sensual side effects the little leaves are indeed a little sister to such a giant as *Cannabis*.

But just because the plant is not a party-goer, is not harmful, and is not abused anywhere in the known world does not mean that it would not be persecuted by those who rule by fear, if they knew of its existence. So in summation we will reiterate the early assessments of the plant and agree that it is a minor psychtropic of well-deserved obscurity.

> *Now say "mum."*

Mum.

The Ally   This plant has a sense of humor!

The Plant

> *garden-green sage*
> > *bitter bitter sage*
>
> *compost sage*
> > *sweet-smoke sage*
>
> *riverbank sage*
> > *shade-leaf sage*
>
> *crenate-leafed sage*
> > *come-to-me sage*
>
> *get-the-willies sage*
> > *whispering sage*
>
> *get-well sage*
> > *get-fooled sage*
>
> *candle-in-a-wind sage*
> > *nobody-knows-it sage*

The Ally   It is when you are really stuck, when you really don't know what to do, when you are nearing the edge of funk and self-destruction, that the leaves are the most powerful and the most precise. And symmetrically, for one not seeking engagement, for one seeking diversion, the plant is not much fun. Outside of her sacred context, *la Pastora* has surprisingly little to offer.

> *It's not a spectator drug.*

Indeed.

History   It seems likely that *ska Pastora* was once much more widespread than it is today. Cultigens generally have long histories, and *Salvia divinorum* is probably no exception. What is not clear is whether the decline of the plant began with the Spanish Conquest, or whether it was already in decline, and, if so, if the reasons were religious or political, or something else.

Gordon Wasson speculated that *Salvia divinorum* was the *pipilzintzintli*, the "Noble Prince" mentioned in Aztec codices. One problem with this identification is that *pipilzintzintli* was said to have both male and female varieties while our *ska Pastora* is, botanically speaking, perfect. The Aztecs were skilled botanists and surely knew the difference between male flowers and female flowers. But it is also possible that the reference to gender is metaphorical, relating to nonanatomical properties of the plant, rather than to dioeciousness. There are some known examples of such use of gender, so Wasson may indeed be correct. It would be extraordinary if

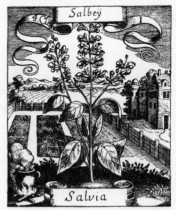

SAGE, FROM VALENTIN'S
KRAUTERBUCH, 1719

a plant of the power and the stature of *ska Pastora* were not well known to the Aztecs.

The Ally

Questing for the muse's spring, up some cold canyon,
stormdrain, up bloodvessels, canyonwalls of
flesh, rhythms surging in the darkness —
the home of the leaves, their nest within
the soul: even consciousness needs a soul. The plants
have consciousness, but no souls. For some of them,
*   that isn't enough.*

How Taken,
The Path of
Leaves

Six to ten or more leaves are chewed into a bolus and kept in the cheeks. The absorption is through the buccal membranes. Siebert's experiments (Siebert 1994) with the juice of the leaves demonstrate conclusively that most, if not all, of the power of the leaves is deactivated in the stomach. In Siebert's experiments, those who swallowed the juice quickly and then rinsed out their mouths with water experienced no entheogenic effects, while the group that simply kept the juice in their mouths and never swallowed it were all affected strongly.

I still prefer chewing and swallowing, if only from a sense of tidiness and tradition. Chewing with your cheeks full keeps the material in motion and insures that all parts of the mucosa are constantly bathed with sage leaf. More than once it has seemed to us that it is the stems, those chewy chewy stems, that finally push it all over the edge.

> *One intrepid researcher called Salvia divinorum "the best-tasting psyche-*
> *delic plant he'd ever eaten." Good point.*

Effects

The effects are different, depending on how the plant is ingested, on whether you meet the ally on the Path of Leaves or by crossing the Bridge of Smoke. And also depending on whether the plant has accepted you. That's metaphorical. Or is it? What neurochemical explanation could account for a threshold that, once breached, will still be open a year later, with no exposure to the plant intervening? Besides, neurochemical explanations are also metaphorical.

> *The plant is self-concentrating.*
> *Your body is the alembic.*

Smoking the dried leaves produces immediate effect. The effect of eating fresh material, while slower to come on, is a deeper and more sustained experience, often with strikingly colored visuals. Drinking tea made from dried leaves falls somewhere in between. (Salvinorin is practicably insoluable in water. The best way to "ingest" dried leaves is to soften them with some hot water, then keep the leaves in the cheeks just as with fresh material.)

Note that while the dosage by ingestion is ten to thirty leaves, the smoking dose amounts to one or two leaves.

> *It's the immediacy, the seamless immediacy . . .*

sometimes it's like it doesn't do much
of anything at all, but how many plants
do nothing with such clarity!

The Plant   There are rumors that the seer's sage may grow wild on some of the less acces-sible plateaus in Oaxaca, but this is unconfirmed. Her people grow the plant be-neath coffee trees, or along streams in ravines. They reportedly do not grow it next to their homes.

at night, it might envelop the house . . .

The plant is very patient.

The Ally   She has many epiphanies. Not all of them are shy, and not all of them are "she." One person encountered the ally as a giant – an immeasurably ancient giant wearing a belt of human skulls. The giant looked directly at this person. The giant wanted to know why he had been summoned. The giant did not want a trivial answer.

The Plant   *checkerboard sage*
        paisley sage
  amazing sage
      calico-ribbon sage
 vortex sage
    owl sage
 shape-shifting sage
     skin-walking sage
 who-are-you? sage
     something-is-moving sage
 get-serious sage
     look-we-have-come-through sage
 on-your-own sage
     she's-leaving-home sage
 metate sage

Class   EXISTENTIA.

Ska Pastora is not a hallucinogen. That is not to say that it does not share some of the characteristics of class *phantastica,* it does. But there are also differences. The "true" hallucinogens all act on the 5-HT2 receptors. While the receptors of di-viner's sage have not been discovered, the experiential evidence points to some new receptor, or to some holographic inundation of mind. And while many hal-lucinogens will help one's golf game (or, as Dock Ellis proved, one's major league pitching), a certain muscular discoordination accompanies the sage inebriation.

On the *Pharmako/Poeia* mandala, I put the little leaves on the path between *phan-tastica* and *inebriantia,* and name it *existentia*. By *existentia,* I do not mean anything Cartesian, nor even David Bohm's separate-from-self implicate order, but mean that which precedes essence.

It's a personal thing. Existence.
        If you can just stop thinking about it.

Salvia divinorum is what you get by crossing an entheogen with an atheist.

Effects   *It's not like being high, it's more like being practical.*

CORRESPONDENCES

ACTIVITY	Domestic Affairs
ANIMAL	Uroboros
ARCHETYPE	Fortune Teller
ART FORM	Lyric Poetry
BODILY FUNCTION	Circulation
BODY PART	Mouth
BUDDHA REALM	Prajna Bhumi
COLOR	Cobalt Blue
COSMIC ENTITY	Singularity
CRUTCH FOR	Indecision
DIMENSION	Fractal
DISCIPLINE	Augury
ELEMENT	World-Stuff
FORM OF ENERGY	Windmill
FORM OF IGNORANCE	Complacency
GEMSTONE	Tourmaline
GEOMETRY	Topology
GOD	The Mother of God

The Plant   In all of our Pharmako/Poeia, this plant is the hidden pearl. Poets, like vintners, love such surprises, and seek them out beyond their better known brothers and sisters: an unknown poet found in a faded chapbook with light in his verses, an obscure vintage the reviewers missed, dust-covered, but filled with mouthfuls of delight. The little leaves, hiding off in the mountains, have successfully avoided the front pages for four centuries.

A Taoist sage, in another range of mountains, after many years of studying
the secrets of alchemy with his master, feeling fully accomplished, descended
the mountain to move into the world. When evening approached, he

*stopped at an inn. The people at the inn marveled at the light that seemed
to hover about him — a sort of magical glow. The sage was chagrined, realizing that his studies were only half completed, and returned immediately to
his teacher.*

To visit the *hojas de la Pastora* is to visit an oracle, and she should be approached
with the same reverence.

> *Caravans of gold, threading their way*
> *from Sardis to Delphi*

Why would someone want to consult an oracle? Why would someone seek a
vision? Or it's like talking to a therapist, to a counselor — the leaves are like the
kalyanamitra, the spiritual friend. They can tell you things.

> *Or make you eat your words.*

It is difficult to speak.

Poesis   Recent studies by Aaron Reisfield (Reisfield 1993) demonstrate that *Salvia divinorum*
is not completely self-sterile, as had been assumed: the plant can produce viable
seeds, though very infrequently. Nor did Reisfield find any significant difference
in the production of viable seeds from flowers pollinated from the same clone
and those pollinated by plants collected from different localities. It is of course
possible that there is little genetic difference between any specimens of *S. divinorum,* even those that today grow in widely separated areas in Oaxaca.

Reisfield's observations strongly suggest that *Salvia divinorum* is a hybrid. The pollen grains of *Salvia divinorum* have low viability, indicative of disharmonious pa-
rental genes. But low pollen viability is only part of the reason that *Salvia
divinorum* rarely sets seed. Even with hand pollination only 2 or 3 percent of the
nutlets mature. Further exacerbating the problem of reproduction, in Mexico,
the plant only flowers sporadically. Flowering seems to require more sun than is
optimal for vegetative growth, so it is only plants growing on the margins of its
normal habitat that flower at all.

The main barrier to fertility, according to Reisfield, occurs after the pollen tube
reaches the ovary. But he was unable to determine whether the infertility was
due to inbreeding depression, a condition not uncommon among plants with a
long history of human relationship; hybridity; or some delayed-action effect of
self-incompatibility. If *Salvia divinorum* is indeed a hybrid, the parents are long lost
in poisonous prehistory — Reisfield knows of no two sages that would account
for the morphological features of *la Maria.*

For you, if you want *ska Pastora,* you will have to get it the same way everyone else
has for the last two thousand years: from a cutting from someone who grows it.

If your shoot is already rooted, or if you live in a humid climate, you can go ahead
and plant it directly. Plant it in shade or scattered light; the leaves don't tolerate
a lot of direct sunlight — I've had some plants do well with almost no sun at all.

If you live in the arid interior, you may have to mist the leaves regularly, or protect them with a humidifier. *Ska Pastora* loves the redwood country, where it gets fog.

The plant will thank you for some feeding. She needs water, lots, but be careful about root-rot in pots. Also, the plants wither if they get root-bound. Protect them from frost.

The Ally

Once you see it, you know it
was there all the time, so why
is it all such
          a big deal? And why
do we keep forgetting?

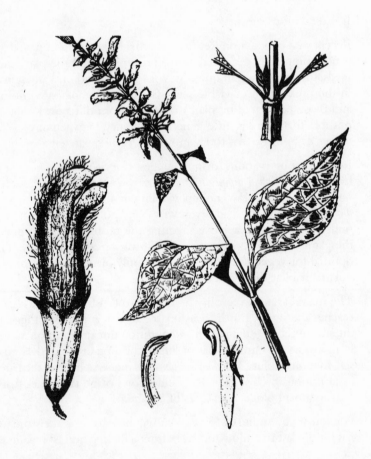

SALVIA DIVINORUM

CORRESPONDENCES

GODDESS	Isis
GRAMMAR	Presyntactical Mammalian
HISTORICAL AGE	Future/Eon
IMAGE	Labyrinth, Hall of Mirrors
LANDSCAPE	Garden
LOGICAL OPERATOR	Identity
MACHINE	Bathyscaph
METAL	Antimony
METAPHOR	Borders
MINERAL	Turquoise
MUSICAL INSTRUMENT	Bull-Roarer
MYTH	Parallel Universe
NUMBER	Complex
OCCUPATION	Poet/Soothsayer
OUT-OF-BODY REALM	Clairvoyance
PERIODIC TABLE COLUMN	Rare Earths
PHASE OF MATTER	Nuclear Condensed
PHILOSOPHER	Anaximander
PHYSICAL CONSTANT	Fine structure constant: $\alpha = 2\pi e^2/hc$
PLANET	Moon
POISON	Terror
PROPORTION	Radial Symmetry
QUARK	*Nen,* The Quantum of Time

On Divination   I used the Bridge of Smoke, laying out the cards. I had smoked lots of times before but this was the first time it really happened. An abyss opened. History opened. The manipulation of the cards by my hands seemed to amplify the effect. The cards fell perfectly. Each one revealed the details and development of my story with a precision that was hair-raising. Then I remembered how Crowley had said that you have to get to know the cards as people. The instant I thought that, the bottom dropped out of the cards, the background of each card became a hole in the table, like an open grave. Then the little figures on the cards moved a little. They shook free and started floating about an inch above the top of the table. They were all standing up and looking at me, waiting for me to ask them something.

The species is well named.

The Ally   It's anti-escapist, the opposite of escaping. It's not likely to be popular. It can be empathogenic, but it's more telepathic than emotional. It lights up the souls of those around us: we hear/know what they really think, what they really want, what they really have done. It's ideal for couples work, for keeping in touch.

On the Darkness   The ally loves the darkness. Light can interrupt and suspend even wildly cosmic and disembodied states, seamlessly returning the petitioner to the mundane. Sometimes it is necessary to turn on the lights to attend to something or someone, a child perhaps. What is amazing is how immediately the interdimensional space reasserts itself when the lights are again put out.

> *The essence of the Path of Leaves is just a few friends sitting around in a dark room, perhaps drinking a little beer or tequila. Some talking. Maybe some singing or chanting. To how many people does that sound like a good time?*

What a joke! No wonder some people can't stop laughing.

> *Or maybe the darkness is to keep others from looking in.*

It may always have been a cultish plant, something on the edges.

> *La Maria is shy. She needs the darkness to illuminate the Logos.*

Or maybe the nighttime tradition is to avoid interaction with the rootless. The ally will take you beyond the little social games that sustain the daylight. You will see the rigidity, but you may not see the importance of sometimes playing along. An uncompromising insistence on the absolute could quickly get boorish.

> *Besides, daytime you have a job and have work to do.*

Effects   Holographic. Even a very tiny amount of smoke can reveal the whole panorama. Dimly, to be sure, but all there, just the same.

The Ally   *There was no me, but there was no not-me.*

The most "Zen" of any plant ally excepting rice.

Effects   Staggering. Lurching. But not like drunkenness: the mind is completely clear. The effect is reminiscent of kava.

On the Logos   The poison has entered the Word. Words become stepping stones, a floating walkway to cross the chasms between.

What we really are is a web of interconnections, the summation of all of our relationships, all the people we know and those we are still to meet. It's not that we are in the web, the web is what we are.

Vowel sounds change the colors; pitch and tone alter the shape of the enclosing space; semantics create texture. Sentences become palpable things, they take visible and tactile form, flying or sinking.

But all in the mind's eye, not in the eyeball: an interactive lucid dream accessible to the will.

> *I saw where thoughts come from, visually. Some were just forming — were seething in a kind of liquid surface, some of them went on and blossomed, became people and conversations . . .*

Poesis Contrary to written lore on *Salvia divinorum,* the leaves can be dried. If you grow the plant, you may only have enough leaves for fresh ingestion in the summer and fall. I cut my plants back in the wintertime — in case it freezes. I have had little success with freezing the leaves, or juicing them and freezing the juice. Maybe it would work. I just find the juice harder to use than the leaves.

But you can dry the leaves, that's the easiest thing to do. The dried leaves carry the smoking-ally.

Effects FIELD REPORT: A MAN, INVENTOR AND PAINTER

"There were things you didn't tell me. It took me a while to learn how to use it. I had to find the right dose. At first I was taking too much, six or seven lungfuls. Two or three is about right.

"It's like heavy *zazen*, like after a very long period of sitting, the place you can get to there. It's changed my life, turned my life around. Things are really going well.

"It's very intense, I call it a reality stutter, or a reality strobing. I think that having been a test pilot, and flying in that unforgiving environment with only two feet between our wingtips, helped to prepare me for this kind of exploration.

"There is something very pagan about it. I don't think you should tell anybody about it. Sex is fantastic. It sensitizes the skin. And it makes you want to go exploring. And sleep is great, I'm sleeping much better. A. said that it relieved her menstrual cramps. And her attitude."

The Plant
> *in-control sage*
>   *smooth-moving sage*
> *snake-skinned sage*
>   *oh-as-little-as-that sage*
> *fooled-me sage*
>   *narrow-nosed sage*
> *weasel-snouted sage*
>   *creeps-up-on-you sage*
> *falls-all-over-you sage*
>   *loves-it sage*
> *just-grows-and-grows sage*

Effects   FIELD REPORT: A MAN, POET AND WRITER

"Hey, all of a sudden that stuff got strong! I used to use it for writing, but I can't do that anymore, it's too strong. But it helps me with some of my business dealings: like it told me how to talk to the producers I had to meet with the next day. I smoke it with my girlfriend. We call it 'the balancer.'"

FIELD REPORT: A MAN, SCULPTOR

"I had heard that it was going to be mild, so I took a lungful and held it in, and was expecting to have to take many more to feel a mild tingle. But it just overwhelmed me. It was so intense, so immediate. I had tunnel vision, I couldn't see anything except this tunnel in front of me, like I was going to pass out. Everything enfolded. I didn't like it. It was too abrupt, too scary. I recall feeling that if someone had walked into the room I wouldn't even have been able to talk to them. It is not subtle."

FIELD REPORT: A WOMAN, PAINTER AND POET

"I smoked it every couple of days for two months. I hate to say this about a plant, but I'm in love with it. It's remarkable. It took six or seven tries before anything happened, almost like it was laying down pathways or something."

my rootlets, my neural rootlets . . .

"Then, all of a sudden, a big whallop, and I mean big. Scary even. It's just remarkable. It is so present, so clear. My life has changed. It has shifted dramatically, and it's because of the plant.

"It is so much what it was, unequivocal. It wasn't like it was a high, it's just Mind. It's so honest! I feel like I was recruited, like I was enlisted."

heh, heh, heh . . .

"It has to do with specificity, the differentiation of form. Every form is filled with its own luminosity of detail. And this is true emotionally also, of my own emotions. Even the days in between the days I smoked I still felt I had this direct access. It's like the feeling after a meditation retreat, the post-*sesshin* feeling.

"I mean maybe I'm making all of this up. Maybe it was just oregano, but I call it 'my sweetheart.'"

The Plant   *green-straw sage*
                       comes-clean sage
                   one-puff sage
                       thin-skinned sage
                   gets-inside sage
                       falls-in-love sage
                   tells-you-she-loves-you sage
                       don't-get-antisocial sage
                   get-to-work-on-time sage

> *lizard-skinned sage*
> *smoke-skinned sage*
> *just-grows-and-grows sage*

Effects   It just gives you where you are. Wherever you are, that is what you get. If you are in darkness, you fly through darkness. The light and the faces you see are the faces that you always carry, the mental faces, lit by the glow of mind. If you are with your lover, the plant is an aphrodisiac.

The Ally   With the leaves there is no place to hide. That is why it is good for finding lost objects or for identifying thieves. It is a poison that illuminates poison: use it to find dis-ease.

CORRESPONDENCES

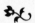

QUANTUM FORCE	Ψ / Schrödinger Wave Equation
REALM OF PLEASURE	Skin
RITUAL EVENT	Birth
ROCK	Ophiolite
SEASON	*Samhain*
SENSE	Sixth
SEXUAL POSITION	Scissors
SIGN	Pegasus
SIN	Lust
SOCIAL EVENT	Exile
TAROT KEY	Moon
TIME OF DAY	Midnight
TOOL	*Phurbu*
VIRTUE	Temperance
VOWEL	High Back /u:/

The Ally   FIELD REPORT, DAYTIME

> *It seemed that as long as I left the quid in my cheek it kept getting stronger. I spit it out about one-thirty. Had an amazing time typing at my computer: it was like the typewriter from the movie "Naked Lunch." M. drove me to the beach. I felt pretty much back to normal. Late in the afternoon we decided to go to a five o'clock movie. We had some time before the movie*

and I strolled through a used book store. A couple of poetry books were on the display shelf. Picked up Tagore. How vacuous! All those high-sounding words but no substance. He had only read about it, thought about it. It was all lies! It was so clear. The book next to it was Housman. Dense, but legitimate. It was there. He did it through clues.

Suddenly I felt completely disoriented. What a fool I was to be out in public. How did I think I could handle going to a movie? The question "How high does it get you?" is meaningless. It's nonlinear. Only the threshold was significant, and the threshold could be so subtle!

Poesis   One of the active ingredients of *Salvia divinorum*, salvinorin, can be extracted from the leaves. Valdes and his group at the University of Michigan isolated 1.2 grams of salvinorin from 5.35 kilograms of fresh leaves, which they dried to 674 grams of milled powder. Valdes didn't report how many leaves he started with, but the leaves that I pick average 2.3 grams fresh, and dry to about 0.45 grams. That works out to between 1,450 and 2,350 leaves to yield 1,200 milligrams of salvinorin, or between 500 and 800 micrograms of salvinorin per leaf. I crumble up several leaves into my pipe, but never smoke more than a quarter or a third of the pipe, which is about one dried leaf. So, back-of-the-envelope, salvinorin is active at ranges of 500 to 800 micrograms, about twenty times more active by weight than DMT (dimethyltryptamine).

Quantitative experiments by Daniel Siebert, Jonathan Ott, myself, and others have since confirmed this arithmetic.

Effects,   Many experience childhood scenes. Parents may be represented abstractly. Ex-
Salvinorin ceedingly fast changes of scene. Ontological revelations.

I have found one salvinorin "hardhead." Under my supervision, the man carefully and properly smoked a full milligram of salvinorin, vaporized in a glass pipe. After a few minutes he shrugged his shoulders, got up, and, trying to be polite, remarked that "maybe there were some visuals."

Poesis   All of the information needed to isolate salvinorin is in Valdes's paper (or, another method, in Ortega's paper). While Ortega and Valdes had to isolate pure crystalline salvinorin quantitatively, simpler extractions would suffice.

But all of this raises some questions. Why do it? On the "Crystal Highway" the ally often shows a more precipitous, and more terrifying, face than she does on the Path or on the Bridge. Many who meet the ally on the Crystal Highway never wish to repeat the experience. The ally is always fast, but on the Crystal Highway she is superluminal. And controlling dosage at the microgram level requires some skill. The raw leaf seems so exquisitely balanced already.

The plant is legal; just grow it. You may learn something. It is plenty strong enough in its fresh or dried form. It is benevolent in that form. When you start dealing with molecules in micrograms, with glass pipes, with overdoses, you are up against possibly serious issues of toxicity. And the sacred leaves of the Shepherdess become a commodity. And then there are the legal considerations.

My advice is to make friends with the *plant*. If you want to socialize, consider smoking *Cannabis*; if you want to get high, try nitrous oxide or smoking DMT. Only if you are ready to walk with an *ally* should you attempt the Path of Leaves or cross the Bridge of Smoke. Just don't blame me if the green beings recruit you, and you become a plant disguised with legs instead of a person.

Effects, Salvinorin: The Crystal Road

I thought that I had measured out 600 micrograms. Later it occurred to me that a substantial amount of the solvent had evaporated in storage, and that each drop was as much as doubled in potency.

The fast drop. A trapdoor. Like on the scaffold of a gallows. The frightening terror of absolute emptiness.

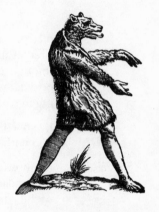

WEREWOLF

His head dropped onto the table and his arms splayed out. The cards flew all over. He fell out of his chair, some vases and books and another chair falling with him. Then his body twitched and I watched him turn into a bear. His whole body grew taut. A deep guttural growl sounded from his throat and he began speaking in tongues. His eyes had completely glazed over. None of it was pretend. I saw the strength: two men couldn't have held him down, if he had run amok.

Trance. Possession. The other side of shamanism, across that terrifying abyss: shape-shifters. There live skin-walkers and werewolves.

Think twice before offering a full moon medicine to a shape-shifter.

Field Report, the Crystal Road

All of the parallel universes were there. My childhood was there, and the death of my son. It was pure terror, all of it swirling through these breaks in time, breaks in what moments are made of. The whole universe was turned inside out. To get back I had to pull it all back through my asshole.

I had to destroy the worlds that I didn't choose to exist in. And some of them tried to stop me from doing that, they kept calling to me, telling me not to do it, that they wanted to exist. We were in the place you are before you are born, and the place you go to after you die. Once you step out of time, once you break through that continuum, all spaces are connected.

That I existed was the most amazing thing. The whole thing was an absurdity, but I couldn't come back unless I accepted it, all of it. All the pain of my life was waiting there, I—'s death was there waiting, but it was like

*I had to choose, it took effort. I had to accept all of it in order to return to
this particular universe.*

Poesis Ortega extracted dried and milled leaves with hot chloroform. He isolated salvinorin from the green residue left over after evaporating the solvent with column
chromatography. He used thin layer chromatography to test for salvinorin in the
fractions, and found it in the sixth and seventh of thirteen. The TLC plates were
developed with 10 percent phosphomolybdic acid in isopropanol (ethyl ace-
tate/hexane, 45:55, Rf = 0.7). Crystallize from methanol, melting point 238–
240°C.

Valdes extracted with ether. He partitioned the dried extract between hexanes
and 90 percent aqueous methanol, saving the polar components in the methanolic fraction.

An excellent product I call "4x" can be prepared by evaporating an ethanolic (or
methanolic) extraction of the dried leaves, and sopping up the oily goo left over
after evaporating or distilling off the solvent with "cleaned" leaves rubbed
through a strainer. Use an amount of cleaned leaf equal to about one-quarter the
original weight of the leaves extracted. The 4x enrichment is suitable for smoking in small pipes.

I've tried "10x" also. In that case, wash out the nonpoplar compounds from the
goo with hexanes, more or less as outlined by Valdes.

Ethnobotany Tea brewed from four or five pairs of leaves is medicinal. Mazatecs use the tea
for headache and rheumatism. It is also said to be good for anemia and problems
of the eliminatory functions.

The Plant The leaves of the moon. With no other plant are preparation and ground state
training so crucial. *Ska Pastora* is a moon doctors' plant. It could typify lunar
medicine all by itself, its light is so pale and white. The lunar medicine is needed
not to avert disaster, as is sometimes the case when dealing with the *phantastica*,
but to hear the words, to comprehend the presentation. "Just this" is not at all
the same thing as "merely this."

> *She will take who you are and run away with it faster than any plant I
> know.*

Effects The word *incredible* gets used a lot.

How Taken, Grow enough leaves to provide eleven to twenty-two leaves, thirty to sixty
Bottom Line grams, for each person. It is traditional to have an extra bundle on hand as a
"booster" for those who desire to return to the trance after their initial voyage.

Arrange the leaves so that the stems all face the same direction. Place them on
the altar. Burn a little incense. Do this in a comfortable room, with cushions,
preferably one that can be completely darkened. In the city, a tarp pinned over a
window will keep out streetlights and such. Start as soon as it is dark.

By candlelight, roll your bundle of leaves into a cigar and chew away until it is gone, or until you can't find your mouth. Or until. Chew well. If you are not going to swallow, or are not going to swallow all of it, provide each person with a nice dish or basket to receive the exhausted quid. But chew long and well. Then blow the candle out. Be accepting. Cleanse your palate with some tequila, or some beer.

Are your eyes open or closed? Are you sure?

After about forty-five minutes, if you. didn't finish all of your leaves, eat the rest. Or eat six or twelve new leaves, if you are inclined. Chanting and singing are appropriate, as is some tobacco. It is easier to get the leaves down if you have fasted half a day before the *velada*. Eat after: at midnight or thereabouts.

Best not to drive, but, if you must, never before you have eaten. Soups go well, and fruits.

Remember: your friends, the darkness, the gathering, and the chewing are all integral parts of the whole experience, and have been so for many, many centuries. The ancestors of two kingdoms await you.

The Ally
> *Sometimes the sage whispers, sometimes it shouts.*
> *Sometimes it tells you to sing, sometimes*
> *it takes your voice, walks off, leaving you*
> *rooted, eyeless, and with the kind of voice*
> *a plant has.*

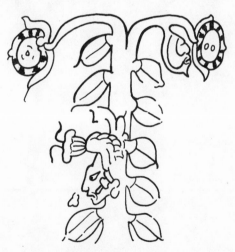

HUN HUNAHPU, FATHER
OF THE HERO TWINS OF THE POPUL VUH,
ACQUIRES PLANT CONSCIOUSNESS;
FROM A LATE CLASSIC
MAYAN VASE

The Plant   Enthusiasm. Entheos.

The plant of the gods, brought within.

> *La planta de los dioses.*
> *La planta amada de los dioses.*

The wise plant, the sage plant,
the plant of the Savioress.

> *La planta sabia.*
> *La salvia de las adivinas.*
> *La salvia sabia.*

We welcome the plant.

> *La planta que salva.*
> *La Salvadora de los sabios.*

We are not different from the plant.
It is we who must save the gods.
It is we who must be diviners.

> *Somos nosotros que debemos ser adivinos.*

ON WILDNESS IN PLANTS

Tobacco, marijuana
  after that
  you are in the jungle . . .

Poetic license, to be sure. Even the wildest plants have a way of being encircled by a shaman's *chagra*. The coca shrub and the opium poppy occur in cultivation more often than not. Still, the main world of plant poisons, the source of the wildness, lies beyond the fences of domesticity.

The wild gods live with the wild plants. Once, all of our gods were plants and animals. The allies are the ancient gods, their wisdom is the ancient substrate of our volition; they are the maternal transmitters of our vision and dreams. Anthropomorphic gods were the children of the plant gods. That is why destroying wild habitat is parricide, because the gods cannot live without their habitat, and it was the gods that made us, and gave us our culture.

The old religion survives on our altars: lettuce, almost wholly devoid of nutritional value, is a symbolic vestige of our earlier life as leaf eaters and is rarely absent from the table. Wild lettuce is a narcotic: a sedative and an analgesic and a medicine of virtue. Augustus, in gratitude to its curative powers, built an altar and erected a statue to *Lactuca virosa*. Almost any edible wild green is richer in vitamins than domestic lettuce. Table lettuce is to wild lettuce what the Protestant's grape juice is to Christ's blood, and plays a similar role. Part of us still knows that we need the Wild Redeemer.

 after that you are in the desert

We need the Wild Redeemer: to seek out its abode. We must fast, or eat locusts, or drink honey from a well, awaiting our interview.

We must claim stones as our sustenance, the earth as our domain. We must leap from the pinnacle of the temple. There is no redemption without a body.

 after that you are in the mountains

E
V
A
E
S
T
H
E
T
I
C
A

ON CAMP FOLLOWERS

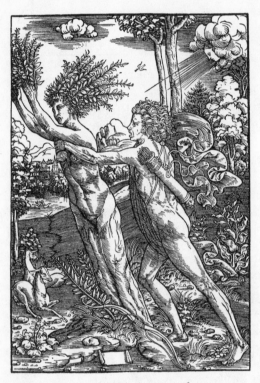

APOLLO AND DAPHNE, EARLY 16TH C.

The Parable of the Barley. The Parable of Hemp. We've met some of our best friends among the camp followers. Some of them we married.

Camp followers are the maenads of the wild part, wild dancers that have fallen under the spell of consciousness. They dance among us: on our garbage heaps and compost piles, and we notice them.

They are maenads or maybe secret agents. We watch their dance and we dance with them. We are both transformed. That's just what happens when plants dance with human beings. We still hear about it in the old stories. Metamorphosis.

The plant changes shape in our arms. She bends and stretches, reforms herself to fit to the pressure of our desire. We change her and the relationship changes our way of life. We take care of her and she takes care of us.

We didn't always live like this. We used to be foragers. Of course, that life had its dangers and its drawbacks also. It had an extremely long and evidently successful history, however – a longer history than since we've turned domestic. Domestic life is OK, but it still depends on the wild. Domestics sometimes forget this – always tragically. We *are* wild. We are part of it. If it dies, we die.

The plant hunter learns to sharpen her senses.
On the lookout: an alert. Are plant-walkers about?
Soul-stealing plants? She tastes
bitter healers, smells sweet-leafed herbs,
finds fiber plants and grain plants,

cold mornings,
mammoth-skin huts.

So we slept with the daughters of gods, and they tamed us.

CANNABIS SATIVA

Common Names	Hemp, marijuana, dope. AKA bhang, ganja, hashish, *mota*, weed, grass, et cetera ad infinitum.
Related Species	*Cannabis indica, Cannabis ruderalis.*
Taxonomy	Of the great dicotyledonous angiosperms: a proud carrier of the distinguished epithet *sativa* in superorder Dilleniidae. Older taxonomies had placed *Cannabis* in the mulberry family, the Moraceae, but the genus is now placed in the Cannabaceae, along with hops. The Moraceae have four sepals and four petals, while the Cannabaceae have five sepals and five petals.
Part Used	Limited only by imagination, but generally the leaves and buds. Unless you are a manufacturer, in which case you want the fiber. Or unless you want the oil, or a nutritious foodstuff, in which case you want the seeds.
	Industrial and agricultural possibilities abound: pulp for paper, textiles, medicines, biomass fuels, construction materials, plastics.
Taxonomy	Considered a monotypic genus for many years. Many botanists, Richard Schultes among them, now recognize three species. Of these, *C. ruderalis* is limited to Central Asia. *C. indica* is distinguished from *C. sativa* by its short stature (under four feet), dense branching, and marbled seed coats. But whether they are distinct species or varieties of one species is of only marginal interest to a plant doctor of our lineage. Our interest is in the plant's resident entity and its psychology.
The Plant	One of the greatest of all camp followers. Wild seeds – eaten, dropped, or thrown away – readily assert themselves on garbage heaps and middens, along trails, anywhere roving bands of human beings leave their characteristic scars on the land.
	Cannabis may be mankind's first cultivated plant, but it has never lost its wildness. Wild populations still exist with all of their vigorous variability, and cultivated strains can return to wild or weedy states with ease.
How Taken	Smoked or ingested: chilams, joints, bongs, brownies – all are effective. In ancient times ointments were used, applied to the skin for transdermal absorption.
The Plant	Dioecious, males and females stick to their own plants, though cases of spontaneous sex change are documented, generally much to the chagrin of the grower.
	The males are commonly sacrificed. The harvested buds are a mass of unfertilized females, infant leaves, meristematic and resinous, stigmas and bracts all stuck together in tight racemes – the smell can travel on the wind for a mile.

The plant has been cultivated for at least ten thousand years. There is no way to know how it was used first: for food, for fiber, or as a visionary power. The seeds yield an edible and useful oil. The herb has been used as a medicament for a variety of ills since antiquity.

In China hemp grows wild and tall, miles and miles of it.

The Ally

> *i called them and they came*
> *out of the woods   the pine and the sabin*
> *and the fir   tramping through the forest*
> *with their roots in the air*
> *at my crazy behest*
>
> *they came along the forest trails*
> *on their heads with glee*
> *to dance at my behest*
> *and there they danced in the clearing*
> *on their heads*
>
> — *Jaime de Angulo, "Marijuana, I"*

Effects   Euphoria. Thought magnification all the way to thought animation; formal structures seen on their own terms; aesthetic experiences, personal and sexual experiences, all brought into high relief. Self and other mix and pull apart. Perspective.

How Taken   Many like to walk in the woods.

The Plant   Latin *Cannabis* is cognate with English *canvas*. *Hemp* is from Old English *haenep*, Grimm's Law consonant shift from the Greek κανναβις. Other Indo-European cognates abound: Old Baltic *konoplja;* Lithuanian *kanãpês;* Persian *kenab,* Old Norse *hampr.* The Sanskrit is *cana, canna,* or *śana,* though other (noncognate) epithets are more common: *bhanga, ganja, siddhi,* and *vijaya. Bhanga* may be cognate with a proposed Old Iranian root *⋆banga,* meaning "psychotropic plant," and ultimately derived from an Indo-European root *⋆bhongo,* relating to divine intoxication, although this is vigorously contested by Martin Schwartz (Flattery and Schwartz 1989).

> *Canna, sweet canna, canna come home with you?*

Non-Indo-European languages yield Assyrian *qunnabu,* Chaldean *kanbun,* Arabic *kannab,* and possibly Hebrew/Aramaic *kaneh.* The Assyrian *qunnabu* was used as an incense in the ninth century BC. Sula Benet's contention that the Hebrew/Aramaic *kâneh bôsm* ("aromatic reed") refers to hemp was dismissed by Ernest Abel because he interprets *bôsm* as "sweet," and claims that Isaiah 43:24 means "sweet-tasting," not "sweet-smelling." And who would ever call *Cannabis* sweet? Most biblical scholars now translate the words as "sweet cane," sugarcane, correcting the earlier mistranslation of "calamus." But in Exodus 30:23 an anointing oil is described as being prepared with myrrh, cassia, and cinnamon, as well as *kâneh bôsm*, and sugarcane in no way fits the bill. It is most likely that *kâneh bôsm*, traded from long distances over the spice routes, was the concentrated form of *Cannabis*, hashish: an ideal incense. Dioscorides also called hemp a reed, undoubtedly because of its tall canelike growth habit.

Cannabis found in the burial of a young woman who died in childbirth near Jerusalem in the fourth century A D attests that the analgesic and medicinal qualities of the herb were known in Palestine. Benet's contention that the ultimate origin of the word *Cannabis* is Semitic is much less tenable. More likely candidates are Scythian or an ancient Finno-Ugric language such as Zyrjan.

References to *Cannabis* use occur in Egyptian papyri as old as 1600 B.C.

The Chinese ideogram for hemp is ma^2, an eleven-stroke radical. The ancient form represents flayed hemp stalks hanging in a drying shed:

The etymologies of some other Chinese words are of interest. *Hemp* plus *eye* combine to form the character for "to see indistinctly," or "to gaze at longingly." *Hemp* plus the character for "spirit" or "shade" creates a devil. Disyllabic words beginning with ma^2 ("hemp") are *narcotic* (*hemp* plus *drunkenness*) and *numb* (*hemp* plus *wood*). Other combinations yield the characters for "signal flag," "to feel with the hand," and (with *stone*) "to polish, to grind." Chinese also has separate ideograms for "male hemp," "female hemp," and "hemp fruits."

In Japanese, "marijuana" is *mayaku*, the kanji being the characters for "hemp" (*ma*) plus kusuri, the character for "medicine." *Kusuri* is an eighteen-stroke character that in Chinese is yao^4 or *yüeh*, meaning "medicine," "medicinal herbs," or "poison." *Yüeh* itself is an interesting character, a combination of the *grass* radical with the character for "music" or "pleasure," the effect produced by music. The primitive ideogram represents a wooden table supporting a drum and two bells.

Plant poisons are herbal music, the music of the grasses.

History, China   The etymologies of the words for hemp in the languages of the people who knew her in her youth are connected mainly to the importance of hemp as a fiber, and secondarily to its visionary virtues. Likewise, the earliest archaeological evidence of *Cannabis* is the impression of hempen cords on clay pots found on

Taiwan dated at 8000 BC. The oldest piece of woven fabric in the world is a frag-
ment of hempen cloth. The medicinal powers of *Cannabis* were recorded around
2800 BC by the great plant-doctor Shên-Nung. Shên-Nung was a great master
of our Way, a man so thoroughly accomplished in knowing his ground state and
being able to return to it that he was able to ingest a dozen different poisons in
a single day and to discover antidotes for each of them.

Shên-Nung recognized the *Cannabis* medicine, and rated it as "superior" for
those seeking immortality, i.e., the alchemical Elixir. At the same time, he warned
against overindulgence, stating that taking *Cannabis* in excess caused one to see
devils. Since later herbalists echoed Shên-Nung's opinion, we should consider it
thoughtfully. "Seeing devils" or "communicating with spirits" is not likely to
mean what the *ayahuasquero* or the doctor of the Poison Path experiences after
drinking *yagé*. Shên-Nung was not a patzer: he conversed with gods and immortals. The great alchemist's warning refers to those so lost in their lunar medicines
that the sun no longer shines from their eyes. This is confirmed by later herbalists
who call the heavy hemp users *necromancers:* fallen shamans lost in the powers of
darkness. Divining with spirits and powers is essential to the poisoner's way; all
the more reason that the warning of our great teacher be taken to heart. Many
Taoists consider *Cannabis* too yin to be useful in creating the Great Elixir.

How to Use   If you are young, you have to learn to say *no.* If you are old, don't be afraid to say
yes. (If you are in between, you are too busy working to get into much trouble
of any kind.)

Effects   A tendency to reverie.

> *find myself drifting*
> *from the text*
> *to other ideas, Dionysus, alive, in*
> *hiding in the hemp plant, the nature*
> *of symbology, the Great Symbol, any game*
> *played with symbols, compared to,*
> *compared to, which*
> *is the essential point of symbology*
> *anyway.*

The Ally   One of the great poisons given to human beings by the hemp plant is paper. Paper was invented in AD 105 by Ts'ai Lun and was made from hemp fiber and
mulberry bark. Bureaucracies often are too sluggish to recognize new technolo-
gies, even one as much to their benefit as paper, and the Chinese Imperial Court
was no exception. Ts'ai Lun had to indulge in a shamanly death, burial, and magical rebirth to get his poison a fair trial. Not having mastered the yogic art of sus-
pended respiration, Ts'ai Lun used the old hollow reed trick to breathe while he
was buried. His friends then burned a quantity of paper over his grave, after
which he miraculously came back to life. Paper won its fair trial, and Ts'ai Lun
became a favorite in the palace.

Along with stone, paper is among the most durable of mediums: gold is melted, iron rusts, but paper (excepting those of the twentieth century) endures. Ts'ai Lun, however, did not endure. When his star of favor fell, rather than face the dishonor of a trial, Ts'ai Lun dressed in his best robes and drank poison.

History, India Hemp, *bhangá* (also *śana*), occurs in both the Rg Veda and in the Atharvaveda. In the Rg Veda the word occurs in reference to soma, but whether *bhangá* refers to "hemp," or to "intoxication," or to "breaking through" is not clear. In the Atharvaveda, *bhangá* is invoked with four other plants in Soma's kingdom (barley, *kusa* grass, *saha,* and soma itself) for deliverance from ill. *Cannabis* is inextricably mixed with the songs and stories of Soma. Here is one.

Once, it happened that the gods lost their powers. Indra himself, king of the gods, began wasting in decline. It is said that the curse of a wise man, a doctor and poisoner of some accomplishment, was the immediate cause. Beyond that, what sin the gods had committed that the good poisoner was able to articulate, we do not know.

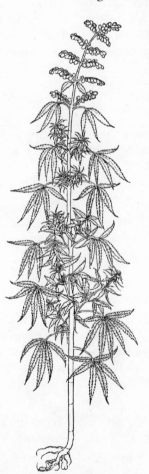

Vishnu agreed to help Indra recover his power. The Elixir, *amrita,* had collected at the bottom of the sea. To get it back, Vishnu told them, they must form an alliance with the demons. Only with the gods and the demons working in concert could the nectar of immortality be recovered. Vishnu added, somewhat under his breath, that he himself would see to it that the demons would never actually receive their share of the medicine.

The great alliance was formed, and the gods and demons used a mountain and a great snake, named Vasuki, to churn up the sea of the Milky Way. Maybe the poison came from the many mouths of Vasuki, as the gods and demons pulled him as a churning rope, or maybe the poison came up because of the prevarication of the gods. Whatever its cause, a great river of poison flooded over the earth and sky, threatening illness and death for gods and animals, men and demons alike. All of them called out to Shiva for help. To save the world, Shiva caught the poison and drank it, but its corrosive virulence turned his throat as blue as that of a peacock.

After that, many good things emerged from the churning sea of milk: the cow, then Varuni (goddess of wine), followed by the tree of paradise with its wonderful aromatic flowers, and finally Soma, the Moon, which Shiva grasped to wear on his forehead. Then Dhanvantari appeared, the inventor of ayurvedic medicine and the physician of the gods. He came bearing a cup of the sacred *amrita.* In the tantric tradition, the *amrita* is the *Cannabis* and milk beverage that the yogis still drink ritually today.

CANNABIS, FROM LEONARD FUCHS'S
NEW KREUTERBUCH, 1543

The *asuras* grabbed the cup of *amrita* and fled. In one story it is Vishnu who is able to recover the ambrosia, by taking the form of a voluptuous woman to distract the demon's attention and then grabbing the cup. In the Tibetan Buddhist version of the story it is Vajrapani who drinks the poison, his whole body turning blue and taking on a wrathful aspect. The demon Rahu had stolen the *dutsi*, the *amrita,* had drunk some of it, and had pissed *hala hala* poison back into the cup. The Buddhas had made Vajrapani drink the poison as punishment for losing the water of life. Vajrapani chased Rahu, caught him, and then severely wounded him with his *vajra*. Some of the Elixir then bled from Rahu's wounds and fell upon the earth, medicinal herbs growing everywhere it fell. One of the plants that sprang up was *bhang,* hemp.

Cannabis became sacred to Shiva, who was then known as Lord of Bhang. By the tenth century *Cannabis* was also sacred to Indra and was called *indraśana,* "the food of Indra." The yogis and *saddhus* call hemp *vijaya,* "victory," to commemorate the victory of the gods over the *asuras.* Shiva's blue throat became known as the "liberator." The gifts the gods gave to man in hemp were said to be courage, delight, and heightened sexual desires.

Effects

> *This will be deducted from your share in paradise.*
> — Dr. J. J. Moreau, quoted by Théophile Gautier

The Plant

She likes forests, she likes open brushland and chaparral. She likes the tropics, she like mountains. She likes Africa, Mexico, China. She likes Alaska. She's cosmopolitan: internationalism is one of her special skills. She knows how to "get around," and needs to – especially this last half century, with every border so determined to keep her out.

Effects

More humor and wit, attention to ideas and innuendo, in the conversation. Or if not, at least rapt attention while you listen. Or, if not, rapt attention for the brief moments you are attentive. Or, if not, at least rapturous inattention.

How to Use

Family gatherings are nice.

History, Europe

Herodotus describes the use of κανναβις by the Scythians in their funerary customs. The Scythian men would huddle in a tent, throw marijuana *spermata* (read "tops") onto a brazier, and inhale the smoke until they sprang out dancing and howling with joy. His account was much pooh-poohed until a Russian archaeologist, S. I. Rudenko, in 1929 discovered censors with hemp seeds still in them in a Scythian burial site in Siberia. He also found evidence that the smoking was not limited to men, nor to funerals.

In 1994 another team of Russian archaeologists in the Altay Mountains discovered the body of a young Scythian woman still frozen in the permafrost. The woman, being called Lady, is thought to have been a priestess. Lady's coffin had filled with water shortly after her burial, and the water froze and remained frozen for 2,400 years. She was dressed in a white hemp blouse and a red wool skirt. She has spectacular tattoos on her arms: one of a highly stylized deer, and another of an antlered griffinlike creature. She was buried with three sacrificed horses, a hand-mirror with a deer carved on its wooden back, and a box of *Cannabis*. *National Geographic* magazine, which recently published a story on Lady, forgot to mention the *Cannabis*, although they described the other items in detail.

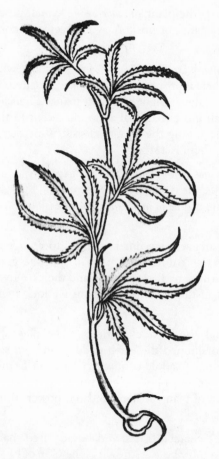

CANNABIS, FROM PETER SCHOEFFER'S
GERMAN HERBARIUS, 1485

Sula Benet points out that the descendants of the Scythians in Eastern Europe still associate hemp with the dead, and serve a soup made from hemp seeds on the Eve of Christmas or Three Kings Day. In another account, in Book I of the *Histories,* Herodotus describes a similar means of intoxication practiced by a people on the Araxes River. *Cannabis* seeds have been found in archaeological sites in Germany dated to 500 BC.

Use of hemp in Thrace is well attested, both by text and by archaeology. Plutarch's description of Thracians getting high by inhaling the smoke from hemp plants thrown onto fire or hot stones is almost exactly like that of Herodotus. The Scythian influence would have been strong in Thrace, and Scythes, though noted by Herodotus to be fiercely hostile to the encroachment of foreign customs into their own culture, freely visited and mingled with the peoples on their borders.

The philosopher Democritus was born in 460 BC in the Greek town of Abdera on the Thracian coast. Abdera had a reputation for being a city of fools, something like a Thracian *Chelm,* but Democritus, the "laughing philosopher," was not one of them. He traveled widely, making long journeys into Egypt and Asia, and devoted his life to scholarship. Besides inventing the atomic theory (along with his teacher, Leucippus), Democritus wrote books on ethics, mathematics, physics, astronomy, art, and literature. He also wrote on horticulture and herbcraft. In *Chirocmeta,* Democritus wrote of several magical plants that various authors have identified with *Cannabis.* One, the *gelotophyllis,* or "laughing leaves," causes laughter and mental phantoms when ingested with myrrh and wine.

Ephippus, a fourth-century BC comic poet, includes hemp seeds in a list of desserts in his play *Cydon.* The list includes *pyramides,* wheat and honey cakes, and may be the first reference to something like marijuana brownies. The next such reference is five hundred years later, in Galen, where he writes about hemp seed cakes. Since Galen describes overindulgence in the cakes as causing a warm and toxic vapor to rise into the head, it is clear that whole tops from the plants were used rather than only cleaned seeds. According to Galen, the cakes were eaten with other desserts to create a feeling of warmth and to stimulate an appetite for drinking. He also mentions that an excess will quench sexual potency: something many men in a state of deep stonedness, being able to find neither their penis nor even their knees, can vouch for.

The Greeks even had a word for smoking the plant: *cannabeizein* – which probably referred to its being burnt in vapor baths, or possibly as an incense. Smoke could be inhaled using hollow reeds.

The first botanical description of *Cannabis* is in Theophastus, 371– 287 BC, who called the herb *dendromalache*. The medicinal properties of *Cannabis* are cited by Dioscorides and by Pliny, as well as by Galen. Still, it seems clear that *Cannabis*, while well known as a textile, was much more marginal as an intoxicant to the Greeks and to the Romans both, at least among the literate classes. Wine better suited their temperaments, and in wine there is a story.

The Return of Dionysus

The true living Dionysus is hiding in the hemp plant, not in the wine bottle. That is where the stranger is. And the strangeness. His vengeance on the society that today persecutes him will be to make them sacrifice their children.

On the Poison Path, we need neither archaeology nor linguistics to recognize that hemp is one of the epiphanies of the Young God: we can spot the god's young companions by their flutes and drums, by their dancing and their tie-dyed colors. We can watch the reenactment of the ancient tragedy as we lock them away in our prisons.

Still, it is not so difficult to let one's mind wander to elder times, to peoples who used stone to carve wood and who worshipped the earth goddess and her son and lover, a long-haired, sometimes effeminate adolescent with a hard-on. Sometimes he rode a panther, sometimes he became a bull. Wherever he went people learned the powers of plants, the magic of plant poisons, and the power of intoxication in its myriad forms.

Traveling was one of the Young God's characteristics, and he acquired many names in his travels. In one part of the country he was known as the God of Nysa, Dionysus. In Egypt he was called Osiris. In another part of the world he was called the Good Omen, Shiva. Whenever the paths of the worshippers of Shiva and the worshippers of Dionysus crossed, they recognized their two gods as one.

Dionysus's home was usually assumed to be Thrace, though it may have been even further east. Thrace was the home of the Getae, whose shamans used hemp smoke to induce visions and oracular trances. Hemp probably came to Thrace through Central Asia and the Caucasus. A very similar route may have been followed by the grapevine. Georgia, at the foot of the Caucasus between the Black

Sea and the Caspian, considers herself the homeland of the vine. It is quite possible that the Western form of the god, Dionysus, carried not only the vine but ganja as well, the favorite plant of his Eastern twin.

Early Greek wine was rarely drunk neat, and was probably never just fermented grape juice. The early Greeks had no way of storing or preserving such a liquid, so they needed strong and preservative admixtures. Odysseus, in the *Odyssey,* defeats the cyclops, Polyphemus, by intoxicating him with straight wine meant to be diluted twenty parts to one before being drunk. This was true poisoner's wine, made with mandrake, opium, hemp, and henbane, with aromatic herbs and spices and resinous trees. By classical times, at Plato's symposium, wine had been considerably tamed, and needed only two-to-one dilution.

One of the names for wine was κρασι, "mixed." Another name for wine was τριμμα, "pounded." Athenaeus said that trimma was a liqueur made of spices, which was drunk by the ancients. The wine drunk during the theater season in Athens was called *trimma*.

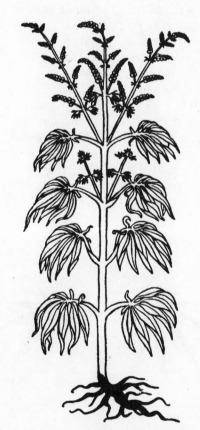

CANNABIS, FROM DIOSCORIDES' ANICIA JULIANA, AD 512

CORRESPONDENCES

ACTIVITY	Agriculture
ANIMAL	Cat
ARCHETYPE	Jester
ART FORM	Harmony
BODILY FUNCTION	Reproduction
BODY PART	Genitals
BUDDHA REALM	Western Paradise
CHORD	Augmented 7th
COLOR	Gold
COSMIC ENTITY	Red Giants
CRUTCH FOR	Stasis
DIMENSION	3D Space
DISCIPLINE	Music
ELEMENT	Wood
FORM OF ENERGY	Biomass
FORM OF IGNORANCE	Procrastination
GEMSTONE	Emerald
GEOMETRY	Hyperbolic
GOD	Dionysus
GODDESS	Sarasvati
GRAMMAR	Language of Birds
HISTORICAL AGE	Neolithic

 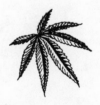

Effects   A tendency to reverie:

> *Greek wines, Egyptian beers, Iakchos:*
> *pilgrims walking to Eleusis.*
> > *Jesus the true vine and Dionysus the wild ivy.*
> *Wine flowing from a spring, a diadem*
> *of poppy capsules on his forehead –*
> > *the Mad One, the "Friendly Stranger":*
> *fucks your wife, steals your daughter,*
> > *leaves death in the house.*
> *He grows vines from the blood of kings.*
> *He is the scapegoat we stone*
> > *on the steps of the temple.*

History   In the Middle East, in the Zend-Avest, Zoroaster calls *bhanga* his "good nar-cotic." He tells of two mortals who drank a cup of *bhanga* and ascended to heaven where they were shown the highest mysteries. *Bhanga* was the link, the connecting thread between realms.

> *Hemp, sweet hemp,*
> *how long will they shun Thee?*

Pharmacology   The major active ingredient is Δ^9tetrahydrocannabinol. Δ^1tetrahydrocannabinol is a synonym for the same compound using a different numbering system. We will hereafter refer to this molecule as THC.

THC wasn't discovered until the early 1960s, by Professor Raphael Mechoulam, who also developed its first synthesis. Seventy to 100 percent of the marijuana high is estimated to come from THC. THC content in the plant varies greatly, from 12 percent in carefully bred, harvested, and manicured buds down to less than 1 percent. In the United States marijuana potency peaked around 1984, with an average of 6.4 percent THC by weight in dry cleaned buds. By 1994 the mean had fallen to 3.4 percent THC.

> *I guess it depends on where you buy.*

The biosynthetic precursor to THC is cannabidiol, or CBD, and is itself often present in significant quantities in harvested hemp. CBD is a sedative and a mild analgesic, and has antibiotic properties. CBD is often called the "body" part of the high, but it is not much of a high at all without the THC. For grass to be good it has to have THC. If it has THC, it can accommodate significant amounts of CBD. Con-noisseurs are able to judge the relative proportions of THC and CBD in smoked samples of marijuana by the effects they experience: how quickly the high comes on, mental lightness versus somatic heaviness, degree of sensory alteration, etc. Tastes vary. Some prefer their grass high on the THC side of the balance, others appreciate the "you're not going ANYWHERE, baby" feeling of the CBD side. Of course, the way things are today in the "free" world, where marijuana and her users are hunted out like witches, your marijuana rarely comes in a package with an analysis printed on the label, so some spirit of adventure is evoked.

On the other side of the biosynthetic divide is cannabinol, or CBN, the degradation product of THC. CBN is psychoactive, but has an order of magnitude less potency than does THC. Again, connoisseurs who have microlaboratories for analysis and lots of time on their hands love to argue about the qualities of CBN, but for most of us it just means that you kept your stash too long and that it has gone flat. That ten-dollar lid you just found under a mattress may as well stay there.

Like vitamins A and E, the cannabinoids are highly lipophilic. That is why you cannot make a good marijuana tea, unless it's buttered. In the body, THC is metabolized quickly, within hours. The metabolites, being as lipophilic as THC itself, get absorbed by fatty cells in the body, and excretion has a significant half-life. Traces of metabolites have been detected in the bodily fluids of heavy *Cannabis* users three to four weeks after their last ingestion. This does not mean that the person is still stoned, or at all impaired: the effects of these metabolites on any kind of performance has not been scientifically demonstrated.

The neuropharmacological actions of THC in the brain are very complex, affecting acetylcholine metabolism, norepinephrine turnover rates, and serotonin and biogenic amine levels. Interactions with many other hormones and enzymes are probable.

The THC receptor in the brain was discovered in the 1980s, and the receptor's endogenous ligand was discovered in 1992. William Devane, its discoverer, named it *anandamide,* inspired by his favorite philosopher, Sri Aurobindo. Devane was working in Mechoulam's laboratory, and Mechoulam is listed as a coauthor of the article that appeared in *Science.* Anandamide evidently has approximately the same strength as THC, but the comparison is based solely on things like adenosine 3',5'-cyclic monophosphate (cAMP) response in petri dishes, the contraction of a mouse's dying vas deferens, and such like. This research is so fresh and timely that new breakthroughs may be announced any day, such as structure-activity studies or synthetic twists of anandamide that are a hundred times as potent. At this time (1994) nobody even knows what anandamide does, or why the brain has such receptors in the first place. All that is known so far is that anandamide receptors seem to be associated with memory functions, higher thinking, motor coordination, and emotion. The receptors are found in many brain regions, which may explain the complexity of some of the effects of THC, and, presumably, of anandamide. Some researchers are mystified and a little embarrassed that the brain produces its own chemicals that do the same thing as "illegal drugs of abuse," such as marijuana and opium. We can only hope that the "why" implicit in their wonder is not solely pursued in the laboratory.

The Ally   *Ahhhh, poisons!*
               Why is it we love them so?

The Plant   Axes of variation: genotype and phenotype. Good seeds, not the kind they grow for rope. Country of origin, latitude, and elevation considered with respect to its proposed site of cultivation. Light, soil, pH, weather, water, and temperature. Humidity. Elevation. North-facing side of the plant versus the south-facing. Fertilizing and pruning. Time of harvesting, month, and the time of day. Skill in curing. Age. Storage.

Effects   *Now in the primeval silence of some unexplored tropical forest I spread my feathery leaves, a giant fern, and swayed and nodded in the spice-gales over a river whose waves at once sent up clouds of music and perfume. My soul changed to a vegetable essence, thrilled with a strange and unimagined ecstasy.*
— *Fitzhugh Ludlow, The Hasheesh Eater*

The Ally   The ally can be a good reading companion. Attention to dosage is important. If there is a lot of the ally there, you need something concentrated, like poetry, or philosophers in the aphoristic tradition, Nietzsche, the pre-Socratics, or maybe Buddhist sutras – something condensed, because forward motion is going to slow to a snail's pace.

But that doesn't matter, because the hand and face of the author emerge from between the sentences, and this is a lot to think about. Personality, sense of humor, his self-image, and his hidden agenda in its depth or in its superficiality are all placed on the table for the ensuing conversation.

Words no longer play a part. . . . The text, at whatever point you pick it up, becomes a voice, the very voice that suits it, and the man speaks behind this voice. The one who wrote it is there, of as little substance as he was, no longer given solidity by the printed character, he is there again, immediately engaged in thinking, in expressing himself, finding his way among his ideas. . . .

Hashish as a hunting dog . . . It sees quicker than we do.
— *Henri Michaux, Light Through Darkness*

Perhaps most astonishingly, hashish even seems able to assist in reading books in languages that one hardly knows: meaning floats up from hidden roots and cognates, while the drift and gist of argument emerge from syntax of sentence and paragraph. I don't believe that this phenomenom has ever been verified scientifically, but the experience is no less wonderful, proof lacking.

Some people like the Ally as an editor and critic – for criticizing their own work – saying that it enables them to see or hear or read their work as others would.

Keeping track of everything, being able to recall it, is trickier. It's kind of like, when you're with her, your memory returns: your identity is there, your projects, your insights, all your answers – except that you are in no shape to make use of them. You have to wait until the next day, when you can lift a pen again, when you can consider the insights at subsonic speed. Unfortunately, perhaps diabolically, the next morning the insights tend to fade away, waiting until you visit the goddess again to reappear.

I keep a pencil handy, as well as my pen, with soft B leads that don't scratch. Shelley wrote all over his Shakespeare folio in pen.

Effects

> Of all that Orient lands can vaunt
>> Of marvels with our own competing,
> The strangest is the Haschish plant,
>> And what will follow on its eating.
>
> — John Greenleaf Whittier, "The Haschish"

Many stories are quite wonderful: tales of insights achieved, blockages cleared. One guy I heard of gets all of his writing done in three months on grass and then quits smoking for the rest of the year. How do you figure it? Someone else smokes and watches TV a lot. It's mostly like a magnified subset of what you usually do, some part of what you usually do anyway, just that you are doing it high.

Several millions of Americans of all classes use this plant regularly, year after year and decade after decade with no grave ill effects. That's just a fact. The tars are the most damaging part of the smoke, but thanks to the public-spirited efforts of marijuana breeders and growers, much less smoke is required today than, say, twenty years ago. Moreover, were it not for misguided laws against "drug paraphernalia," people could have access to inexpensive and efficient filters to further reduce the toxicity of the smoke.

Still, some damage and harm are inevitable in any endeavor. Let's get together and figure out what the problems are, where the harm comes from, and try to find some way to mitigate the damage. Unfortunately, you have a "moral" problem yourself, so you're not interested in helping. You are only interested in punishing.

The Ally

Cannabis is a great potentiator: it enhances and synergizes with many other medicines – almost anything, it seems. Interaction of THC with ether is documented. Researchers report that *Cannabis* enhances the effects of nitrous oxide, and also of *Salvia divinorum,* especially on the Bridge of Smoke. Some even like marijuana as a way to come down from psychedelics.

When engaged in the psychoanalysis of an ally, however, one must be careful about mixing, as the sum is often greater than the parts. At the same time, the *Cannabis* ally has a way of masking the effects of certain other poisons, especially alcohol, and probably cocaine, enabling or even encouraging excess. Some evidence suggests that marijuana and alcohol together impair driving skills more than the alcohol would alone. Many drug fatalities are the result of mixing multiple poisons.

CORRESPONDENCES

IMAGE	Ships with Sails
LANDSCAPE	Mountains
MACHINE	Calliope, Organ Grinder
METAL	Copper
METAPHOR	Lake
MINERAL	Jasper
MUSICAL INSTRUMENT	Guitar
MYTH	Bacchae
MYTHIC HERO	Coyote
NUMBER	Integers
OCCUPATION	Farmer/Smith
OUT-OF-BODY REALM	Overflowing Joy
PERIODIC TABLE COLUMN	Halogens
PHASE OF COITUS	Fantasy/Looking
PHASE OF MATTER	Supersaturated
PHYSICAL CONSTANT	Hubble Constant
PLANET	Venus
POISON	Diffidence
PROPORTION	Harmonic Mean
QUARK	Strange

History

Hashish rode to Damascus in caravans, trotted horseback to Alexandria, walked on to Tangiers and Marrakesh. Hemp sailed to Jutland, smoke drifted across Africa: bangi, canna, dagga, Zanzibar, Mozambique to East Africa, Lake Victoria, Malawis, south to the Bantu, Hottentots, and Bushmen, to the Pygmies, Zulus, and through the Riamba cult in the Congo, the gourd water-pipe its inseparable companion.

Adapted to xeric heat by resin-covered leaves, *Cannabis* made itself at home in desert mountains. Islamic reaction to hashish was mixed: from prohibition to toleration to, as with the Sufis, love. Hashish, even where not completely socially acceptable, is rarely included in the Koranic indictment against alcohol.

Hemp sailed to Europe, and to the colonies. George Washington grew it, and pulled his male plants. Credible evidence (Conrad 1993) suggests that he smoked it, and was knowledgeable enough to be able to compare it to hashish, when some came into his possession. Jefferson considered it a superior crop to tobacco, and advised his countrymen to cultivate it. By 1850 *Cannabis* was America's third largest crop.

Effects
When you first begin smoking it you see things in a wonderful soothing, easygoing new light. All of a sudden the world is stripped of its dirty gray shrouds and becomes one big bellyful of giggles, a spherical laugh, bathed in brilliant, sparkling colors that hit you like a heat wave. Nothing leaves you cold any more; there's a humorous tickle and great meaning in the least little thing . . .

    — Mezz Mezzrow, Really the Blues

The Ally
If a man wishes to rid himself of a feeling of unbearable oppression, he may have to take to hashish.

    — Friedrich Wilhelm Nietzsche, Ecce Homo

The *Cannabis* ally may be contraindicated for depression. It has the possibility of helping, but it may not be strong enough to get you back together, and then you will be worse off than before. If your ally can't get its job done, it falls back upon you like an enemy. Be certain that between yourself and your ally there is enough strength to succeed before you sign on. So, OK, how do you know if you have enough strength? Well, intuition maybe. Well, OK, you don't know. That's why we call it poison.

Effects
I returned to hasheesh, but only when I had become hopeless of carrying out my first intention — its utter and immediate abandonment. I now re-solved to abandon it gradually — to retreat slowly from my enemy, until I had passed the borders of his enchanted ground, whereon he warred with me at vantage. Once over the boundaries, and the nightmare spell unloosed, I might run for my life, and hope to distance him in my own recovered territory.

    — Fitzhugh Ludlow, The Hasheesh Eater

History
The laws against marijuana use have a great deal more to do with racism and religious bigotry than with public health. The opium laws present some analogy, in that originally it was only the smoking of opium, the Chinese method of in-gestion, that was outlawed, not the use of laudanum. Likewise, the first marijuana laws were directed against "Hindoos," "Syrians," and "Mexicans of the lower classes." The scientific input of pharmacists and doctors kept marijuana out of federal and military law much longer than such rational voices were able to pre-vail at the state level. Between 1915 and 1927 the majority of the United States passed antimarijuana laws.

1897: HASHEESH ANTICS: IT WAS A WILD ORGY

Class interest also played a part in the new drug laws. Marijuana users were viewed as being lower class as well as dark-skinned, as being ruffians and ne'er-do-wells. The fear of a general revolt from the lower classes was the nightmare shadow that no amount of gentility could completely wipe away. Perhaps the bourgeoisie could not understand how or why the poor would endure such obvious social inequity year after year without doing something about it. Evidently their own commitment to morality and the social contract was based more on expediency and self-interest than belief, and they were afraid that the "new" drug marijuana might reveal the shamlike nature of their hegemony in a revolutionary light. They feared that the "new" drug would break the thin veneer of civilized restraint and turn men with nothing to lose into desperadoes running amok: killing, raping, and pillaging – and maybe even in the "better" neighborhoods . . . an understandably frightening apparition.

All of the threads of the drug hysteria – the fears of foreigners, the religious bigotry, the worker's fear of competition, the fear of revolution – were exacerbated by the Depression. Baseless stories of "reefer madness" multiplied in the newspapers, the Hearst papers in particular. Insanity, uncontrollable sexual lust, violence, and suicide were all presented as effects of marijuana in "true" articles in the Hearst press. Hearst's paper and timber companies had recently developed a new way to bleach wood pulp for paper making. About the same time, a machine was invented for extracting the fibers from hemp, which suddenly made the *Cannabis* plant potentially serious competition in the paper business.

In 1930 the Hoover administration created the Federal Bureau of Narcotics with Harry J. Anslinger as its first commissioner. The bureau was part of the treasury department, because it was recognized that the only constitutional foundation for the federal government to involve itself in private commerce was through taxation. (The Harrison Act of 1914 was also written as a tax law.)

1923: MARIHUANA MAKES FIENDS OF BOYS IN 30 DAYS
1923: HASHEESH GOADS USERS TO BLOOD LUST

The new bureau was a response to scandals and corruption in the old bureau, the Prohibition Bureau, which had formerly been in charge of enforcing the Harrison Act. Following a Weberian law of growth, the new bureau sought greater and more terrible enemies to justify and expand its existence, and Harry Anslinger focused on the killer weed, marijuana. An ax murder in Florida by an overtly psychotic man was paraded out as a marijuana murder, because the man "had been known to buy doped cigarettes." Maybe someone remembered the Lanfray "absinthe" murders of 1905. The propaganda campaign was so transparent and outrageously ludicrous that it would have been comical had it not been successful enough to create devastating and tragic results. The Marijuana Tax Act was passed in 1937 by legislators who knew little, or even nothing, about what it was they were prohibiting.

1934: A NEW DRUG MENACE AT THE UNIVERSITY OF KANSAS
1937: THE WEED OF MADNESS

In case you think that such yahoo tactics are the quaint stuff of history, your author recently saw a full-size billboard along a freeway in Oakland, California, that said, in large letters, "Drugs can kill!" Beside this message was a pair of lips holding a large marijuana cigarette. Now listen, four hundred thousand to half a million Americans die every year from smoking tobacco cigarettes. If you search the records of centuries of marijuana use by hundreds of millions of users, you might be able to find a documented casualty somewhere, but, in spite of the many millions of dollars spent by the government in an effort to prove the *Cannabis* plant an enemy of public health, your search will not be easy!

Toxicology The toxicity of drugs is measured by the LD50, the dose that is lethal for fifty percent of the subjects. The LD50 for *Cannabis* is unknown – no one has ever found it. In September 1988, DEA (Drug Enforcement Agency) administrative law judge Francis Young said that *Cannabis* is, "in its natural form, one of the safest therapeutically active substances known to man."

The issue of toxicity for a *poisoner,* however, is a much subtler issue, one to which we will return later. First we must consider toxicity in its grosser aspects, and consider the charges brought against marijuana by the Prohibitionists and their fellow travelers.

One of the first indictments against marijuana in the United States, and given as a reason that it should be outlawed, was that there was no other drug "that would produce the pleasurable sensations you would get from *Cannabis*" (Charles Fauns, 1911, U.S. House Ways and Means Committee, in Abel 1980). Like masturbation in the nineteenth century, pleasure alone was enough to identify the presence of the Great Tempter. It is instructive that the first three entries in the following list of the ill effects of marijuana were, indeed, also applied to masturbation.

- Marijuana produces abundant pleasurable sensations
- Incites sexual immorality
- Causes insanity
- Incites the user to commit murder
- Makes people jump from high buildings
- Makes people listen to jazz and wiggle their hips when they dance
- Leads to more dangerous drugs, like heroin.

Of these charges, only the first has withstood the test of scrutiny. That does not stop those whose business it is to spread fear from bringing back out all the other charges – does not stop them today, nor will it tomorrow.

In the 1970s it appeared that marijuana would be legalized. President Nixon's drug commission recommended decriminalization in its final report. President Carter also favored decriminalization, and said before Congress that "penalties against possession of a drug should not be more damaging to an individual than the drug itself." The ensuing backlash is a lesson in the power of propaganda. Congress held hearings to which only antimarijuana witnesses were invited, and Senator James Eastland proclaimed that the nation was undergoing a marijuana "epidemic" in which civilization would bog down under the weight of "a large population of semi-zombies." It was a replay of the 1930s.

One of the leaders of the Prohibitionist backlash was a former OSS and CIA employee, Gabriel Nahas. Nahas had worked with Lyndon Larouche in a propaganda coverup of Kurt Waldheim's war crimes (Waldheim had been a Nazi officer during World War II). When Waldheim succeeded in becoming the secretary-general of the United Nations, he appointed Nahas to the Narcotic Control Board, and placed him in charge of all United Nations grant money for *Cannabis* research. It was a controversial appointment, not only because Nahas was poorly qualified professionally, but because he had already been caught by his colleagues in presenting a fraudulent report of a marijuana death in Belgium. Nahas gave out the money selectively, and in the late 1970s a number of "new studies" began appearing, stating that marijuana was indeed dangerous after all, that it was not a "soft" drug, and that the marijuana that your children were smoking was many times stronger than whatever you may have smoked in the sixties. The new charges against marijuana were:

- It causes chromosomal damage.
- It damages the immune system.
- It causes brain damage.
- It causes decreased testosterone levels in males.
- It causes "amotivational syndrome."
- It causes damage to the lungs.

All of these alleged effects except the last have been seriously challenged if not refuted. Heavy smoking, of anything, definitely impairs pulmonary functioning.

The report of low testosterone levels in marijuana users was refuted by a follow-up study. More studies, since, have found both for and against. The decrease, however, even when found, rarely falls below the "normal" range of variation. Ditto chromosomal damage: some found some, others did not, but in no case was it dangerous.

Nahas himself was part of the team that reported immune system damage involving T-cell lymphocytes. Blood taken from marijuana users and grown in petri dishes exhibited lower resistance to disease. As with the testosterone research, some follow-up studies were able to replicate Nahas's findings, while others refuted them. No study has shown any higher incidence of cancer or disease among actual marijuana users than among a control group. On the contrary, many regular users not only enjoy excellent health but also report absence of colds.

The report of organic brain damage was so flawed that it could be called fabrication. This leaves "amotivational syndrome." I'd answer that one too, but, really, why bother? It's just too much trouble.

A much more challenging thesis is Nahas's belief that the subjective effects of marijuana are inimical to successful civilizations, whereas those of the legal drugs – alcohol, tobacco, and caffeine – are not.

The Poison
Path

Method, we believe in you!
You glorified all of our ages.
We have faith in poison.
We will give our lives completely, every day.
For this is the ASSASSIN*'s hour.*

> *– Arthur Rimbaud, "Morning of Drunkenness"*

Interestingly, Nahas cites Moreau as his reference for his summary treatment of marijuana's psychological effects. Dr. Jacques-Joseph Moreau was the founder of the *Club des Hachichins.* The purpose of the Hashish Club was to investigate the nature of madness, using hashish as a psychotomimetic. It was Moreau who gave hashish to Baudelaire and Gautier. Balzac and Flaubert also both attended meetings of the club, at least as observers. All participants were required to keep notes.

Moreau discovered a correlation between the effects of increased dosages of hashish and the progressive stages of mental illness. This evidence led him to the belief that mental illness was not a matter of physical damage to the brain, the current belief of his time, but that mental illness was chemical in nature. No finer application of the *poison way* had been recorded in European history, at least since Paracelsus. How Nahas is able to read the work of those gifted doctors and conclude that the Ally, if not imprisoned or destroyed, will bring about the collapse of Western culture is appalling.

> *It is right then, that sophisticated persons, and also ignorant persons who*
> *are eager to make acquaintance with unusual delights, should be clearly*
> *told that they will find in hashish nothing miraculous, absolutely nothing*
> *but an exaggeration of the natural. The brain and organism on which hashish*
> *operates will produce only the normal phenomena peculiar to that individual*
> *– increased, admittedly, in number and force, but always faithful to their*
> *origin. A man will never escape from his destined physical and moral*
> *temperament: hashish will be a mirror of his impressions and private*
> *thought – a magnifying mirror, it is true, but only a mirror.*
>
> *– Charles Baudelaire, The Poem of Hashish*

The Ally   The Ally plays over the day's tape, and tomorrow's tape. The Ally fills in appropriate blanks, brings up pointed questions, can prompt you to resolutions. That you rarely keep these resolutions, especially if one of them is about laying off the Ally for a week or two, in no way detracts from their truth.

Sometimes things can get silly.

Effects

Suppose you're the critical and analytical type, always ripping things to pieces, tearing the covers off and being disgusted by what you find under the sheet. Well, under the influence of muta you don't lose your surgical touch exactly, but you don't come up evil and grimy about it. You still see what you saw before but in a different, more tolerant way . . .

 − *Mezz Mezzrow, Really the Blues*

How to Use

So much depends upon dosage. So much depends upon intent. So much depends upon context.

I take haschisch with some followers of the eighteenth-century mystic Saint-Martin. At one in the morning, while we are talking wildly, and some are dancing, there is a tap at the shuttered window; we open it and three ladies enter, the wife of a man of letters . . . caught in our dream we know vaguely that she is scandalous according to our code and to all codes, but smile at her benevolently and laugh.

 − *W. B. Yeats, Autobiography*

One plant person I know said, "Smoking it occasionally makes you wise; smoking it a lot turns you into a donkey."

The Ally

Like the *ska Pastora* ally, the *Cannabis* ally can assist with augury. In fact, that is one of its greatest strengths. But the euphoria is very seductive. The *little leaves,* they are for professionals: who would keep doing that for pleasure? But the ganja ally soothes. In her palace she presents you with many delights: pleasant sounds and bright colors, graceful movement, hilarity and poignancy, all of which can distract the aspirant from the true goal − the Queen herself.

The Queen is the vatic whispering of crossing branches in a tree, knots in the warp of time where the obvious no longer hides beneath the expected. She can advise you. Usually fairly soundly, in my experience. Still, as with any ally, it doesn't hurt to follow the custom of the Persian kings and to wait for a second opinion in the light of the next morning.

Marijuana and the Poison Path

We have noted the absence of marijuana fatalities, and the relative pharmacological safety of the plant. But as doctors of the *ancient art,* just as we are not deterred because a particular poison is fatal if used incorrectly, neither are we impressed nor lulled because another poison is subtle and sweet.

I was even all dressed in my biking clothes; smoked some bong and never left the house.

Skilled poisoners avoid habits. Many have dropped *Cannabis* from their pharmacies completely, others limit their partaking to special occasions. We are (most of us) not *saddhus.* Our governments and neighbors ban nudity as well as *Cannabis.* We know the feeling of "morning fog" − a dullness in the morning. We know that she who gives dreams also takes them away. We know about quitting.

It was like two weeks of PMS.

The *Cannabis* ally has a way of pretending that she's not doing anything. One psychedelicist told me that he was taking Prozac and had quit all other drugs – his daily marijuana evidently not counting. In truth, experienced ganja smokers adjust and lead quite ordinary-looking and often successful lives. They write books, they play music; they sell real estate, and they sell corporations. Some practice law and others practice medicine. They design computers and they build houses; they teach and they preach.

> *Then there are the brain surgeons and the airplane pilots . . .*

Some of them get high every day. But just as tobacco and heroin habitués need their ally to feel normal, so the hemp smoker can confuse his intoxication for the *ground state* – a mistake the doctor of our lineage ought never make.

> *He who has recourse to poison in order to think will soon be unable to think without poison.*
>
> *– Charles Baudelaire, Artificial Paradise*

Some of the confusion is the result of governmental propaganda that declares any and all use of *Cannabis* to be abuse. Even novices of the Poison Path know that this is nonsense. But with so many preposterous lies being disseminated the real boundaries tend to get lost. Socialization creates boundaries, but the socialization must be based on actuality. No one who begins the day with a drink can long deny that he has an alcohol problem. But how many pot smokers who start out every day with a joint think that they are abusing marijuana?

> *Nobody will acquire the habit but the destined drug-slave; and he may just as well have the hashish habit as any other; he is sure to fall under the power of some enchantress.*
>
> *– Aleister Crowley, "The Psychology of Hashish"*

Thus spoke the famous drug fiend, the "wickedest man on earth."

Chemistry   The principal active ingredient in marijuana and hashish, Δ^9tetrahydrocannabi-nol, oxidizes into cannabinol, CBN. The degradation rate is increased by heat, light, and air. Hashish that is three or four years old will have little THC remaining in its outer layer, though the inner part of the ball may still be potent.

In fresh material, almost all of the THC is present as tetrahydrocannabinolic acid: THC.COOH. This form of THC is inactive. It must be decarboxylated to THC by drying and heating. Pyrolation accomplishes the decarboxylation, as does cooking. Eating fresh marijuana will produce little effect. THC.COOH can be decarboxylated by heating it on a cookie sheet in a preheated oven for five minutes at 200°F or for ten minutes at 120°F.

The base form of THC may be extracted and concentrated into hash oil with any number of solvents, such as acetone, alcohol, hexanes, or methylene dichloride. Evaporate the solvent to recover the oil. If alcohol was used as the solvent, the oil may be redissolved in a nonpolar solvent such as petroleum ether and the polar compounds washed out with water in a separatory funnel or its equivalent.

If the hash oil is high in CBD (cannabidiol), the CBD can be "isomerized" into THC by dissolving the oil in anhydrous ethanol or methanol, adding a drop of concentrated sulfuric acid for each gram of oil and refluxing over a water bath. At 100°C the reaction takes about two hours. When the reaction is finished, dilute the alcohol with an equal quantity of water and extract the oil with petroleum ether or hexanes.

Effects A certain sallowness. A dullness that verges on the sultry. A gradual erosion of confidence, and argumentiveness resorted to as a defense.

That mostly all disappears after a few weeks of abstinence: a ruddy vivaciousness returns and the world starts looking better and life seems easier.

How to Use, Tetrahydrocannabinol is a bronchodilator, and some studies, as well as anecdotal
Asthma evidence, suggest that marijuana smoke, or, perhaps better, a marijuana aerosol could be effective against asthma. High-quality pot would reduce the amount of smoke required, as would pot doped with hash oil. We hope that some other country that has left it to science rather than to the police to determine whether or not marijuana has medicinal benefits may provide asthma sufferers with more research in this promising area.

Poesis A fine recipe for hashish fudge is in the *Alice B. Toklas Cook Book*. Alice says that the fudge

> *might provide an entertaining refreshment for a Ladies Bridge Club or a chapter meeting of the DAR. . . . Euphoria and brilliant storms of laughter; ecstatic reveries and extensions of one's personality on several simultaneous planes are to be complacently expected. Almost anything St. Theresa did, you can do better . . .*

Recipes for hashish or marijuana brownies abound. The one and only crucial step is the making of the ghee, the hash butter. Once you have ghee, you can make anything that uses butter, even buttered toast. One stick of butter to an eighth of an ounce of marijuana is a satisfactory rule of thumb. Sauté the herb in the butter over medium heat, then strain out the remaining solids.

Attention to dosage is important. It is easy to overdue it, and even veteran heads do not always find that experience to be pleasant. And take care that the brownies (or cake, or whatever) are not eaten by naive innocents. I know of one case where a group of siblings with their families were visiting their teetotaling minister father over the Christmas holidays. Someone had baked a batch of particularly strong dope brownies, and was in the act of passing them around to the brothers and sisters when their ministerial father, who had a sweet tooth, walked through the room. Seeing the brownies, he quickly ate several, definitely more than two, before anyone could think of a way to stop him. He then retired to his study to prepare for the upcoming Christmas Eve service, which was beginning shortly. His children awaited his return with not a little apprehension.

Fortunately, all turned out well. The pastor returned home beaming, exuberant over the service, exclaiming how the "spirit" had been there, and how it was just about the best Christmas Eve service he could remember.

Effects   Patterns emerge: visual patterns, larger structures and conversations in music, insights into others, and insights into self. Sensory enhancement: new tastes, new sounds, colors with a spiritual glow.

High weirdness. Things happen most uncannily. Paranormal phenomena: out-of-body experience, synchronicity to the point of seeming telepathy.

Sex is affected also: other worldly, this worldly, her worldly, his worldly, one-worldly. Two voices singing one aria, creation and improvisation in one long, stretching, eternal now. Tactile sensations exist in their own space: accessible to both but owned by neither. Genitals and other bodily parts expand, become the whole body, the two of you climbing over them like Lilliputians.

How to Use   FIELD REPORT: A STUDENT

> *I used it to learn organic chemistry. If I memorized the reactions both straight and high, they stuck and I never forgot them.*

Effects   The experience of a lively pot party – everyone talking with great animation, the conversation filled with colorful non sequiturs and nobody noticing or caring – can be disconcerting to the uninitiated. Sentences begin with one subject and end with another. People saying opposite things congratulate each other in agreement. For those already inclined to blather, marijuana is a gift from God: it encourages one's strong point and simultaneously quiets the critic among the listeners.

The Ally   For some, it's a social animal. For others, it's like salt to sprinkle onto canned entertainment, to make it tasty. For some, it's just an everyday fact of life, a crutch they've used for so long they can't imagine life without it.

How to Use   Experienced potheads are able to adjust and drive automobiles convincingly. Results of tests for impairment have remained ambiguous in spite of tremendous political pressure to find against the herb. Doctors of our Way, who have, alas, outgrown the protection of the special angels who watch out for the young and foolish, avoid driving under any sort of intoxication if at all possible.

Pothead skiers and snowboarders generally favor smoking up while on the lift, though a significant minority condemn the practice as dangerous to self and others. In any life-threatening situation, such as skiing, rock-climbing, surfing, or diving, it seems obvious, O Young Men and Women of the New Age, to weigh the risks most carefully. Few of you will, I fear.

The Ally   Some doctors prefer to take it alone, to socialize with their thoughts, with a book, or with nature.

Poesis   The cannabinoids can be extracted from the herb or from the resin with alcohol. If the herb is used, it should be briefly baked to complete the decarboxylation of the THC. Cold alcohol will extract adequately in two or three weeks. Refluxing will do the job in a hurry. The tincture is sometimes called "green dragon."

The Ally   *Cannabis* demands flexibility, but not morality. Hypocrisy passes the gates freely, larceny giggles as it steals. And, though it may take a special effort, the violent can still crack heads. It has long been a favorite of soldiers.

Effects   FIELD REPORT: A SUCCESSFUL REAL-ESTATE BROKER

> *I smoked it every day for twenty-five years. It gave me confidence. I never got sick, either. It was when I quit that I started getting colds.*

How to Use,   *Cannabis* can cut both ways in matters of insomnia: the excitement of the mental
Insomnia   effects act as a stimulant to some. Still, many users report that they take marijuana to sleep. Recent studies suggest that the cannabidiol, CBD, is the hypnotic part of *Cannabis*, and therefore those desiring a sleeping ally (and there are many) would do well to seek out high-CBD strains of *Cannabis indica*.

Effects   That astute and intrepid *poisoner* Aleister Crowley investigated hashish carefully. Crowley, much like Baudelaire before him, described three effects of hashish: the "volatile aromatic" effect, the "toxic hallucinative" effect, and the "narcotic" effect. Of the first, Crowley says:

> *One is thrown into an absolutely perfect state of introspection. One perceives one's thoughts and nothing but one's thoughts, and it is as thoughts that one perceives them. Material objects are only perceived as thoughts; in other words, in this respect, one possesses the direct consciousness of Berkeleyan idealism.*

It is in this stage that Crowley concentrated his work: preparing himself, finding minimal doses, extending the meditation as long as possible, etc.

At a higher dose, he describes the second stage, the "hallucinative" effect, where the images of thought pass so quickly that they appear to be external instead of internal.

> *The Will and the Ego become alarmed, and may be attacked and overwhelmed. This constitutes the main horror of the drug; it is to be combated by a highly – may I say magically? – trained will.*

In the "narcotic" effect, he says, one simply goes off to sleep.

In "The Psychology of Hashish," published in the *Equinox,* Crowley attempts to map the insights and experiences of hashish to the five Buddhist meditations on the *skandhas,* perceptively noting where they coincide and where they differ, and with consummate integrity clearly states where his own knowledge ends and speculation and hearsay begin.

As I said, there is but one remedy; we are all more or less subject to this wandering of thought, and we may all wisely seek to overcome it; that remedy is to train the mind constantly by severe methods; the logic of mathematics, the concentrated observation necessary in all branches of science, the still more elaborate and austere training of magic and meditation.

The Ally Potheads and lushes are like cats and dogs. The cat, cool and composed, awareness bristling out like fur, watches the dog jumping up and down, tail wagging in dissolute abandon, tongue hanging and dripping idiotically, sees the whole creature huffing and puffing like some huge oaf. All the dog knows is that if that smart-ass cat ever forgets to look over his shoulder he's going to lose a mouthful of fur.

Effects It can inhibit dreaming. Some war veterans take it to stop their bad dreams.

CORRESPONDENCES

QUANTUM FORCE	Photon
REALM OF PLEASURE	Oral/Lips
RITUAL EVENT	Confirmation
ROCK	Serpentine
SENSE	Hearing
SEXUAL POSITION	Indescribably Intricate
SIGN	Draco
SIN	Gluttony
SOCIAL EVENT	Arrest
TAROT KEY	Magus
TIME OF DAY	Midmorning
TOOL	Tripod
VIRTUE	Tolerance
VOWEL	Low Back, ɔ

Marijuana and Civilization According to James A. Munch, who worked closely with Harry Anslinger for many years, Anslinger worked so diligently to try to arrest leading jazz musicians in the 1940s because he felt that they were "role models" for young people. But beyond that, he didn't like jazz and considered it degenerate. He once wrote in a memorandum that swing had been invented by a pot-using musician, and he didn't like swing. In Munch's words, the effect that the musicians were after from marijuana was a lengthening of their sense of time, so that they would be able to put more grace notes into their music than if they simply followed the written score. Munch complained that a regular musician would just play a piece of music the way it was written, but that a musician who used marijuana would work in about twice as many notes, would "jazz" it up.

fearing change, they grasp the letter

And we remember Lyndon Larouche campaigning against rock 'n' roll.

Employers fear change in their workers, governments fear change in their citizens, churches fear change in their parishioners.

Change in the order, the order that is written and dependable. They don't play it the way it's written, and are therefore much worse than the ordinary criminal: they are heretics and blasphemers. The War is a religious war.

Casual drug users should be taken out and shot.
        – Daryl F. Gates, Los Angeles Chief of Police, to Senate Hearing, 1990

How to Use, Medical Uses

Marijuana may be the most effective antinausea *pharmakon* known. For some people it is the only effective remedy against epilepsy. *Cannabis* is effective in treating glaucoma and is useful in the treatment of multiple sclerosis. It seems to be the only relief for certain kinds of chronic intense pain, pain that is not relieved by morphine.

For people with AIDS, and cancer patients undergoing radiation or chemotherapy, marijuana can be a savior, relieving nausea and stimulating the appetite. The obstinancy of the United States Drug Enforcement Agency in insisting that marijuana has no medical value reminds one of the priests who refused to look through Galileo's telescope to see the mountains on the moon.

The whole earth is in Revolution.

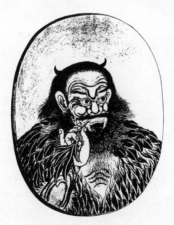

SHEN-NUNG

Many women find marijuana an ideal medicine for menstrual cramps. The use of marijuana as an aid to childbirth was attested to at least sixteen hundred years ago. Marijuana's usefulness in mood disorders needs to be explored with the same scientific and psychiatric methodologies that were given to Prozac.

No poison is risk-free. Still, two thousand people die each year in the United States from aspirin, and that is two thousand more than die from marijuana.

The Ally   *It puts just a little different perspective on things, and that little shift is enough to break out of a brooding cycle, that something that seemed big is not overwhelming. I get some distance, then I can deal with it.*

Effects   Confusion and paranoia. Many quit the Ally for this reason. Many who don't, should. Especially young people who haven't developed their solar medicine. The answer is the judo way, to back off, to hit it from the side instead of head-on. Back off, come down, limit your dosage and your situations. Learn to say no. Be a doctor of the Poison Path and observe from the outside for a change. Learn something about *ground state training.*

Poesis   Bhang is a relatively mild beverage, offered to Shiva by pouring some over his lingam, and by being drunk by his devotees. Shanta Sacharoff, in *Flavors of India,* gives this recipe.

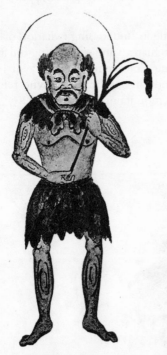

SHEN-NUNG

2 cups water
1 ounce marijuana
4 cups warm milk
2 tablespoons blanched, chopped almonds
⅛ teaspoon garam masala (cloves, cinnamon, cardamom)
¼ teaspoon powdered ginger
½ to 1 teaspoon rosewater
1 cup sugar

Pour the boiling water into a teapot and steep the marijuana for seven minutes, strain through muslin, squeezing out as much water from the herb as possible. Set water aside. Grind the herb in a mortar with two teaspoons warm milk, squeeze the milk out into a bowl. Repeat four or five times until you've used about ½ cup of milk. Add chopped almonds to the herbal mass and grind as before with more warm milk. Squeeze as before. Repeat several times and then discard the pulpy remains. Combine milk and water and add garam masala, dried ginger, rosewater, sugar, and the remaining milk. Chill and serve.

The Ally   It fills me with cravings.

Effects   FIELD REPORT: A MAN, A FORTY-YEAR-OLD JEWELER AND SCULPTOR

> *Cannabis has always been a mixed blessing for me. It is great for shaking out the cobwebs and mental constructs that my mind digs, allowing me to jump out and see a greater view, yet if only I could remember those great realizations! If I repeat the ritual, I just fall deep into another rut which seems to brings my daydreams forward, robbing my slumber of dreams, and all need to actualize anything is moot, because it has already been seen and passed on to another daydream. I think it can be a big trap, perhaps more suited to those who are mega type A and need forced relaxation of their drive.*

The Ally   A struggle with despondency, which the ally begins to be a part of. Solar medicine is important. Physical exercise, some kind of physical training regimen helps immensely. If it gets bad you need to clean up. The ally itself will tell you to lay off. But it's hard to remember that the next day. After she has already said that a bunch of times I think she stops trying. Sometimes a new ally can help.

How to Use, Migraines   Substantial anecdotal evidence claims that marijuana can prevent or decrease the frequency of migraine headaches. The great William Osler concurred, stating that *Cannabis indica* is probably the most satisfactory remedy for migraines available. The medicinal virtues of *Cannabis* were much more widely known and employed in the late nineteenth century than in the late twentieth century: consider the loss as "collateral damage" of the War on Drugs. Users claim that marijuana works best as a preventative, that once the migraine begins, it is too late.

Effects   FIELD REPORT: A MAN, A FIFTY-YEAR-OLD PROGRAMMER AND POET

> *I smoke it in the evenings but not usually at work, unless I'm designing, working on architecture. For organizing the big picture it's great, but it is not good for details. Once I got high with a friend at lunch and then found out that I had to spend the afternoon debugging hexadecimal. That was a nightmare.*

Ally, the Poison Path   We are all intoxicated. We were born into an insane asylum, a world crazymaking. We believe what we see and hear. The real myth is the myth of sanity, of rationality: it's a disease that is eating away at the earth. All the poisons flow from our denial. We deny our madness, we forget our crimes, we dismember the corpse, we imprison our children. We need poison to poison the poison, to remember the sacred nature of intoxication, the green body of the young god.

The Plant   *Cannabis* will outlast us. It will colonize the empty scars we leave behind us.

The Ally

> *It began with the laughter of children . . .*
>   – Rimbaud, "A Morning of Drunkenness"

DIE GIFTKÜCHE

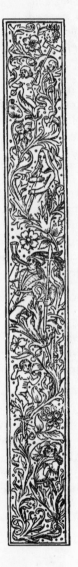

Poetry as a Way: animating the plant is folly, but letting the plant animate you is wisdom, to paraphrase Dōgen.

We are in Hell's Kitchen here – dark alembics bubble their poisonous fumes. With powerful acids and reductions the flux crystallizes: a temporary energy well. To be cleaved in the mind.

Knowledge is evil. "Wise as serpents." Angels with minds like knives, prideful and satanic. Rebellious. Religion relegated to faith, fruits and berries left to the Devil. The Protestants open a secret door for alchemy but still execute "witches."

> Lost in substances. Materiality triumphing over spirit, the poison as empire.
> When "just this" reduces to "merely this."

What's going on? Are these atoms immoral? Naked shapes and seductive twists, acetylating, Mara dancing, Maya dancing, Shiva.

Jesus is of course a *pharmakos*. Who gathers up all the poison of the world and takes it with him to be nailed to a cross where it can no longer harm us. Or so He thought. A powerful sorcerer. It is said that if you believe in Him you are freed of all those poisons He placated by returning them to their Father.

> He is the Salamander, born of fire and tempered in fire,
>   baptized in sulphurous fumes.
> We burn him as a heretic.
> He absorbs the poison and acquires a many-hued patina:
>   a peacock's tail shining like the Moon-Crested's throat.

One of the poisons the Savior took with Him was Moral Law, that the world might be free for Love. But someone removed a nail, and Moral Law is preached again. Never believe *all* of the claims of *any* sorcerer.

> (*Except this one, of course.*)

> We live in a state of intoxication already. Like revelers drunk on mandrake,
> we believe what we see. Dreams and reality intertwine. Seeing phantoms,
> we destroy cities, lay waste entire countrysides.

We deny the god, that he has come, and loose poisons upon the world. A war of poisons. Fighting is the nature of poisons. We deny their sacred shrines within our bodies and they pour out upon the world. To tame them you must name them, and be able to call them.

His venom becomes the great Medicine.
He quickly consumes his venom,
For he devours his poisonous tail.
    – The Book of Lambspring

You have to recognize the poisons to be free of them. They are ethereal, but certainly related to molecules in a most odd, surprising, and natural way. Pharmacology is close to the atomic level – so that a great deal of confusion and ambiguity can result when poison is investigated metaphysically. Not clear that's a bad thing, of course.

On the other hand, if the tryptamine won't cross the blood-brain barrier,
why not stick a methoxy group onto the phenyl side, maybe at five, to re-
duce the polarity? And while you're at it, add a methyl group to that alpha
carbon to hide the amine. Even monoamine oxidase might be fooled.

Subtler poisons are so pervasive that their scale is global or universal – yet they operate in history. No need for quantum mechanics here – or for an excursion into materialism, be it ever so mystical.

The alchemical retort, the alembic:
    pharmacy, drug laboratory. We sit,
watch our breathing, or run, eat, make love.
We eat leaves, we burn leaves, we grind seeds
and ingest them. We move atoms, alter
wave functions. Terrible smells of corruption.
Books of formulae. Books of verse.
The poisoner's workbench.

There are many poisons about. Often they enter us unbidden and unnoticed. The subtlest poisons can live within us indefinitely, like quiet parasites. (Tobacco, to cite one contrast, is so exceedingly strong and obvious that its dangers are entirely avoidable.)

"All things contain poison," our beloved Paracelsus wrote, "there is nothing without poison."

Cigarettes, books, apples.
    Windows, walls.

All poisons are potential allies.

I have drunk poison whiles he utter'd it.

    – Shakespeare, Much Ado about Nothing

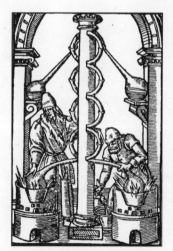

AN ALCHEMIST AT WORK

REVERIES ON
THE GREEN MAN ~
MISCELLANEOUS PLANTS

Go backward. From Amazonia, *Curipira,* the Master of Animals, a dangerous spirit whom every shaman must meet and be able to charm with words and songs, must be able to bargain with. He wears no clothes, has shaggy hair, has a huge penis, has large green fanglike teeth. His green feet are attached with the heel in front. So track backward.

To a tavern in England, green face on the hanging sign, green hat, green Robin, Robin of the Wood. Maybe Jack-of-the-Green, the foolish son who never worked but gets the girl anyway.

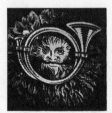

"THE GREEN MAN AND
FRENCH HORN," SIGN
ON PUB, LONDON

Backward, then to church. Gothic arches rising from a head of leaves, a head with foliage growing from its mouth and eyes, ivy and oak, or acanthus. At Exeter there are twenty carvings of the Green Man on the interior of the cathedral. Two of them sprout *Artemisia,* beautifully intricate wormwood leaves that wrap up and around the column.

At some cathedrals the Green Man shares the tympanum with the prophets. At others, hidden behind the saints, he bears the weight of civilization on his shoulders, his stone head carved into the base of the columns and arches. Almost always, foliage grows from his mouth as well as over his face. Leaves are his words. He speaks leaves, vines, and supple stems.

*Leonotis
leonurus*

This South African plant is known as "lion's tail,"or "wild dagga," *dagga* being a term for marijuana. The name "Lion's tail" perhaps comes from the form of the inflorescence; how the lion's ear got involved is not clear. The Hottentots smoke the resin and the flower buds. The plant contains several phenolic compounds, $C_9H_{10}O_5$, $C_8H_{10}O_5$, two diterpenes, $C_{20}H_{28}O_5$ and $C_{20}H_{28}O_3$, and 0.4 percent marrubin oil.

METAPHYSICA

Leonotis leonurus grows easily from seed, and will grow to more than two meters in height. In the mint family, the plant has the opposite leaves and bilabial flowers characteristic of the Lamiaceae. The flowers are orange and quite beautiful, and wild dagga is now grown mostly as an ornamental. A decoction of the leaves is used as an emmenagogue and purgative in Mauritius. In South Africa the decoction is used for a wide variety of conditions, both external and internal, including asthma.

My compatriots and I have tried to substantiate the reported narcotic and inebriating effects of the smoke with mixed, mostly unspectacular results. One plant person, however, found the smoke very relaxing and "clarifying."

❍

Backward, Roman masks, Bacchus. Bakta. Bakti. A path with heart. Shiva, perhaps.

Hang out at the theater, but not with the comedians. Hang out at the Mysteries: Dionysus and the Great Goddess, traveling together. Child of the Great Mother, god of wild earth, with snakes in his hair; the conqueror whose armies bear flutes and green staves, *virga,* defeating all opponents with love and dancing. Women wearing ivy leaves, women nursing wolf cubs at their breasts.

> *Hirsute, the Hairy Man. The Wild Man.*
> *Der Wald: forest. Sylvan. Savage.*
> *Green is Osiris, whom we remember.*

The Wild Man is the Natural Man: man without civilization – he is the projection of our imagined essential nature, what we would be like without police departments to subdue us. The medieval Wild Man was considered stupid: the rationale for feudalism. You need the nobility because people on their own are too stupid to feed or clothe or house themselves. The Wild Man today is the savage: the rationale for the police state. You need the police and prisons because people in anarchy are vicious beasts, dog eat dog, man eat man. At the very least they murder their father.

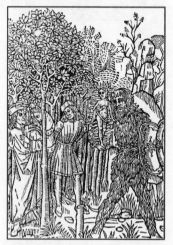

But the Green Man is the projection of the Tree of Life, the life force. He is sap, fertility, semen, perhaps helpless and foolish but not stupid. He is the Natural Prophet, the Primal Word. He is creative but oddly passive. Yin-like.

A projection of essential nature without civilization and without humanity: vegetable life. Before morality. He is not the Tree of Good and Evil, he is the other tree. The Sun-Tree.

We think of Dionysus.

THE AUTHOR MEETS THE WILD MAN, FROM DIEGO DE SAN PEDRO'S CARCEL DE AMOR, 1493

> *When Laura was a little girl in Illinois, she and her friend would catch*
> *fireflies and pull off the abdomens and stick the glowing part of the bodies*
> *onto their arms and legs and the backs of their hands. They would wave*
> *their arms in the darkness, dancing.*

Dionysus, dismemberment his birth and his death. The madness he brings is not immoral, but pre-moral, a child's absorbing delight in beauty and wonder.

Dionysus as the revealer of mysteries, whose worshipers wear huge beards made of leaves. An army of women carrying musical instruments. They march toward a bloodless victory in India. Pan and Silenus both sign on for a tour of duty. The women accept them. The unconquerable army rides forward on donkeys.

Dionysus as panther, hunter. Animation, vital force. Not immoral, but amoral.

> *The cat keeps playing with the mouse. He backs off, pretends to ignore it,*
> *so that the mouse will try to run. Then he bats it, throws it around, then*
> *waits for it to revive again.*

He is the god of excess, the god of sacred inebriation, on the wild side of the fence. Jesus was the true vine, but Dionysus kept the wild ivy.

> *They planned her birthday out in detail. Not that she was new to drinking*
> *or bars: she had had a fake ID for two years. But it was a rite. They had*
> *drivers, had friends chosen to carry her when she passed out, even had the*
> *couch all made up with sheets and a blanket, with the forethought of plastic*
> *and newspapers on the rug, a vomit bowl ready, ibuprofen ready. And it hap-*
> *pened just like that. I watched them carry her in.*

Panther, magpie, cymbals: Dionysus is the red-purple line, the way of sexuality and sensuality, the way of poisons.

> *Why are perfectly accomplished saints and bodhisattvas attached to the red-*
> *purple line (the line of passion and sexuality)?*
> *   – Shōgen*

Don't forget that it was Dionysus gave Midas the gift of gold, the golden touch, the Great Stone. So Dionysus was a Master Alchemist. Somewhere he had a forge, and a crucible.

> *It is either under the influence of the narcotic draught, of which the*
> *hymns of all primitive men and peoples tell us, or by the powerful ap-*
> *proach of spring penetrating all nature with joy, that those Dionysian*
> *emotions awake, in the augmentation of which the subjective vanishes*
> *to complete self-forgetfulness.*
> *   – Nietzsche, Birth of Tragedy*

◑

Leonurus
sibiricus

This plant is called "Siberian motherwort" or "marijuanilla." According to Emboden (1979) it is smoked in Malaysia as a marijuana substitute. Díaz (1975, 1979) reports the same practice from the highlands of Chiapas. The closely related common motherwort, *Leonurus cardiaca,* may have similar properties. Motherwort is unusual in the mint family for the presence of three alkaloids. It is not clear whether or not the alkaloids are responsible for the psychotropic effects of the plants.

I find the effects to be more sedative than euphoriant, but the sedative effects are distinctive. The plant might fare better as a tobacco or after-work drink substitute than as a marijuana substitute. I would certainly add it to any herbal smoking mixture aiming in the sedating and tranquilizing direction.

⊙

Green is Osiris. "L.S.", in the Birmingham *Post* in May of 1925, speculated that the Green Man common on British tavern signs is Osiris, a legacy of the Romans. If, indeed, of classical descent, the Roman Green Man was more likely Attis, the

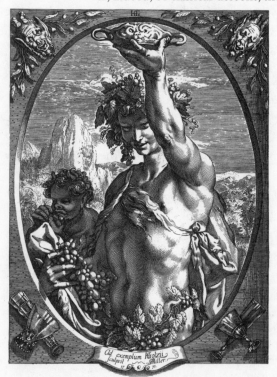

self-castrated lover of Cybele who hung himself on a pine tree. Like Osiris, Attis was green, and like Osiris and Tammuz, another form of the "dying god." The same author claims that the Axe and Bottle on tavern signs is also of Egyptian origin, the axe being a hieroglyphic symbol for divinity, and "neter," the bottle, the vessel from which Nu pours the nectar of immortality.

Osiris was the original John Barleycorn, the slain god whose body, the chaff, is scattered to the winds at threshing time. Like his mythological descendant Dionysus, Osiris also went to India, conquering by teaching art, sculpting, music, and the arts of beer- and wine-making. Osiris is sometimes portrayed with ears of wheat sprouting from him – a corn god.

"BACCHUS," GABRIEL MULLER (18TH C.), AFTER HENDRIK
GOLTZIUS (LATE 15TH– EARLY 16TH C.)

The jealous Set cut Osiris into fourteen pieces and scattered them. Isis gathered them up and put them back together, but she never found his penis. His penis had been eaten by a crab. So she made one, fashioned one out of wood.

If Osiris is the flooding Nile, that which renews Isis, the land, and keeps her fertile, then Set is dryness, desertification. Set seems to be winning.

Lactuca virosa   A minor sedative. Wild lettuce was once used to adulterate opium, and has long been used as an opium substitute for minor pain, cough, and insomnia. The dried latex is often dissolved in wine, or dissolved in alcohol as a tincture. The latex can also be smoked the way opium latex is, and I have reports from experienced opium smokers who have derived some satisfaction from it. The dried latex is called lactucarium, and is listed as a hypnotic, sedative, expectorant, anodyne, and diuretic. An alkaloid comprising several percent of the weight of lactucarium is called *lactucin,* and is said to be molecularly analogous to morphine. If opium is available, it is superior to lactucarium in every way I can think of.

Lactuca virosa is of European origin, but is widely naturalized as a weed in the United States. Also naturalized is *L. serriola,* the prickly lettuce. *L. canadensis* is a widespread North American species. All of these species, as well as garden lettuce, *Lactuca sativa,* contain lactucarium, though it is strongest in *L. virosa.* Wild lettuce bears a strong resemblance to dandelion, and inhabits some of the same locations. Both are in the chicory tribe of the Compositae, in sub-tribe Crepidinae. But the ray flowers of wild lettuce are pale yellow, or even cream or bluish, while dandelion rays are yellow. And the pappus, the fine bristles so characteristic of dandelion fall off of the wild lettuce achenes separately. Also, the achenes (the seeds) of wild lettuce are slightly flattened. Both plants have milky sap.

Jeanne Rose (1983) says that mixed with camphor and applied to the testicles, lactucarium suppresses sexual dreams. Unless she publishes her methodology, I would consider that claim to be "hearsay."

Aphrodite made a bed of lettuce leaves to bear away the body of Adonis.

○

Dionysus as the Divine Child. Son of a single mother, a love child, like Jesus.

> *Wherever you find a lot of women together, like at the Mysteries, there is*
> *bound to be one —*

Mothers of Devouring Love and their little child gods: the darling boys who can't grow up. Some of them turn nasty. Dionysus didn't want to be like his father, became the only Olympian to stay faithful to his wife. (Just because Hephaestus never actually got it into Athena doesn't mean he wasn't guilty).

> *And I am desolate and sick of an old passion.*
> *Yea hungry for the lips of my desire:*
> *I have been faithful to thee, Cynara! in my fashion.*
> *— Ernest Dowson*

Black Virgins began appearing in Europe in the eleventh and twelfth centuries, at the same time as the great proliferation of the Green Man. Cathedrals were often built on the sites of shrines to Isis and the Divine Child Horus. Divine Child Christ. The father hiding in the foliage.

Fir tree, yew tree, ivy, vine.

◊

Argemone mexicana   The Mexican prickly poppy, or "chicolote," is another opium substitute, as is *Argemone polyanthemos,* from the Southwest. Moore (1989) says that an ointment prepared from the latex is effective topically for sunburn, and that an infusion relieves cramping from diarrhea and nervousness from PMS or caffeine excess.

As with all such plants, care must be exercised. Cases of poisoning have been reported from *A. mexicana,* and also from a Hawaiian speices, *A. glauca,* and an Indian species, *A. alba.* All of these *Argemone* species contain isoquinoline alkaloids, such as protopine and berberine, both of which also occur in *Papaver somniferum.*

◊

The Green Man was carved into wood and stone, accepted great loads— supporting fountains, arches, cathedrals. Leaves poured from his mouth, spiraled up the columns.

He came with the May. He came bearing summer. On one portal at Chartres cathedral, there are three Green Men: an oak Green Man, a vine Green Man, and between them an acanthus Green Man. They are the wild, the cultivated, and the boundary, the between place where camp followers and the semi-domesticated plants live, the plants that have not lost all of their poisons.

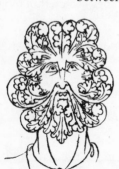

GREEN MAN BY VILLARD DE HONNECOURT, A 13TH-C. ARCHITECT (PERIOD OF CHARTRES CATHEDRAL)

Many Green Man heads have a devilish appearance: a grin, a touch of foolishness, like they have an inner joke, an inner knowledge that sets them off from the demons, gargoyles, and saints. Or two heads will be huddled together, like two sages, with leaf hair and leafy beards, looking like druids, given special and privileged admittance to the Holy House. Or sometimes a mason or an architect would carve his own face as a Green Man, a worldly and human visage sharing the aloof and stylized company of the immortals.

There are some Green Women also. At Briode, there is a mermaidlike figure with her tail split to the crotch, reminiscent of *yacu mama* of Quichuan Amazonia, tails covered with branchlets and leaves instead of scales and fin.

At St-Bertrand de Comminges, a naked female angel squats and gives birth to a Green Man head. Or not quite an angel, Lilith: harpy-like, with wings but no arms, birdlike feet as in Bosch. But a face so kind and benevolent, even in the act of birthing . . .

○

Eriodyctyon   Yerba santa.
californicum

Red Barnes, the legendary recluse and hermitic prospector of Trinity County, California, called this plant "mountain balm," and added dried leaves to his smoking mix to stretch his tobacco. He also used the "camphor plant," *Salvia sonomensis,* which he said gave you "mentholated" tobacco. (He added the camphor plant to his Copenhagen snoose also, and said that it was strong enough to make him woozy.)

I drink an infusion of the leaves as a decongestant for colds. The chemistry of yerba santa is a particularly complex mixture of flavonoids and other compounds, so I don't think the herb's effectiveness is just my imagination.

GREEN MAN BY
HANS WEIDITZ, 1521

Following Barnes, I frequently add mountain balm to my own smoking mixtures. I find something deeply soothing and comforting about it, but it may just be because it is one of the very first plants I ever collected, and is closely associated in my memory with so many hot days on the trail in the Trinities,

> *the pungent incense of the doug fir and the cedar; the cold streams, the*
> *water, the swimming holes.*

Smoking yerba santa actually may not be so smart: it is so full of resins, oils, and waxes.

> *Once in a while won't hurt. . . .*

Look for it on serpentine outcrops.

○

Dionysus is poison. He is the liberator from madness and likewise the cause of madness. Heraclitus said that Dionysus was the god of death, Hades, and excused the obscene phallic songs of the worshipers because of the divine nature of their inspiration.

Dionysus is the *pharmakos,* the fertility scapegoat who descends into the underworld and brings forth spring. He is the wanderer, the hump-backed flute player, Kokopeli, scattering seeds from his pack. Or again, Cernunus, with an erect cock. Or *Amanita muscaria,* red head breaking through the vulva, foreskin stretched, a sanguinary infant at the moment of birth.

○

Lagochilus   Another reputedly inebriating mint. Like *Salvia divinorum, Lagochilus inebrians*
inebrians   contains no alkaloids. The tincture is official in the Russian pharmacopoeia, used

for hypertension and other nervous disorders. Lagochilin, $C_{24}H_{44}O_6$, 1 to 3 percent of the plant, is a diterpene and a sedative in humans at doses of thirty milligrams. It is unknown if lagochilin is responsible for the alleged narcotic and hallucinogenic properties of the plant.

The plant grows in Central Asia.

o

Serotonin, dopamine

> *naked dancers in torchlight.*

Dionysus lives in children, but we hunt him down and root him out. We demand civility, even in celebration, but the head goes on singing. We deny the god. We legislate and stigmatize. We go mad.

We deny our own intoxication. Opposite of remembering, we forget. We deny the sacred nature of inebriation, see only the profane and thus deny the spring. And so we dismember. We kill and analyze: lyse. Like the crab, we dismember. Like Pentheus we imprison the worshipers, not seeing that they are our own children. Is this not madness?

The head goes on singing.

o

Apocynum cannabinum & Apocynum androsaemifolium

I treat these two plants together because they are so similar, and, in fact, are reported to hybridize (Moore 1979). *Apocynum cannabinum* is called "Indian hemp," a most suggestive name that actually refers to the plant's use as a fiber. *Apocynum androsaemifolium* is called "bitterroot," or "dogbane." These two plants are the major representatives of the Apocynaceae in temperate North America, the family richest in alkaloids of any plant family in the world. Both plants are cardiac stimulants. Moore (1979) states that *A. cannabinum* is significantly more dangerous than *A. androsaemifolium,* and that the plants are not to be used interchangeably. Duke (1985) concurs that the two plants must not be confused.

In spite of the widespread use of *Apocynum androsaemifolium* by American Indian tribes for a wide variety of ailments, Duke states frankly that he is afraid of this cardiotonic plant. As Duke's many years of research have proved him to be a man not easily frightened, I have put my own longstanding interest in both of these plants on hold, pending more chemical and biological studies.

o

Greenness is viridian: verdant, verdure,
the creative force of nature,
the Creator in, not of, not apart from:
Viriditas.

> *The word is all verdant greening, all creativity.*
>   – *Hildegard of Bingen*

Jesus is "Greenness Incarnate," born of Mary who is *viridissima virga,* the greenest of the green supple branches.

> Latin *virga:* flexible branch,
> related to *virgo,* virgin.

The greenness is all, the link between microcosm and macrocosm.

> *The soul is the freshness of the flesh, for the body grows and thrives
> through it just as the earth becomes fruitful through moisture.*
>   – *Hildegard of Bingen*

Green is the moist force: υγρα φυσις, *ugra phusis,* moist essence, the epithet of Dionysus.

Sin is drying up, the dry and cold that hardens the heart. Wetness and fire are the work of the spirit. The Elixir as Heavenly Dew.

Vala: moist envelope of the soul.

> *Come forth O Vala from the grass & from the silent Dew
> Rise from the dews of death for the Eternal Man is Risen*
>   – *Blake, Four Zoas 126:31–32*

The vital moisture: animal sperm, semen,
    "slime," Latin *virus,*
    the poisonous sap or juice of plants, *virulent.*
The poison in greenness, the poison of life,
    penetrating and suffusing the body of the world.

Green Man as the Divine Imagination,
the Divine Word,
    His Words are leaves.

❍

Hedera helix   As stated earlier, ivy was the plant most commonly associated with Dionysus and later with Bacchus. An early Council of the Church forbade the use of ivy wreaths because of its pagan associations. What Dionysus was doing with the ivy is not certain. Ruck (Wasson et al. 1986) suggests that it was the wild nature of ivy that was represented, ivy being the wild vine while the grape was the domesticated vine. Grieve (1971) thinks that the ivy wreath came from the custom of binding ivy around the head to prevent drunkenness.

And, interestingly, ivy was commonly added to wine. (The ale admixture was ground ivy, a different plant, *Glechoma hederacea.*) The addition of ivy to wine, in all probability, was for its narcotic properties. In addition, according to Duke

(1985), ivy, like ground ivy, is also an antiseptic, and therefore may have functioned as a preservative. But one wonders about ivy: what else does, or did, it do?

An astounding list of herbal properties are ascribed to ivy, many of them contradictory, such as being both a vasoconstrictor and a vasodilator. Ivy leaves were drunk to alleviate drunkenness, and ivy has been used on several continents as a narcotic. It is called a stimulant and also a sedative. Ivy is so high in saponins that the leaves can be used for washing wool. Other herbal uses are for rheumatism and as an emetic. Lewis (1977) lists vomiting, diarrhea, and nervous depression as the symptoms of ivy poisoning.

❍

The Green Man holds snakes, or has snakes growing from his head with the leaves, green of the sacred groves. Sacred groves, sacred temples.

Many Indian temples begin as wayside shrines, gradually accumulating size and importance. The simplest wayside shrine consists of a tree, a stone, and a snake.

The serpent is the *pharmakon*. When the Hebrew tribes were being poisoned by snakebites, Nehushtan, the bronze serpent, befriended them. Moses raised the metal serpent up on a cross, and all those who gazed at it were saved.

Hezekiah later destroyed Nehushtan, and cut down the sacred groves of Asherah.

The fiery madness had returned.

St. Patrick rid Ireland of snakes by poisoning the earth with his staff. He protected himself with magic, black magic, curses. He used "The Deer's Cry" against "spells of women and smiths and druids; against every knowledge forbidden to the souls of men."

The Christian saints and missionaries cut down the sacred groves. Tree worship was particularly difficult to *uproot*. Living, rooted trees were suspect generally, being of little use to a sky god and probably even belonging to rivals. Perhaps because of the cross, Christianity was unable to incorporate or assimilate the Sacred Tree into its traditions, as it had so many other pagan beliefs.

The cursed cross.

St. Boniface cut down the sacred oak of Thor, and used the wood to build a cross and a chapel. So fanatical was the man that the only way the Frisians were able to halt his destruction was by killing him, in 755.

The power of the Word: the victory of Christianity over paganism is also the triumph of literacy and a cosmopolitan worldview; it is the triumph of the Apocalypse. The Apocalypse is both their power, the source of their fanaticism and also their great disease. It is their Great Poison.

The Apocalypse is a *new* kind of poison that attacks eternity and creates history.

Revolution, a New Age, the Final Conflict, the Millennium.

Crowding all that need for newness into one apocalyptic moment:
    – Norman O. Brown, "Love Hath Reason, Reason None"

The poison rubs a callous on the heart. The heart is a beating thing, like a drum, creating and sustaining the eternal moment. The Apocalypse is static. It stands outside of time and rubs a blister like a bad seam. Justice and righteousness crowd out love, a cauldron of sulphur with no mercury. Those poisoned by the Fixed Time are driven more by fear of the old gods than by faith in the new One. A new level of superstition and intolerance appears, directed at the earth itself.

Time is saturn.
Fixed Time is the sulphur of saturn.

Christianity's final solution to the Tree of Knowledge was to cut it down. It is not clear that that has changed.

❍

Genista
canariensis
[Cytisus
canariensis]

Based on field reports from Michael Harner, James Fadiman investigated the properties of Canary Island broom, *Genista canariensis,* a shrubby member of the bean family (Leguminosae, or Fabaceae), and published his findings in *Economic Botany* in 1965. *Genista canariensis,* like all species of broom, is not native to North America, but was introduced from the Canary Islands. Other species were introduced from the Mediterranean. According to Fadiman, a Yaqui shaman learned about the properties of broom after being instructed to smoke the blossoms of the plant by a *plant teacher* during a trance. The preparative technique is to age the blossoms for ten days in a sealed glass jar, then to dry them and smoke them.

Fadiman's paper was published thirty years ago, and surprisingly little has been added to our store of knowledge since that time. It is indeed with chagrin that this reporter is unable to supply you with a first-hand account of the effects of this promising plant. So many plants, so little time. I will try to remedy this omission in Book Two of *Pharmako/Poeia.*

My major obstacle has been in obtaining the blossoms. Although Scotch broom (*Cytisus scoparius*) and French broom (*Genista monspessulana*) are both common and aggressive invaders of the California landscape, Canary Island broom is not, in fact being rather rare. Identification of the various species requires taxonomic skill; botanical keys cite the relative elongation of

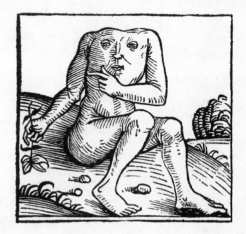

A WELL-DEVELOPED PLANT PERSON

the racemes, the presence or absence of a few hairs on the back of the banner, and the length of the leaflets. In Canary Island broom the leaflets are five to ten millimeters long, while in French broom they are ten to fifteen millimeters. If your taxonomic experience is like mine, the length of the leaflets of the plants you collect will be precisely ten millimeters.

Five species of *Genista* occur in California, along with three species of *Cytisus*, as well as *Spartium junceum,* Spanish broom. The taxonomy is further complicated by the promiscuous tendencies of broom to interbreed, so much so that most of the California plants are hybrids.

Given this state of affairs I think it is not unreasonable, nor insulting to Mr. Fadiman, to double-check his assertion that the plant he collected in Palo Alto is indeed *Genista canariensis,* especially as *The Jepson Manual* lists the western transverse ranges, not the San Francisco Bay Area, as being the plant's habitat. It is quite possible that French broom is as effective as Canary Island broom and that French broom, rather than Canary Island broom, is the plant that Fadiman tested.

Fadiman also tested Scotch broom (*Cytisus scoparius*) and Spanish broom (*Spartium junceum*). For all three plants, the blossoms were aged in a sealed, sterile glass jar. Fadiman mentions that whereas the flowers of Scotch broom and Spanish broom faded, the Canary Island broom flowers retained their yellow color. The aged flowers were then dried and rolled into cigarettes and smoked. Subjects reported that *G. canariensis* was the most pleasant and effective. After inhaling one cigarette, subjects reported feeling relaxed and good about themselves, and friendly toward the others in the room, the effects lasting about two hours. With larger doses, several cigarettes, the subjects also reported intellectual clarity and flexibility, along with physical ease, psychological arousal, and alertness. In some cases heightened awareness of color and closed eye imagery were reported.

All parts of Canary Island broom contain cytisine, the poisonous alkaloid also found in the mescal bean, *Sophora secundiflora,* of which I will write more in Book Two. Richard Evans Schultes (Schultes and Hofmann 1980) says that hallucinogenic activity for cytisine has not been demonstrated. But the use of the mescal bean as an entheogen is well documented, dating back at least 8,000 years. It is also quite possible (and I think likely) that the reported effects of *Cytisus canariensis* are not due to cytisine, but to some other substance, such as a terpene.

All of the brooms deserve more study. Christian Rätsch (1992) states that Yaqui magicians also use the seed capsule to prepare a divinitory drink used for time travel (effects which are likely to be from cytisine and the other alkaloids). He also writes that the blossoms are mixed with marijuana for an aphrodisiacal smoke used in sexual magic circles.

In the field, *Spartium* can be distinguished from the other brooms by its round stems and simple (undivided) leaves, which are less than an inch long. Scotch broom is best recognized by its strongly five-angled stems. The leaves of Scotch broom are ternately compound (divided into three leaflets), and rather sparse—sometimes the plant looks as if it were leafless. Both French and Canary Island broom have ribbed stems, but not as deeply angular as in Scotch broom. Like Scotch broom, French and Canary Island broom have ternately compound leaves. As stated earlier, the leaflets of French broom are generally ten to fifteen millimeters, while those of Canary Island broom measure five to ten millimeters.

The most important diagnostic feature of the brooms may be the *banner*. All of the brooms have yellow flowers, with the distinctive pea-flower shape common to most legumes. The two inner petals of the flower are usually joined together and are called the *keel,* the two petals that enclose the keel are called the *wings.* The *banner* is the top petal, which is usually bent upright (reflexed). The banner of Scotch broom measures fifteen to eighteen millimeters. The banner of French broom is ten to fifteen millimeters and is *glabrous* (hairless). Canary Island broom has a banner ten to twelve millimeters long and is glabrous *except for a V-shaped hairy area from the base to the tip.*

Be careful that the flowers do not mold during the aging. Some people report headaches after smoking prepared broom flowers, and mold might be the culprit. Note that *Cytisus canariensis* is a synonym for *Genista canariensis.*

○

Green as the outlaw, outside the law. It just grows by itself, with or without our approval. Green Man as the barbarian, the Wild Man beyond the wall.

> *Only barbarians are capable of rejuvenating a world laboring under*
> *the death throes of unnerved civilization.*
>   *– Engels*

Robin Hood; Robin of the Green, King of the May. Jack the Fool, who met the Green Man of Knowledge. Wild strobe lights, dancing. A Green Man raving all night, taking his seat the next morning in Parliament.

The Maypole at Merrymount. The counterculture arrived in the New World shortly after the Pilgrims. Thomas Morton was the co-owner of a company that brought a group of indentured men to Massachusetts in 1625. They built their settlement a few miles from Plymouth. The purpose of the company was profit. When the reality of the prospects in the Massachusetts wilderness became apparent, Morton's partner shipped out for Virginia, where he planned to sell off the indentured men, leaving Morton in charge in his absence.

Morton, who was a poet, made a speech to his men telling them that they had nothing to lose but their chains, and why not rebel, declare themselves free men, and learn to live as the Indians did – that far from being the abode of the Devil, as the Pilgrims saw it, the New World wilderness was the Garden of Eden.

They set up an anarchistic community and named it Merrymount. Morton had pagan leanings and told the company stories of the old gods. They set up a

Maypole and invited the local Indians to a celebration. The men found the Indians friendly, ready to have a good time, and ready to trade. Morton's men showed the Indians how to fire muskets, and found that the Indians would make a good trade in furs in return for muskets and powder.

Stories of the parties and the mixing with Indians got back to Plymouth, and Miles Standish made a surprise raid with some soldiers and kidnapped Morton. Standish had provided the Indians with their first generic term for white Europeans (*cutthroat*). when he had invited two leading chiefs to a council inside his fort and then had them both murdered with swords. Standish wanted to lynch Morton on the spot, but some of Standish's men convinced him that Morton had important friends in England and that there might be repercussions. Instead he chained Morton to a tree on an island to await the next ship for England, assuming he would starve to death. The Indians fed him.

◐

Humulus   Hops. Hops is best known to us because the flowers are added to beer as a pre-
lupulus   servative and bitter flavoring agent. It was the extraordinary bactericidal properties of hops that first allowed beer to stay fresh long enough to be transported, making beer the prime impetus behind the formation and spread of the Hanseatic League (DeLyser and Kasper 1994, Kasper 1994).

But hops has other herbal powers: it is a powerful soporific. A bitter hops tea at bedtime is effective against insomnia and in alleviating stress. Hops pillows have been used to aid sleep for a thousand years. Hops is also used to stimulate the appetite and, according to Jeanne Rose (1983), to ease delerium tremens. James Duke (1985) says that while he personally would not hesitate to drink a decoction of hops, chamomile, and valerian as an herbal sleeping potion, he would never recommend it to anyone else. It is not clear from the text if his reticence is related to the bitter taste or to other properties of *Humulus lupulus*.

Young hops shoots may be eaten like asparagus, and were so by the Romans.

Nothing that I have read or experienced gives any merit to the stories of hops being grafted onto marijuana plants; supposedly resulting in a THC-containing hops plant that you could grow in your front garden. On the other hand, grafting marijuana onto hops rootstock might indeed result in a perennial marijuana.

◐

Romanesque Green Man: Hrabanus Maurus (784–856) identified the leaf with sexual sin. Carvings of the Great Goddess appear on churches, her legs spread, giving birth to vegetation. Sexual scenes also, leafy men and women with exaggerated genitalia.

The Christian devil. The Christian shepherd-god.

The Green Man grows hooves, an even-toed ungulate, big-horn sheep pecked into basalt.

Smell of the forest in summer, pine trees, Pan's semen, dripping down cracked furrows of bark, thick with terpenes.

> *Metamorphosis into a tree. A fall, into the state of nature. The spirit, the human essence, hides, buried in the natural object; "projected." Great Pan is dead. Ovid's Metamorphoses, the death of the gods, and the birth of poetry.*
>
> Norman O. Brown, "Daphne" (*Apocalypse and/or Metamorphosis*)

Great Pan is dead — the Tree felled and bucked, limbs piled to burn, *the limbs of Osiris.*

> *No god, that men can conceive of, could possibly be absolute or absolutely right. All the gods that men ever discover are still God: and they contradict one another and fly down one another's throats, marvellously. Yet they are all God: the incalculable Pan.*
>
> — D. H. Lawrence, *Reflections on the Death of a Porcupine* (quoted in Merivale 1969)

Pan. Everything. Panic, the fear of emptiness and infinity. The head is not sprouting, but devouring — the Green Man who consumes even enlightenment.

The Way of Poisons: *metanoia, kensho;* OWNING the Green Man. Welcoming the stranger: "The least of these, my brethren."

All we consume is the Buddha.

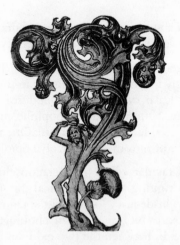

THE GREEN MAN AS DAKINI

NITROUS OXIDE

Common Name	Laughing gas.
Related Substances	Other nitrogen oxides, NO and NO_2; nitrogen itself, N_2; ammonia, NH_4; oxygen, O_2; carbon dioxide, CO_2.
Chemistry	N_2O: two atoms of nitrogen, one atom of oxygen.
How Taken	Inhaled. Professionals, such as anesthesiologists or dentists, carefully mix it with oxygen and use pharmaceutical-grade gas. Others get it how they can: whippets, said to be fairly clean, or racing tanks, said to be technical-grade and to contain impurities. If you are fortunate enough to have a pharmaceutical tank, make the extra effort to get a scuba regulator. Whippets usually go into balloons.
Effects	The wah-wahs.
How Taken	Never inhale gas directly from a tank or cannister: expanding gas is very cold (Charles's Law) and can freeze your throat. Most of the (rare) injuries and fatalities associated with nitrous oxide use are from things like tanks falling over, people standing up and falling over unconscious, dropped cigarettes – from stupid things like that. Or even more stupid, people putting bags over their heads or turning on a tank in an enclosed space, and then dying of anoxia.
	Nitrous oxide supports combustion as well as oxygen does, in matters of open flame, but that does not go for your bodily respiration. YOU still need oxygen. Be sure you get it.
Effects	The calculus of abstraction. Infinite series as the nature of consciousness. Relation. Ratio. Discrete versus continuous. The identity of quantization and possibility.
Pharmacology	Anesthesia in general is not well understood. The anesthetic action of gases and solvents probably involves their solubility in the fatty membranes of synapses. As deep-sea divers learn, even nitrogen will dissolve in synaptic membranes if under enough pressure. Nitrous oxide is lipophilic and dissolves easily in fats, which is the reason it is used for whipping cream. One recent study claims that the anesthetic properties of nitrous oxide involve opioid receptors.
	That such spectacular effects of metaconsciousness derive from so simple a molecule is intriguing. And the radical differences between N_2O and NO_2 underscore the inadequacy of simplistic rationalistic approaches to alchemical theory. Nitric oxide, NO_2, is a brown, choking, poisonous gas and a major component of smog. In between the two oxides is NO, nitrogen monoxide, recently discovered to be one of the most important and ubiquitous neurotransmitters in

the body, involved in smooth muscle mediation generally, and in penile erection particularly.

The Plant
> *A product of decomposition, nitrogen cycling,*
> *air to plant to earth to air:*
>> *transmigration of elementals,*
> *anaerobic reduction: nitrogen*
>> *moving through green, finding*
> *brief lodging in amino, nucleic acids.*
>
> *Nitrogen is the temper.*

Soil bacteria that feed on ammonium-rich ash and detritis from plants excrete nitrous oxide. Burning biomass, such as in brushfires and forest fires, also releases nitrous oxide into the atmosphere, but recent studies suggest that this mechanism is a minor factor in the measured global increase of N_2O in the atmosphere. Clear-cutting and slash-and-burn agriculture, as would be expected, also feed nitrogen-oxide emitting bacteria. But most researchers believe that it is the burning of fossil fuels that is the most significant factor in the build-up of atmospheric N_2O.

$N_2 \rightarrow NO_3$
> *Alliance between plants and bacteria.*

$NO_3 \rightarrow$ amino acids
> *Plants.*

amino acids $\rightarrow$ proteins
> *Plant seeds, fruits, and flowers, eaten by animals.*

proteins $\rightarrow NH_4$
> *Death.*

$NH_4 \rightarrow NO_2, N_2O, NO_3$
> *Aerobic and anaerobic soil bacteria.*

A few nitrates are created by lightning.

Toxicology
New evidence suggests that chronic exposure to low levels of nitrous oxide increases infertility in women. The mechanism is unknown. A single exposure to a large concentration of N_2O has not been linked to decreased fertility.

Heavy prolonged use of N_2O has been linked to central and peripheral nerve damage. Vitamin B12 is inactivated by nitrous oxide, which is needed by the enzyme methionine synthase in order to function. Dietary B12 supplements may or may not aid recovery from the neuropathy. Dietary methionine is more likely to be helpful. The nerve damage, or most of it, is reversible with abstinence from the gas. The first sign of the neuropathy is a tingling in the fingers or in the feet.

J. F. Nunn (1987) reports that exposures of less than half an hour appear to be safe, while exposures of over two hours are likely to interfere with the methionine synthase in the liver, a condition that will then last for several days. Nunn's study thus indicates that the toxicity of N_2O can build up over a period of up to three days, implying that judicious users should wait at least that long between heavy sessions. It is not clear how long an exposure is required to disrupt DNA synthesis to the point of nerve degeneration, but, considering the decades of nitrous oxide use and abuse, and the rarity of the condition, it is likely that many days of heavy exposure are the danger here, not an evening of inhaling balloons. People have undergone dental work requiring two hours of nitrous oxide anesthesia twice a week for months at a time.

Nitrous oxide should not be used by pregnant women, nor fertile women seeking that condition. Ditto all the other *poisons,* but in particular the vitamin B12 deficiency associated with prolonged use of N_2O increases the risk of bearing a child with an open spinal chord or an undeveloped brain.

Effects	*pulsations,* *that's the first thing:* *pulsations of light and sound.*
The Ally	Basic things, like the difference between one and zero, become immensely significant.
The Plant	*Nitrogen is the temper,* *a buffer to oxygen,* *lest we burn too whitely.*

We all breathe the same air. We live on a nitrogen planet. Nitrogen is our primary substrate, the ocean we feel within and through. Little bits of it oxidize in bacteria, a chicken-and-egg problem: combine with carbon, carbohydrates, nitrogenous bases for DNA, or with amino acids for proteins.

Cyanide is just CN, carbon and nitrogen – no oxygen. Lacking the elemental poison itself, cyanide can't abide those who possess it.

Alkaloids are plant ambassadors to the animal world, passing the proteinacious frontiers with a nitrogen passport.

    Nitrogen is wind and movement,
        plants with nitrogen grow legs, or wings.

History   Nitrous oxide was discovered in 1772 by Joseph Priestley, the discoverer of oxygen, nitrogen, and ammonia, and perhaps the greatest chemist to appear since Paracelsus. Alchemy was dead by the eighteenth century, but Priestley is clearly aligned with the best of the old tradition: he was a Unitarian minister and a philosopher as well as an experimental scientist. He was a student of languages: he studied Chaldee and Syriac, and could read Arabic as well as French, German, and Italian. Priestley is mostly remembered because of his discoveries of oxygen and nitrogen and for laboratory techniques for working with gases, but he also published ten volumes on theology, the history (and corruption) of religion, and metaphysics, as well as several books on color, light, and electricity. He met Lavoisier on a trip to France, and it was from Priestley that Lavoisier learned how to prepare oxygen.

Priestley's father lived in Yorkshire, was of the Nonconformist Party, and raised his son in that tradition. Priestley's whole education was in "alternative" schools. He never attended a university. In spite of a severe stutter, as a young man Priestley supported himself by teaching school. He corresponded with Benjamin Franklin and taught his students and himself electricity and chemistry. He also wrote political tracts, supporting the American Revolutionary cause and later that of the French.

The Ally
> *more reckless close to the edge*
> *but it is more than self-destructive impulses,*
> *it is the very*
> *the very very*
> *energy*
> *that creates what it is*
> *you are starting from to begin with, ahhh,*
> *right!*

At the age of thirty-four Priestley moved with his family to Leeds. His house was next door to a brewery, and it was in experimenting with those *poisons* that he began his career as a chemist. He collected the gas bubbles coming up from the brewing vats and discovered that they would extinguish a candle flame. He learned to prepare this "fixed gas" himself and invented soda water, for which he was given a gold medal by the Royal Society. He invented the pneumatic trough to collect pure gases, and was the first to collect hydrogen chloride gas, bubbling it through mercury instead of water.

It was at Leeds that he conducted the experiments that led to the discovery and characterization of nitrous oxide, oxygen, nitrogen, ammonia, and hydrogen chloride gas. There is no record that Priestley ever inhaled nitrous oxide, but he did inhale oxygen. He proved that oxygen was the part of air that supported life when he was unable to resuscitate a mouse that had collapsed fifteen minutes after he had placed it in a bell jar, while another mouse in a jar of oxygen remained conscious over twice as long, and revived after being rescued from the jar (Priestley warmed it in front of his fireplace). Priestly deduced that oxygen was richer than common air and correctly intuited that it would be beneficial for cases of morbidity where a person was short of breath. He also sensed that pure oxygen would be too rich to breathe all the time, that one would "live out too fast."

Priestley included plants in his gas experiments, discovered that plants breathe, and that their respiration was opposite and complementary to animal respiration – that, indeed, it was plants that saved animals from dying of their own exhaled poisons. He deduced the role of plants in absorbing carbon dioxide from the air and assimilating the carbon into organic living forms, thus founding biochemistry.

While Priestly was attending a banquet of the "Constitutional Society" on July 14, 1791, to commemorate the anniversary of the storming of the Bastille, town conservatives, encouraged by the government and the mainstream church, burned down his house and his laboratory, destroying his books, manuscripts, and everything he owned. The French offered him asylum, but Priestley finally chose to emigrate to America. He died in Pennsylvania, a friend of Washington and Jefferson.

> It's the instant of going
> into or coming out of
> existence that is
> important – to catch on
> to the secret of the magic
> box
>
> – Allen Ginsberg, "Laughing Gas"

History   The gas baton was passed to Thomas Beddoes, a doctor, chemist, poet, and, like Priestley, a pamphleteer of antiwar politics. It was because of his political views

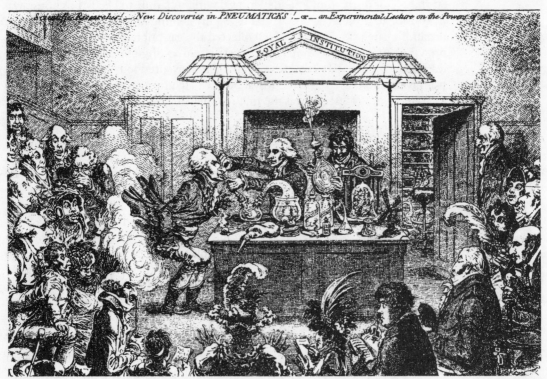

SIR HUMPHREY DAVY EXPERIMENTS WITH NITROUS OXIDE

that he was forced to resign his chair in chemistry at Oxford. Beddoes moved to Bristol and founded the Pneumatic Institution. Priestley's friends Erasmus Darwin and James Watt were visitors and supporters, as was Priestley's son. Beddoes took on a twenty-year-old self-educated student of chemistry named Humphrey Davy as his assistant and associate.

Davy had already disproved a theory that nitrous oxide was the disease-spreading contagious gas created by decomposing flesh. He perfected the preparation of nitrous oxide and performed many experiments with it, including extensive inhalation by himself and many others. He reported his findings in a six-hundred-page book.

> *"Ha! Ha! Ha!" said Inflammable Gass. "He was the Glory of France. I have got a bottle of air that would spread a Plague."*
> – *William Blake, "An Island in the Moon"*

Davy was something of a poetaster, and both Samuel Taylor Coleridge and Robert Southey visited the institute and became his friends. Coleridge liked Davy's poetry, and said that if he were not the first of chemists, he would be the first of poets. Southey was less generous, but did say that Davy had all the elements of a poet, just lacking the art. Southey and Davy experimented with laughing gas together numerous times, exploring great cosmic raptures. Some of the imagery is in Southey's long poem *The Curse of Kehama*:

> *. . . trees of light growing in a soil of ether.*

Coleridge, though his association with opium is better known, tried laughing gas and ether also. He attended Davy's lectures to get new metaphors, and to witness the colors of burning metals and gases.

Davy's experiments with nitrous oxide established his reputation, and he was given a position as a lecturer in chemistry in London. Davy became a great chemist. He used electricity to prove that lye and potash were compounds, not elements, and he discovered and isolated the real elements that they contain: sodium and potassium. He discovered boron and barium and calcium. He was the first chemist to isolate strontium and magnesium. He proved that a diamond was pure carbon by burning one with electricity. He also invented the safety lamp used thereafter by miners, and refused to take a patent on his invention.

Dr. Beddoes and the Pneumatic Institute didn't fare as well. The experiments with laughing gas had attracted many visitors, including women. The combination of women and radical politics with wild explorations of consciousness aroused a conservative backlash, and use of the gas by the general public was curtailed.

> *Nothing exists but thoughts. The universe is composed of impressions, ideas, pleasures and pains.*
> – *Humphrey Davy, under N_2O (1799)*

The Ally

> It beats,
> it walks, beats.
> It gets closer to the edge,
> cuts through what it has been told,
> and says no, forget the safety factor.
> Forget the safety factor,
> I want the stuff that's going to take me over the edge.

History

Perhaps the best-known experimenter with nitrous oxide was William James, and on the evidence of the importance of those experiments for his spiritual development and career, we claim James as a doctor of the *poison path*.

> *Our normal waking consciousness, rational consciousness as we call it, is but one special type of consciousness, whilst all about it, parted from it by the flimsiest of screens, there lie potential forms of consciousness entirely different. . . . No account of the universe in its totality can be final which leaves these other forms of consciousness quite disregarded.*
>
> — *William James, The Varieties of Religious Experience*

In 1882, James was struggling with Hegel, and had just written a paper admitting defeat, or the impossibility of the union of opposites. A small book by another philosopher, Benjamin Blood, called *The Anesthetic Revelation*, prompted him to try nitrous oxide. The results of his experiments forced James to add an addendum to his paper: with the stimulus of nitrous oxide Hegel evidently became something of a paper tiger. In his own words, good and evil were reconciled "in a laugh." James wrote that under the influence of the gas, identification of opposites stream through the mind torrentially:

> *I have sheet after sheet of phrases dictated or written during the intoxication, which to the sober reader seem meaningless drivel, but which at the moment of transcribing were fused in the fire of infinite rationality. God and devil, good and evil, life and death, I and thou, sober and drunk, matter and form, black and white, quantity and quality . . .*
>
> — *James (1882)*

Benjamin Blood, whose writings impressed James favorably, explored the nature of existence through nitrous oxide for over fifty years. He published books and pamphlets until the end of his life, when he was in his eighties, and came as close as anyone to founding a religious-philosophical cult based on the insights catalyzed by the gas.

> *The Anesthetic Revelation is the Initiation of Man into the Immemorial Mystery of the Open Secret of Being, revealed as the Inevitable Vortex of Continuity. Inevitable is the word. Its motive is inherent — it is what has to be. It is not for any love or hate, nor for joy nor sorrow, nor good nor ill. End, beginning, or purpose, it knows not of.*
>
> — *Blood, The Anesthetic Revelation*

Blood claimed that his insight into the nature of what is gave him moral sustenance and equanimity for the rest of his life. He believed that the "anesthetic
revelation" provided experiential confirmation of Jesus' saying "My Father and
I are one." Blood was quite certain that with the aid of the gas one would be
"beyond instruction in spiritual things" – a mystic:

> *Now for the first time, the ancient problem is referred to empirical resolu-
> tion, when the expert and the novice may meet equally on the same ground.*

Benjamin Blood foresaw an anesthetic revelation revolution, in which thousands
of people ("hundreds every secular day") would receive a consciousness-changing
sacrament and would "date from its experience their initiation into the secret of
Life."

Astute pupils of the poison way should find much to consider in the good doctor's
vision: something in it should have a ring of familiarity. Did the anesthetic revelation fail? If it did, why? Is it that not everyone achieves the apotheosis attained by
Benjamin Blood? Or is it perhaps that there is more to a path than the revelation
that begins it? Or perhaps the fruits of the anesthetic revelation are still being
harvested, and the alchemical philosopher was more successful than he dreamed.

> *I strongly urge others to repeat the experiment, which with pure gas is short
> and harmless enough.*
> – *William James*

The Ally   *trying to think,*
                   trying to maintain
                   that, politely, there,
                   that that which
                   keeps questioning
                   is really smarter than that
                   which is saying
                   that it's not

Class   METAPHYSICA.

Marked by attention to the ultimate dialectic of being. According to philosopher
Xenos Clark (in Shedlin 1992):

> *Mr. Blood and I agree that the revelation is, if anything, non-emotional. It
> is utterly flat. . . . The real secret would be the formula by which the "now"
> keeps exfoliating out of itself, yet never escapes.*

We must, however, understand the term *nonemotional* as not excluding hilarity,
which by all accounts seems to be the most appropriate and characteristic stance
to metaphysical ontology.

History   Laughing gas appeared in the United States in the 1840s. Doctors and other side-
show artists (the differences were not always so clear) toured the country giving

demonstrations of the gas complete with audience participation. The men inhaling the gas at sideshows would dance around, hoot, howl, jump, or fight – whatever was expected of someone wildly "inebriated."

A National Institute on Drug Abuse monograph refers to the people who toured with these shows as "charlatans," but it was one of them, Dr. Gardner Colton, who finally got the medical establishment to pay attention to Davy's work and to use N_2O as an anesthetic. A young dentist named Horace Wells, who had attended one of Colton's lectures, was the first to extract a tooth from a patient under nitrous oxide. Gardner Colton administered the gas. Wells continued to use nitrous oxide on his own patients until he committed suicide in 1848, but the medical establishment mostly ignored or disbelieved his claims. The first dental clinic devoted expressly to dental extractions under laughing gas wasn't opened until twenty years later, by Gardner Colton.

The Ally
> *There are no differences but differences of degree between different degrees of difference and no difference.*
>
> *– William James (1882), reflecting on Hegel,*
> *   after inhaling nitrous oxide*

Effects
The revelatory properties of the gas are largely dulled by alcohol. This is surprising, considering the synergism of ether with nitrous oxide and that alcohol is likewise a hydrocarbon solvent. Evidently the semipolar nature of the ethanol molecule works at some neuropharmacological cross-purpose to more strictly nonpolar solvents.

Psychonauts (Ernst Jünger's term) report that nitrous oxide's revelatory effects are multiplied by *Cannabis* and vastly multiplied by plants or substances of class *phantastica,* such as psilocybe mushrooms or LSD. Not surprising.

Poesis
Nitrous oxide can be prepared by heating ammonium nitrate, but it is not a good idea to do so unless you are a handy chemist. For one, NH_4NO_3 is explosive. For another, the reaction can yield other nitric oxides, which you have to wash out with sodium bicarbonate and activated charcoal, as you definitely do not want them in your lungs.

The Ally
Nitrous oxide has been criticized on the grounds that the perceived profundity of its insights are only seeming. One example that is often trotted out is a ditty by William James, containing, he thought, the essential key to the secret of human society:

> *Higamous hogamus,*
> *   woman's monogamous;*
> *Hogamus, higamus,*
> *   man is polygamous.*

But actually, if you think about it enough, it's kind of hard to top.

Matters of State and Liberty

Nitrous oxide is a restricted substance. One effect of the restriction is that the poor, the young, and the less educated inhale toluene, butane, or gasoline instead, all of which are significantly more dangerous than nitrous oxide. Restrictive measures in England were sparked by suspicion that sexual improprieties were taking place at the Pneumatic Institute, and by the generally radical politics of those frequenting the institute. In the United States, nonmedical use of N_2O was prohibited long before there were any known health risks associated with the gas, the inebriation it caused being sufficient proof of its sinfulness.

> *Free laughter. Giggling. Revelations.*
> *Maybe*
>   *a smart-alecky grin.*

Getting high is against the law.

The Ally

> *it's the whatever-it-is*
> *that what's doing it. that what just keeps*
> *going forward, the creative aspect —*
> *that creates what's going on*
> *out of what wouldn't be.*
> *I'm trying to think that there is something about it*
> *is more than Thanatos —*
> *something about exploring edges, the edge*
> *of death herself, itself, herself, the edge:*
> *something more libidinous and sexual about it,*
> *going out to the edge and walking around it*
> *more like cunnilingus —*
> *edge and oblivion, the spaces between*
> *vision, blackness, consciousness, waking and dream,*
> *between breaths, a dancing forth,*
> *one is a ripple, one is a runnel.*

❍

> *For in this Period the Poets Work is Done: and all the Great Events of Time start forth & are concievd in such a Period Within a Moment: a Pulsation of the Artery.*
>
>   *— Blake*

THE POISON PATH II

> *With the very poison, a little of which would kill any other being, a man*
> *who understands poison would dispel another poison.*
>
> – *Hevajra Tantra*

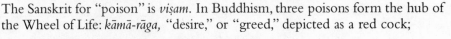

The Sanskrit for "poison" is *viṣam*. In Buddhism, three poisons form the hub of
the Wheel of Life: *kāmā-rāga*, "desire," or "greed," depicted as a red cock;

> *a grasping quality: reaching out, to attain: meristematic*
> > *shoots after light, fungal hyphae seeking nourishment;*
> *or hanging on, grasping backwards, clinging.*

**INNER CIRCLE
OF THE
BUDDHIST
WHEEL OF LIFE**

dveṣa, "hatred" or "aversion," a green snake; and *moha*, "ignorance," "folly," "de-
lusion," represented as a black hog. They chase each other and bite each other's
tails. Each poison is dependent on the others, and the whole cycle of birth and
death is dependent upon them.

> *the snake's tongue flicking, smell*
> *is tasting the air, repellents*
> > *as important as attractants:*
> *amines of corruption, pheromones of disease,*
> > *bitterness in leaves*

In rain-forest canopies the trees avoid each other: branches of each tree filling in
just up to the others, like pieces of a jigsaw puzzle, but a little space between, just
enough to foil crawling insects.

> *Some say the black hog is the mother of the other two;*
> > *others disagree, saying that greed and hatred*
> > *are equally fundamental.*
> *Some say that all sentient beings can obtain buddhahood;*
> > *others are less charitable,*
> *as much as charity has anything to do with*
> > *the veracity of spiritual laws.*

o

> *What shocks the virtuous philosopher delights the chameleon Poet.*
>
> – *John Keats, letter to Woodhouse, 1818 (in Durr 1970)*

The Poison Path is the narrow way, the twisting path, or no path at all. *You* could
make it, O Nobly Born, you just might survive, yes, but who could follow you?
Better to send them down the big road, well trodden and paved; this Poison Path

is no shortcut. The Poison Path is best suited to tricksters and magicians who, if the stories are to be believed, come back to life after getting killed.

◐

A special transmission outside the scriptures.

Poisonous dharma, poisonous datura, why be surprised that they grow together? A poison-filled cobra, what's he hiding? Medicines and powers, oak tree in the yard, a turtle-nosed snake.

> *Even today, right here, people are losing their lives, bitten by this snake.*
> — Hekigan Roku, The Blue Cliff Record

The poison becomes pervasive, and poisons the path itself.

◐

> *Socrates compares the written texts Phaedrus has brought along to a* PHARMAKON: *a "drug" or "medicine," — a philter which acts as both remedy and poison. . . . This charm, this spellbinding virtue, this power of fascination can be — alternately or simultaneously — beneficent or maleficent. . . . Operating through seduction, the* PHARMAKON *makes one stray from one's general, natural, habitual paths and laws.*
> — Jacques Derrida, Plato's Pharmacy

The primary poison is the Word — the *Pharmakos* — the one who stands-in-for. All other poisons function through this one, the signifying poison. Signifying monkey. Jesus should have been stoned, not crucified.

Pharmakos also meant "poisoner," and "sorcerer," and "magician." Plato banned the *pharmakeus,* the shaman, from his Republic in 480 BC. The Chinese kicked the shaman out of the government in the first century, along with her whole family.

Standing-in-for, the Logos. Morphine wearing the mask of endorphin, tetrahydrocannabinol dressed up like anandamide. Molecules standing in for stimuli: sensation symbolized on the cortex, rhodopsin a metaphor of light. Intellect is mediated and mediator, a mapping of pattern to patterns of ions, ratio, concentration of amines, layers of neurotransmitters themselves in flux, charged and shaped by emotion and memory. Mind acts it out, moves mountains, changes its own environment, altering the very reactions that led to the alteration.

and that's a good trick

Patterns, likeness of pattern, and some analogous likeness of likeness: the swelling of sound in adagio and its neuronal reflection. The great bead game, poetry is poison — echoes of phonemes, ghosts standing in for ghosts.

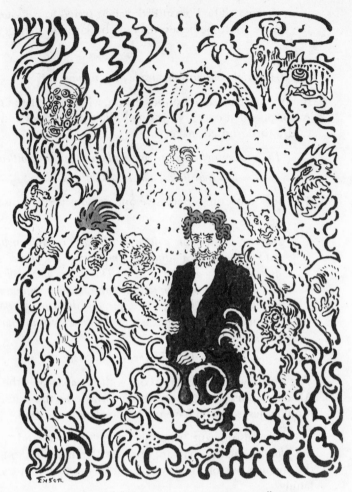

JAMES ENSOR, "SELF-PORTRAIT WITH DEMONS," 1898

Poison as defilement: *kleśa,* the ten defilements, the seven deadly sins, the speck of dust that spoils the immaculate mirror, *Ālaya,* the "Store-Consciousness." The fly in the ointment is Beelzebub.

In the *Lankāvatāra Sūtra* the *kleśa* is an uninvited guest, the one who doesn't fit in or belong, Dionysus, perhaps, or a furry critter with pointy ears, Coyote, or maybe two gods, wandering together among mortals, disguised.

> *If the Tathāgata-garbha or Ālaya-vignāna were not a mysterious mixture of purity and defilement, good and evil, this abrupt transformation (parāvṛtti) of an entire personality would be an impossibility. That is to say, if the Garbha or the Ālaya while absolutely neutral and colourless in itself did not yet*

*harbour in itself a certain irrationality, no sentient beings would ever be a
Buddha, no enlightenment would be experienced by any human beings.*

    – D. T. Suzuki, The Lankāvatāra Sūtra

The *Ālaya* is the Ally.

●

The defilements are graffiti on the white wall of the Great Warehouse. Or maybe
the storehouse walls are transparent, and the apparent graffiti our discrimination,
itself the coloring – pigments, makeup – Empedocles' cunning artist mixing and
applying his polychromatic *pharmaka* to votive offerings, creating men and
women and trees. The Creator made the World from poisons.

> *Krankheit ist wohl der letzte Grund*
> *Des ganzen Schöpferdrangs gewesen;*
> *Erschaffend konnte ich genesen,*
> *Erschaffend wurde ich gesund.*

> *Disease at bottom brought about*
> *Creative urgence – for, creating*
> *I soon could feel the pain abating,*
> *Creating, I could work it out.*

>   *– Heinrich Heine (in Freud, "On Narcissism")*

●

There is no point to calling that defined as impure as being pure, or is there? "All
the intrinsically pure defilements." All co-created, co-dependent impurities of
thought and brain, flying at us like angels, or emerging from their own arising: a
leaf, a horn, a dream, a voice that passed and dropped a word.

We are not trying to say that they are nice, these poisons, but "nice" is a relative,
not a god.

> *Poison eyes, poison ears, poison songs:*
>   *dreams within a dream.*

We hope we have not poisoned the world in vain.

●

> *The intent of our teaching is like a poison-smeared drum. Once it is*
> *beaten, those who hear it, near and far, all perish. That those who hear it*
> *perish is surely true. But what about the deaf?*

>   *– Zen Master Shiqi Xinyue, "Stone River" (in Cleary 1990)*

GLOSSARY

✣

ACETYLATE: To attach one or more acetyl groups (CH_3CO) to an organic molecule with a reagent such as acetic anhydride or acetyl chloride.

ALBEDO: In alchemy, the "whitening" stage that follows the nigredo (q.v.) or "blackening" stage, and precedes the citrinitas (yellowing) and rubedo (reddening) stages.

ALEMBIC: An alchemical retort used for distillation.

ALKALOID: A nitrogenous compound commonly found in plants as a secondary metabolite. Many alkaloids are poisons thought to serve as protection against herbivores. Alkaloids are a rich source of pharmaceuticals. Morphine, cocaine, caffeine, quinine, and strychnine are all alkaloids.

AMYGDALIN: Also called laetrile, a cyanogenic glycoside in the seeds of of peaches, apricots, and especially bitter almonds. According to the *Merck Index*, it is not effective as a cancer treatment.

ANALGESIC: A medication that reduces or eliminates pain, such as morphine or aspirin.

ANANDAMIDE: A neurotransmitter that binds to the same receptors in the brain as does tetrahydrocannabinol, the active constituent of marijuana.

ANGIOSPERM: A flowering plant, plants with covered seeds, the largest class within the phylum of vascular plants, as opposed to gymnosperms, plants such as conifers that have naked seeds.

ANHYDROUS: Without water, dry. And we mean it.

ANODYNE: An older name for an analgesic, an agent that reduces or eliminates pain.

ANOXIA: Without oxygen, especially in the pathological sense; i.e. suffocation.

ANTHELMINTIC: A poison that will dispel worms.

ANTHROPOPHILIC: The community of plants, both wild and domestic, closely associated with human beings.

ANTHROPOPHYTIC: The plant communities adapted to living on land scarred, altered, improved, or ruined by human beings; often called "weeds."

ANTIATHEROGENIC: Reducing or eliminating the buildup of fats inside the arteries.

ANTITUSSIVE: Reducing or alleviating coughing.

ARRHYTHMIA: Irregularity in the force or rhythm of the heartbeat.

ASCOMYCETE: A sac fungus; a member of the class of fungi producing spores inside of an ascus, or sac, including yeast, truffels, and morels, but not gilled mushrooms.

ATHANOR: The alchemical furnace, usually a large affair, used for digestion and other cooking. In a more general and metaphorical sense, the place where you sit and cook until the work gets done.

AUTONOMIC SYSTEM: The motor nerves and ganglia not under voluntary control, such as the heart, glands, and smooth muscles. The autonomic nervous system is divided into the sympathetic and the parasympathetic systems.

BICYCLIC: A molecule containing two fused rings. Also, characteristic of the interest of velodrome habitués.

BIPHASIC: Characterized by two phases of action.

BUTANE: C_4H_{10}, an aliphatic hydrocarbon used in cigarette lighters and as a liquified petroleum cooking gas. Propane is C_3H_8.

CAPNOMANCY: Divination by smoke.

CATHARTIC: Purgative, or laxative: purifying.

CHLOROPLAST: A membrane-bound, chlorophyll-containing organelle found in algae and green plants; the site of photosynthesis.

CHOLINERGIC: Receptor sites and neurons activated by acetylcholine.

CLONODINE: An adrenergic agonist used in shaving soap and experimentally to ease alcohol and nicotine withdrawal.

COGNODYSLEPTIC: Causing an alteration in mental functioning distinct from stimulants and depressants.

CULTIGEN: A plant with no known wild or uncultivated counterpart.

CYANOGENIC: Capable of producing hydrogen cyanide, usually by hydrolysis.

CYTASE: An enzyme that dissolves cellulose.

DAKINI: The symbol of the inspiring power of consciousness in Vajrayana Buddhism, usually depicted as a naked and wrathful dancing female figure.

DIASTASE: Enzymes that convert starch into maltose sugar.

DICOTYLEDONOUS: Of the subclass Dicotyledonae, one of the two divisions of the angiosperms, the other being the Monocotyledonae. Dicotyledonous plants have two cotyledons (initial leaves) and the vascular bundles are in rings. Monocots, such as lilies and grasses, have a single initial leaf and scattered vascular bundles.

DIOECIOUSNESS: The state of being dioecious; having the male and female flowers on separate plants.

DIPLOID: Having two sets of each autosome (any non-sex chromosome), abbreviated ($2n$). Most higher life forms that reproduce sexually are diploid. Human beings are diploid, having a full set of chromosomes from each parent. Diploid hybrids, crosses between two different species, are generally sterile. For a hybrid to be fully fertile, it must be polyploid, perhaps tetraploid ($4n$), having two sets of chromosomes from each parent.

DISTILLING: As in distillation, boiling off a volatile substance, such as alcohol, from a mixture or solution of several compounds, such as alcohol and water, and then collecting the volatile part in a separate receiver by condensation.

DITERPENE: Terpenes that have four isoprene (C_5H_8) units. Terpenes are unsaturated hydrocarbons common in the essential oils of plants.

DIURETIC: Increasing the flow of urine.

DROSS: The black residue left after smoking opium, containing morphine and a mixture of partially oxidized morphine derivatives. I've never seen a good chemical analysis of opium dross. Questions of the pleasure and safety of smoking dross are matters of debate.

ECTOMORPH: In the system of W. H. Sheldon, a body type characterized by a lean and slender build.

EIDETIC: Characterized by vivid visual images.

EMETIC: Causing vomiting.

ENDOGENOUS: Originating within an organ or part.

ENDOMORPH: A body type characterized by soft body development originating in the endoderm. Rubenesque.

ENTHEOGEN: Generating god within. A term proposed by Carl Ruck, Jeremy Bigwood, Danny Staples, Jonathan Ott, and R. Gordon Wasson, as a replacement for such terms as *psychedelic, hallucinogen, psychotomimetic,* and a host of other words used to denote the plants and substances of the *phantastica.*

EPILEPTISANT: Causing epilepsy or epileptic reactions.

EPINEPHRINE: Adrenaline, a hormone produced by the adrenal glands.

ETHANOLPHILIC: Attracted to alcohol, alcohol-loving.

EUPHORIANT: A substance producing euphoria, feelings of blissful pleasure.

EXOTERIC: Relating to the external, suitable for non-initiates.

FEBRIFUGE: Antipyretic, an agent that reduces fever.

FLAVONOIDS: Naturally occurring phenolic compounds, often colored, such as coumarins and anthocyanins. Many flavonoids are biologically active. Research into the pharmaceutical usefulness of flavonoids is continuing.

GENOTYPE: The genetic constitution of a cell or organism, as contrasted with its phenotype, the outward, observable properties.

GLYCOSIDE: Large organic molecules common in plants that can be broken up to produce sugars, usually through hydrolysis.

HALOTHANE: A nonexplosive synthetic anesthetic.

HARMINE: A β-carboline found in the ayahuasca vine (*Banisteriopsis caapi*) and in Syrian rue (*Peganum harmala*) along with hamaline. Both harmine and harmaline are monoamine oxidase inhibitors (MAO-Is).

HERMETICISM: A philosophical school based on the writings of Hermes Trismegistus, and associated with magical and alchemical traditions.

HEXANE: C_6H_{14}, an aliphatic hydrocarbon and a major component of gasoline.

HOMEOSTASIS: Physiological equilibrium, and the tendency to return to same.

HOOPA: An indigenous people living in northwestern California.

HORDEAE: The barley tribe of the grass family.

HYDROCARBON: A molecule composed of hydrogen and carbon, such as methane, ethylene, acetylene, and paraffin.

HYDROLYSIS: A chemical reaction of a compound with water, the H and -OH parts of the water molecule attaching themselves to the dissociated parts of the reacting compound.

HYDROXYL: An -OH functional group in organic molecules, designated by the prefix "hydroxy."

HYDROPHYTE: A plant adapted to water or wet environments.

HYOSCYAMINE: A poisonous tropane alkaloid related to atropine and scopolamine common in many plants of the nightshade family.

INFLORESCENCE: The flowering part of a plant.

ISOMER: A compound having the same molecular formula as another compound, but differing in structure.

ISOQUINOLINE: Alkaloids such as morphine and papaverine that contain a C_9N double ring.

KAVALACTONE: Any of a number of compounds related to kavain, with various substitutions, found in the many varieties of the kava plant.

KEFIR: A beverage of fermented cow's milk.

LACTIFER: a glandular process or group of cells in a plant that produce latex.

LAETRILE: Amygdalin (q.v.)

LIGAND: A general term for a molecule that binds to a receptor.

LIPOPHILIC: Nonpolar molecules having an affinity for fats and lipids, and generally insoluable in polar solvents like water.

LYSE: To dissolve or loosen or break open; in cells often catalyzed by an enzyme.

LYTIC: Producing lysis, the breakdown or disintegration of a molecule or membrane.

MAZATEC: An indigenous people living in central Mexico, Oaxaca.

MERISTEMATIC: Relating to the undifferentiated cells undergoing division in the growing tip of a plant.

MESOMORPH: A body type with stocky, powerful musculature, cf. ectomorph and endomorph.

METABOLITE: A product of metabolism, thus the breakdown products of drugs in the body.

METHIONINE: An essential amino acid not synthesized by the human body, important in biological methylations.

MOXIBUSTION: A Chinese therapeutic technique in which smouldering herbs are applied to specific points and meridians on the body, related to acupuncture.

NEPENTHE: The drink (νηπεζφές) that Helen served to Telemachus's companions when he was visiting Menelaus, said to bring the forgetfulness of all past ills.

NERVINE: A substance acting as a general tonic for the nerves.

NEUROHORMONE: A hormone secreted by or acting upon the nervous system.

NEUROPATHY: An abnormality of the nerves, especially degeneration.

NEUROTOXIN: A poison that acts upon the nervous system.

NEUROTRANSMITTER: A chemical secreted by an electrically excited neuron into a synapse, that then binds to specific receptor sites on the membrane of the postsynaptic cell. It's actually a little more complicated than that sounds. A single mammalian motor neuron can have more than 10,000 synapses on its surface, and there may be 10,000 different classes of neurons in the brain of a vertebrate. *The ten thousand things.* And synapse can be a verb.

NIGREDO: The "blackening," the first stage of the alchemical process, concerned with eliminating all the non-essential in order to arrive at the *prima materia*, the original matter.

NORNICOTINE: An alkaloid found in tobacco and in pituri, closely related to nicotine (nicotine has a methyl group on the nitrogen in the pyrrolidine ring, nornicotine does not) and similar in its properties. Nornicotine is an effective insecticide.

ONEIROMANCY: Divination by dreams.

OPIOID: Related to opium. The receptor sites in the brain that bind with morphine are called opioid receptors.

ORGANOLEPTIC: Involving the use of the sense organs. The old flavorists relied upon organoleptic testing almost exclusively, and had to train for many years to refine the sensitivity of their noses and palates. Since the invention of the gas chromatograph the art has declined.

PALMATE: In botany, a leaf that is divided into leaflets from a single point at the base. Like the fingers of a hand. Like a *Cannabis* leaf. By contrast, a pinnately compound leaf is divided along an axis, like an acacia leaf.

PAPAVERINE: An alkaloid occurring in small amounts in the opium poppy. Papaverine is a vasodilator, especially of the smooth muscles.

PARASYMPATHETIC SYSTEM: The part of the autonomic nervous system mediated by acetylcholine that stimulates digestion and, with a generally inhibitory effect, restores the body to normal functioning following emergencies.

PEPTIDE: An organic molecule composed of two or more amino acids linked by peptide bonds formed between carboxyl (-COOH) groups and amino (-NH$_2$) groups. Peptides are common byproducts of protein digestion.

PERICARP: In a plant, the wall of the ripened ovary, or fruit.

PHARMACOKINETICS: The process by which a drug is absorbed, distributed, and metabolized by the body.

PHENANTHRENE: An aromatic hydrocarbon composed of three linked benzene rings, and the alkaloids such as morphine and codeine that contain such a group.

PHENOLIC: Containing a hydroxyl (-OH) group linked directly to a carbon atom on a benzene ring. In phenols, the hydroxyl group tends to be acidic rather than basic.

PHENOTYPE: The outward, observable part of an organism, its expression, rather than its genetic makeup (the genotype).

PHYLOGENY: The evolutionary history of a taxonomic group.

POACEAE: The grass family, also called the Gramineae.

PROTEINACIOUS: Containing, or relating to, proteins.

PROTOPLASMIC: Protoplasm is an old, now obsolete, word that biologists used to denote all of the life-stuff inside of a cell before they discovered its constitution in more detail. The word has been largely replaced by *cytoplasm*, denoting all the living stuff inside of a cell except for the nucleus.

PSYCHOANALEPTIC: A drug that produces excitation.

PSYCHODYSLEPTIC: A clearly biased word meant to denote any drug that creates a qualitative alteration of mental functioning, distinct from psycholeptics and psychoanaleptics.

PSYCHOEULEPTIC: Just trying to work within the system. I don't really like the *-leptic* words: *lepsis* denotes seizure, as in *catalepsy*. But if *they* can have psychodysleptics, *I* can have psychoeuleptics, drugs that enhance the functioning of the brain and the nervous system.

PSYCHOLEPTIC: In the system of Delay and Deniker (1961), a drug that induces depression.

PSYCHONAUT: A word first used by Ernst Jünger to refer to explorers of inner space.

PSYCHOTOMIMETIC: A word that means "mimicking psychosis," used by early LSD and mescaline researchers to refer to such drugs. While entheogenic substances can certainly illuminate the general spiritual principles involved in paranoia and other psychological states, few still believe that LSD produces a useful clinical model of such states. As a term to denote the *phantastica* generally, "psychotomimetic" is extremely biased.

PSYCHOTROPIC: Turning or affecting the mind; a neutral and useful term that could be applied to all of the plants in this book.

PUTREFACTIO: In alchemy, a part of the nigredo stage: the dying and rotting of preconceptions.

PYRIDINE: An aromatic ring compound found in coal tar, analogous to benzene, except that the ring contains one nitrogen atom and five carbon atoms, instead of the six carbon atoms of benzene. The word is applied to alkaloids such as nicotine that contain a pyridine ring.

PYROLATION: The act of burning something. Smoking tobacco is ingestion through pyrolation.

QUICKSILVER: Mercury, the metal, and by extension the alchemical principle.

RADIOLARIAN: Marine protozoans with distinctive radially symmetrical silicaceous skeletons.

REFLUXING: Boiling a liquid in a container with a condenser attached, so that the liquid returns to the boiling chamber. In an extraction under reflux, the hot solvent is continuously recirculated through the matter to be extracted. An old-fashioned coffee percolator is a reflux extractor. Technically, the term *percolation* refers to simply pouring solvent through porous matter and a filter.

RIPARIAN: Relating to the banks of a river or stream.

SADDHU: A Hindu ascetic. Some saddhus smoke large quantities of *charas* (marijuana) to worship Shiva.

SCOPOLOMINE: Also called hyoscine; a tropane alkaloid related to atropine, common in *Datura* and *Brugmansia* and other members of the nightshade family.

SEDATIVE: Having a soothing and calming effect, relieving anxiety.

SESQUITERPENE: Unsaturated hydrocarbon compounds common in plants containing three isoprene units, $C_{15}H_{24}$. Cf. diterpene.

SESSHIN: "To meet the mind," an intensive meditation training retreat in Zen Buddhism, varying in length but commonly lasting seven days.

SETACIOUS: Characterized by bristles or stiff hairs, setae.

SOLANACEAE: The nightshade family, containing potatoes, tomatoes, eggplant, jimson weed, belladonna, and many other alkaloid-rich plants.

SOMATIC: Relating to the physical body, rather than to the mind, the environment, or a particular bodily organ.

SOPORIFIC: Inducing sleep.

SPASMOLYTIC: Tending to facilitate or induce spasms, especially of the smooth muscles.

SPODOMANCY: Divination from ash, such as divining from the shape of the ash on the end of a cigar.

STUPEFIANTS: Agents that tend to stupefy or dull the senses.

SYMPATHETIC: The sympathetic nervous system is part of the autonomic nervous system (cf. parasympathetic system). Mediated by epinephrine or norepinephrine, the sympathetic division is centered in the midportion of the spinal chord and excites many bodily functions for flight or fight emergencies.

SYNCRETISM: Combining various different and distinct systems of thought or belief into a new hybrid system.

SYNERGISM: Interaction of several agents or forces that results in an effect greater than the sum of the parts.

TAXONOMY: The science and study of systematic classification, especially of biological organisms. The great saint of the discipline is Carolus Linnaeus, to whom Erasmus Darwin wrote a charming book-length poem. According to one eccentric philosopher who writes about love, Dionysus, and the psychoanalysis of history, taxonomy is the mark of an "anal retentive." Novelist Jim Dodge once said that his personal idea of hell was to be trapped in a room with two taxonomists on speed. In my experience, at such times, the atmosphere is immensely silent, the only sound being softly popping neurons.

TERPENE: Common constituents of essential oils, containing some number of isoprene units, $CH_2:C(CH_3)CH:CH_2$. Q.v. diterpene, sesquiterpene.

TETRAPLOID: Containing four sets of chromosomes ($4n$) in the nucleus. Tetraploid hybrids, in contrast to diploid (q.v.) hybrids, are usually fertile.

THALAMUS: A mass of gray matter in the posterior part of the forebrain that relays sensory impulses to the cerebral cortex.

THUJONE: An isomer of camphor found in the essential oils of wormwood, sage, cedar, and tansy; one of the major active ingredients of absinthe.

TOLUENE: A flammable solvent, $CH_3C_6H_5$, used in high-octane fuels and model airplane glue.

TRANSDERMAL: Through or by way of the skin, as in transdermal skin patch, where the medicine is absorbed through the skin rather than being taken orally or by injection.

VAS DEFERENS: The main duct through which semen is carried from the epididymis to the ejaculatory duct. The vas deferens is very sensitive to electrical and chemical impulses, and after surgical removal is often used in pharmacological testing.

VATIC: Oracular, said of seers.

VERMIFUGE: Something that expels intestinal worms.

WORT: A plant; also, the infusion of malt that is fermented to make beer.

WORTCUNNING: Plant knowledge, herbcraft.

XERIC: Adapted to, or characterized by, an extremely dry environment.

ZAZEN: Sitting meditation, especially as practiced by the Zen sect.

REFERENCES

I. COMMENTARY

On the Nature of Poison

The seminal text is de Angulo (1926). More details on Pit River shamanism appear in de Angulo (1950), which was republished by Turtle Island in 1973. Additional material is in de Angulo's unpublished papers at the University of California, Santa Cruz, including portions of *La Psychologie Religieuse des Achumawi* in English.

See also Freeland (1923) for Pomo concepts of doctors and poisoners.

On poison and spiritual practice, we assume that the reader is fully familiar with the various warnings, precepts, and outright condemnations against using certain, some, or all drugs within a spiritual discipline. That is our beginning point. That, in spiritual practice, one should avail oneself of traditional methods and teachers seems almost too obvious to restate.

Plant People

Prusinkiewicz and Lindenmayer (1990) cover the mathematical generation of plants. The book has a comprehensive bibliography. Goethe would have found this book of extreme interest.

Riedlinger (1982) presents a fascinating account of Sartre's mescaline experience, and its subsequent effect on *Nausea*.

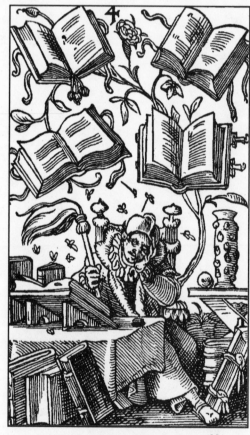

READY TO HARVEST, JOST AMMON, 1588

Plants as   Some of the stories and images are based on material from Mamallacta (1990),
Teachers   Miller (1990), and Gallegon (1988). The role of plant teachers in Indian and Mestizo belief systems in Peru is discussed by Luna (1984, 1986) and Luna and
Amaringo (1991). Quichua shamanism is discussed in Whitten (1976, 1982). The
latter book has a chapter on the role of ceramics in shamanism by women.

More general introductions are found in ethnographies from around the world,
too numerous to list here. Ethnographies that focus on particular plants, such as
Lophophora, will be listed in the sections dealing with the particular plant. Two
other books particularly relevant to South American shamanism are Reichel-
Dolmatoff (1975) and Taussig (1987). But I take issue with Taussig for positing
"magic aids hegemony" as a law of the universe. The position of magic and the
magician is more ambiguous, like that of lawyers.

The Nature   Background texts on shamanism and spirit helpers are numerous, but Lommel
of the Ally   (1967) and Coyote Man (1973b) are of particular note.

With the term *ally*, Castaneda (1968, 1971, 1972), though highly problematical
(see De Mille 1976, Noel 1976, and Fikes 1993), is inescapable. Best to consider
Castaneda's use of *Yaqui* and *Mescalito* as unfortunate slips in otherwise inspired
fiction. Ditto the datura sections. A literary parallel may be found in James Mac-
pherson's *Ossian* poems, which had an important effect on the Romantics, including Goethe.

De Angulo poem quoted from Pendell (1975).

The Mad   For a pharmacognosy text, I prefer Evans (1989) to Tyler (1981). Lewis and Elvin-
River Plant   Lewis (1977) is a must. Stuhr (1933) is very difficult to find, but is filled with anecdotal pointers of the herbal properties of so many species of plants that for the
serious plant hunter of the western United States it is worth some trouble to obtain. Duke (1985) is expensive but reliable, the closest to a "definitive" text that
I know of. None of these books mentions *Prunus emarginata*.

The   Abandon every hope ye who enter here.
Great Work;
Sun Medicine   Primary alchemical texts are much more widely available today than they were
/ Moon   twenty years ago, but . . . but what?
Medicine

A few good ones: Paracelsus (1967), *The Hermetic and Alchemical Writings;* Waite
1990, *The Hermetic Museum.* Several translations of Hermes Trismegistus are available. The Chambers translation (Trismegistus 1975), originally published in 1882,
has an index and more footnotes on the Greek than does Mead (1964), though
Mead presents a much more even and elegant translation. Outstanding is a new
book by Copenhaver (1992). Copenhaver translates the *Corpus Hermeticum* and
Asclepius, which come to about ninety pages, but includes one hundred fifty
pages of intensely scholarly notes (almost line by line), more than eighty pages
of introduction and bibliography, and sixty pages of indexes: one Greek, one

Latin, and one general. The elegance of Mead's style alone saves the great translator's book from complete obsolescence.

By the seventeenth century alchemy had lost its experimental edge, and began its slide into a Pythagorean rationalism with no praxis, pretty much where it stands today. John Dee was perhaps the last of the alchemical line who was first a scientist. Dee was a spiritualist, but also a mathematician, cartographer, and inventor. According to plant person and hermeneutic scholar Paul Lee (1994), Dee's inventions contributed to the defeat of the Spanish armada. Dee, his countryman Robert Fludd, and Michael Maier in Germany were all associated with the Brotherhood of the Rosy Cross, an international movement that was more political than spiritual, bent on resisting the Jesuits and the Counter-Reformation (Yates 1972).

But how could Rosicrucian physics compete with Galileo, or with Kepler? Johannes Kepler was the true bridge between the two traditions, achieving the seemingly impossible task of encapsulating a Copernican solar system inside of nested Platonic solids. "Geometria est archetypus pulchritudinis mundi" (Geometry is the archetype of the beauty of the world). Pythagoras could hardly have argued. In the appendix of *Harmonices Mundi,* Kepler attacked the ideas of Robert Fludd, sensing, correctly, that Fludd had abandoned the empirical (Pauli 1955). In the intellectual battle that followed, Fludd's arguments have an oddly modern, "New Age" sound to them; readily dismissive of mere measurements, especially those not in conformance with the beauty of a preconceived spiritual order.

Perhaps the finest book of the Rosicrucian alchemists is Michael Maier's *Atalanta Fugiens*, republished recently by Phanes Press (Maier 1989), complete with a cassette recording of Maier's alchemical fugues.

The Pythagorean/occult alchemical tradition was revived by Carl Jung (1967, 1968, 1976), who applied it to the individuation process. Continuing from Jung, Fabricius (1989) presents a wonderful collection of plates and drawings from various hermetic texts, and an extensively footnoted and indexed commentary based on depth psychology, including discussion of LSD experiences.

The occult/magical alchemical tradition is summarized in Burckhardt (1967) and Burland (1967). McLean (1989) presents thirty alchemical mandalas, any one of which could serve as the basis for a whole system, and describes each one in detail. Fulcanelli (1971) connects alchemy with Gothic cathedrals and cant. Two historical books are Waite (1970) and the new Patai (1994) on Jewish alchemists.

The experimentalists represent one last alchemical thread. They are found today among Rosicrucians and Steiner groups, and spin-offs such as Frater Albertus's Paracelsus Research Society in Salt Lake City. Some of these groups believe in biological transmutation (Hauschka 1966, Kervran 1972) . Kervran believes that certain plants (yeast, for one) can transmute sodium and oxygen into potassium: $^{23}Na + ^{16}O \rightarrow ^{39}K$, to cite just one example. Hauschka's vitalism goes even further, claiming to have measured fluctuations in the weight of sealed ampules of seeds, before and after germination, as well as changes in the elemental content of their mineral ash.

Using algebra, some arithmetic, a table of isotopic weights, and Einstein's mass-energy equation, I calculate that even Kervran's minimal transmutation yield of two milligrams of potassium in three days (he claimed that some flasks yielded ten or a hundred times this amount) would produce 46 million BTUs of energy. That corresponds to 375 watts of continuous power over three days, a hot little flask, indeed.

Before summarily dismissing such results as pseudoscience, one should remember the stir created in the physics community by Martin Fleischmann and B. Stanley Pons when they announced their own discovery of cold fusion in Salt Lake City in 1989. In the weeks following their announcement, prestigious laboratories from around the world reported replication or partial replication of the Pons/Fleischmann findings: excess energy, unexplained neutrons. This was Nobel Prize stuff, and theoreticians stepped forward to propose obscure mechanisms to explain what had been a theoretical impossibility the week before. I was ready to cast palladium electrodes myself. As more and more nay-sayers published negative results, some wondered if *intent* might be crucial to the mysterious experiment. I find it comforting that there are physicists who are not such confirmed skeptics that they cannot occasionally go gaga.

One last matter of the plant work. Gregg and Philbrick (1966), in their book *Companion Plants,* describe a Steiner group invention called the "sensitive crystallization" technique – for divining whether two kinds of plants "like" each other, are "allies." The technique involves three petri dishes each containing supersaturated copper chloride solution. A drop of the juice of the first plant to be tested is added to one of the petri dishes, a drop of the second plant to another, and a drop from each plant into the third dish. According to the book, each plant imposes a distinctive crystalline signature onto the pattern of the growing crystals in the dish. If the two patterns of the plants being tested reinforced each other in the third dish into a grander, stronger, and more symmetrical design, the plants were said to be "allies." Conversely, if the two patterns disrupted each other, the two plants should be planted away from each other in a garden. This was the first meaning of "plant ally" that I came across.

The technique was also said to be able to display the relative "health" of biological organisms and fluids. Realizing that the experiments, if true, provided convincing empirical evidence for vitalism, I got as far as buying the petri dishes and reagent grade copper salts. I can't remember why I never got around to the experiments—maybe because I was living in the woods and didn't have a laboratory. These days I only believe in scientific things, like communicating with plants directly.

The best book on the spagyric art, the vegetable work, is Junius (1985). In the forthcoming companion volume to *Pharmako/Poeia,* if we cannot make use of spagyric technique, we may nonetheless avail ourselves of its obfuscation.

Bulrush Bye (1979) lists a monograph on *bakana* by himself and D. Burgess as "in preparation" for the Harvard Botanical Museum Leaflets. It has not been published, to my knowledge.

Ott (1993), in *Pharmacotheon,* reports that *piri-piri* is parasitized by *Balansia cyperi,* a mushroom. Plowman et al. (1990) found ergot alkaloids in *Balansia* collected in the Amazon and in the United States on *Cyperus.* It is quite possible that *Balansia* also infects *Scirpus atrovirens.* Raffauf (1970a) reports harmaline type β-carbolines in *Scirpus.* The combination on an MAO-I with entheogenic amines could be extremely potent.

Methodology I; The two most important reference books on hallucinogenic/entheogenic plants
Methodology II are Schultes and Hofmann (1980) and Ott (1993). Schultes and Hofmann is the old standard; Ott's book is more up-to-date and contains a wealth of detail on certain plants not found in the older book. Ott's knowledge is encyclopedic and eccentric, and *Pharmacotheon* may have the most extensive bibliography on his subject ever collected.

The matter of terminology is not settled. Schultes uses *hallucinogenic,* Hofmann still uses *psychotomimetic,* while Ott is the leading champion for *entheogenic.* Others use the dreaded word, *psychedelic.* I prefer to waffle, as mood and context strike me. Mushrooms may be entheogens, but LSD, according to my young informants, is still psychedelic.

Entheogen is an excellent word, well formed and with attested classical foundation. But I strongly object to Wasson's statement that we must use it because, unlike *psychedelic, entheogen* is "unvulgarized by hippy abuse." The desperate campaign to trivialize the sixties as just a bunch of stupid, idealistic "hippies" has been underway for more than twenty years now. This Orwellian rewriting of history has been embraced by a number of intelligent people who should know better. Placing flowers into loaded rifle muzzles is neither vulgar nor trivial.

Rätsch (1992) is broad in scope, containing many psychoactive plants that are not hallucinogens (nor "entheogens"), and each plant is referenced for further reading. A very nice book, recently reprinted in paperback, and an important addition to any poisoner's library.

For general herbals, Duke (1985), though expensive, is probably the most complete and is usually available at good libraries. Grieve (1971) is an excellent source for traditional uses and folklore. Rose (1983) is more contemporary and is also quite good. For coverage of wild plants of the western United States, I trust Moore (1979, 1989, 1993). I've heard that S. Foster's *Herbal Bounty* is good, but it is out of print and I haven't seen it. You also need a book on poisonous plants, such as Fuller and McClintock (1986).

Rinzler (1990) covers the medicinal properties of kitchen herbs.

Ground State Calibration

The world experts here are probably the Buddhists. The Dhyana, or Zen school, in particular, has spent a thousand years ironing out the wrinkles in their grounding practice. The Pali text *Satipatthana-sutta,* the "Discourse on the Practice of Recollection," is a basic text from the lion's mouth. Contemporary books on beginning practice are widely available; qualified teachers somewhat less so. Basic techniques are covered in Aitken (1982), Hanh (1987), Beck (1989), Kapleau (1965), and Suzuki (1970). Similar approaches are to be found in *vipassana* ("insight") and tantric texts.

On Reading the Dhyana Sutra

What I must learn is that all substances lack true substance;
To linger on the No-Residue is to make fresh Residue.
Forget the Word even while it is spoken, and there will be nothing you do not understand;
To tell your dream while still dreaming is to pile vanity on vanity.
How expect the flower-in-the-air★ also to produce fruit?
In mirage waters how suppose you will find real fish?
The suppresssion of movement is Dhyana; Dhyana itself is movement;
'No Dhyana, no movement' – that is the Truly So.

     – Po Chü-i, translated by Arthur Waley

         [★flower-in-the-air: specks in the eye, illusion]

Thanatopathia; Tobacco; Pituri; Killing Time

The Macumba song is from Bramly (1975). Bramly is a journalist, not an anthropologist, and had enough integrity to get personally involved in his subject matter.

The outstanding book on tobacco and shamanism is Wilbert (1987), highly recommended. The pharmacology of nicotine is covered in Julien (1988) and Lewis and Elvin-Lewis (1977). Rocio's story based on Gallegon (1990).

Klein (1993) presents a cutting and insightful study of our love/hate affair with tobacco, with a refreshing whimsical edge. Claiming that his book is for "academics or fools," Klein draws on literary, philosophical, and cinematic sources to build his playful case. I especially liked the way he apologized to all those who supported and defended him through his long, non-publishing academic career, only to be presented at last with the prickly, politically uncomfortable *Cigarettes Are Sublime.*

The advertising slogans, and some beautiful posters, are in Heller (1994).

The best articles on pituri are in Watson (1983a, 1983b).

Phenomenological Taxonomy of Psychotropes

See Eddington (1928) for his analysis of the limits of scientific inquiry. I don't think any of the new books on quantum physics and mysticism have surpassed these lectures that Eddington delivered in 1927, the same year that Heisenberg published his famous uncertainty inequality, $\Delta p \Delta q \; h/2\pi$.

Díaz's system is described in Díaz (1979), an excellent article on Mexican "psychodysleptic" plants. Lewin (1931) is a seminal book for the whole field. Lewin published the first chemical paper on peyote. But it was Arthur Heffter who, after being unable to determine by animal experiments which of the several alkaloids he had isolated from the cactus was the active one, performed self-experiments and was therefore the first person to experience the effects of purified mescaline and establish that it was the primary active alkaloid in peyote.

Other ideas on systematics are in Emboden (1979), Fischer (1971), Govinda (1981), and Metzner (1974).

Occult correspondences are based on too many sources to list, but a good start is Govinda (1960), Trungpa (1973), Crowley's "Liber 777" in Crowley (1973), Iamblichus (1988).

Inebriantia;   First off, *wine* is the common name for a product of the grapevine, *Vitis vinifera*,
Yeast;   not for the plant itself: please indulge my simplification. Ditto for *beer* and *Hordeum.*
Wine;
Beer;   Roueche (1960) is a concise and well-researched general history of alcohol. A
Aqua Vitae;   more detailed history, concentrating on wine, is Younger (1966). McCarthy
the Alcoholic (1959) is recommended, particularly for the essays on wine and drinking in the
Muse   classical world. Wykes (1979) is a popular history of beer and brewing, mostly in
                 England. Two excellent books of quotations about drinking are Mortlock and
                 Williams (1947) and Digby and Digby (1988). Hannum and Blumberg (1976)
                 present a comprehensive history of brandies and liqueurs. See Goodwin (1990)
                 for alcoholism among writers.

Animal intoxication is described in Siegel (1989), in an otherwise mostly disagreeable book. Siegel has made a career of studying the "drive" for intoxication among animals. He describes, without the least moral repugnance, an experiment in which two monkeys are placed in a pyramid-shaped enclosure filled with water except for the very apex – just enough air for one monkey – and how the two monkeys fight for the air space until one or the other drowns. In the follow-up experiment, two other monkeys are given LSD, before being placed in the death cage. On acid, both monkeys drowned, each one supposedly deferring to the other: "No, you take it," "No, please, you," etc. The moral that Siegel draws from this is that "with LSD, there are no survivors."

Maybe because this kind of "science" is music to the ears of the Drug Enforcement Administration (DEA), Siegel was one of the few researchers during the Reagan years to receive funding to do research with schedule I controlled substances on human subjects. Siegel testified for the DEA in its effort to schedule MDMA, dismissing the many claims of the drug's therapeutic potential as being "just like those formerly made for LSD."

The Louisiana quotation in the *Hordeum* chapter was recorded by Marina Bokelman.

On the origins of agriculture, besides Anderson (1952), see Renfrew (1973).

Watkins (1978) discusses the role of barley in an Indo-European ritual drink that may have included lysergic acid amides, as suggested in Greene (1992).

On henbane in ale, see Rätsch (1992).

A compelling account of the effects of alcohol on the Iroquois and Huron in the seventeenth century is Edmonds (1968). The paper on the Aymaru drinking custom is by William E. Carter, in Du Toit (1977).

Timor Mortis: William Dunbar; compare also Kenneth Rexroth's "Thou Shalt Not Kill," in his *In Defense of the Earth* (New Directions, 1956).

Aether,   Much of the pharmacology is from Blumgarten (1944). The history of ether use
Fossil Fuel   is found in Brecher (1972), Blum (1969), and High Times (1978). Allen Ginsberg's poem is in *Reality Sandwiches,* Ginsberg (1966).

National Institute on Drug Abuse (NIDA) Monograph 129 contains up-to-date information regarding toxicity of hydrocarbon solvents.

Mead and   Gimbutas (1974) mentions the bee goddess. Kerenyi (1976) writes of bees, honey,
Divine   and mead in more detail. Younger (1966) has a few paragraphs on metheglin. Also
Madness   see Virgil, *Georgics, IV.*

Balché use is described by Rätsch (1992).

On the   The Nahuatl poem is from Leon-Portilla (1992).
Seduction of The Rilke line is from the "Second Elegy" in the *Duino Elegies.* For "Sam-
Angels   mael/Sam-el," see Davidson (1967).

Absinthe   The best book on absinthe in English, on which much of my historical material is based, is Conrad (1988). The book is filled with literary history, anecdotes, and reproductions of some of the many paintings inspired by the *la feé verte.* If you buy only one book, get this one.

On *Artemisia,* see Gary Snyder's beautiful poem "Earrings Dangling and Miles of Desert" (Snyder 1991). It will appear in *Mountains and Rivers without End,* a striking example of poetic convergent evolution. More on the mythology of wormwood is found in an article by Albert-Puleo (1978).

I think the thesis presented in Arnold (1988, 1989), that van Gogh became addicted to terpenes by drinking absinthe, and for that reason licked his paintbrushes, is untenable. There is no corroborating evidence that an absinthe habit (Arnold uses the word "addiction") leads to a craving for other terpenes. Nothing in van Gogh's paintings resembles the visual effects produced by absinthe, but the swirling colors may indeed reflect the effects of heavy metal poisoning. On the other hand, impressionism generally may indeed reflect the brightening and mottling effects of absinthe on the perception of color.

More recipes are in Dick (1903), Rack (1863), and Delahaye (n.d.).

I have recently learned that there is an absinthe society in the United States, whose members meet from time to time to exchange lore and homemade liqueurs. Reports I have heard of Portuguese absinthe sound as if it is of very low quality, probably made from alcohol and essential oils. I've seen some absinthes that merely steep wormwood in alcohol, without distilling it. On the other hand, the absinthe being served now in Prague sounds like the real thing, though my informant saw no absinthe spoons and drank his potion neat.

Calea
zacatechichi

More information on *Calea* is in Duke (1985), Schultes and Hofmann (1980), and Ott (1993).

Euphorica;
Opium;
Heroin and the
Nature
of Addiction

Thomas De Quincey is almost a cliche, but worthwhile. There are two versions of *Confessions.* The original (De Quincey 1950) was published by Heritage Press in 1822 and is less than half the length of the revised version Dent published in 1856 (De Quincey 1982), and is in almost all cases the more cogent of the two. Baudelaire (1971) devotes the last half of *Artificial Paradise* to discussing De Quincey's work. Cocteau (1958) is a worthy successor to those two classics.

The prehistory of the poppy plant is studied in Merlin (1984). A very fine botanical work on the genus *Papaver*, including keys, is Grey-Wilson (1993).

Chemical properties of the opium alkaloids are in Bentley (1954) and Small and Lutz (1932). Atal and Kapur (1982), published in India, contains articles on the chemistry, biochemistry, pharmacology, and extraction of the alkaloids, and on cultivation of the poppy. Nice book. Also published in India is Husain and Sharma (1983), covering cultivation, international markets, harvesting, poppy straw extraction, and alkaloidal extraction from opium. Addens (1939) focuses on the legitimate opium trade, but has some information on extraction. Small press books dealing with cultivation and harvesting include Drake (1974), Griffith (1993), O (1979), and the recently published Hogshire (1994).

Social history is found in Aldrich (1979), newspaper clippings from 1859 to 1950 dealing with narcotics and marijuana; Berridge and Edwards (1987), about nineteenth-century England; Courtwright (1982), which claims that the mean economic status of morphine users was declining even before it was outlawed; Hayter (1988), the classic study of the romantic poets who used laudanum; and Palmer and Horowitz (1982), which presents writings on the drug experience by women. Latimer and Goldberg (1981) is a more general history.

McCoy (1972) looks at the role of the United States government in the heroin trade in Southeast Asia. This book also describes the acetylation reaction. *Ramparts* and Browning (1972) contain essays on other political aspects of the heroin trade. Westermeyer (1982) is an interesting and well-researched account of opium use in Laos.

Detzer (1988) is the story of a social worker who gets addicted to poppies, with good descriptions of scrounging for poppies in the Pacific Northwest.

In the matter of addiction and recovery, I like Lydon (1993), filled with scenes and events of the sixties and seventies that will evoke many stark memories in those old-timers who survived that epoch. The question of addiction in a more general sense is in Leonard (1989) and other books in the bibliography. Other accounts of the narcotics problem are addressed in Brecher (1972), Blum (1969), Kohn (1987), and Krivanek (1988).

That leaves fiction (Algren 1949), semifiction (Burroughs 1959), and nonfiction autobiography (Pepper 1979). All good.

On the price of alcoholism in the United States: the U.S. Public Health Service in 1990 estimated the cost of alcoholism to society to be 130 billion dollars ($130,000,000,000.00). Thirteen percent of this figure consists of direct health care costs, and 60 percent is lost wages and productivity. It is difficult to put a dollar figure on the violence and abuse that occur inside alcoholic families. Few of these costs would result from the same level of societal addiction to narcotics. Eliminating the 16 billion dollars of direct health costs would be a double savings, for that sum would be deducted from the costs of health care and added to the money that would be available for other expenses. The absence of narcotic abusers from mental health hospitals is well documented. On the amount of lost wages and productivity that would be caused by ten million Americans' being addicted to narcotics, we have little information. But it should be noted that William Halstead, the "father of modern surgery," was a morphine addict all through the most productive and creative years of his life.

But this is all moot speculation. Before any such experiment occurs, you will be reading this book in translation from an extinct tongue.

Kava Kava   *Kava: The Pacific Drug,* by Lebot, Merlin, and Lindstrom (1992) is the best book on kava, by far. The book is the second volume of a projected series called *Psychoactive Plants of the World* from Yale University Press, general editors Richard Evans Schultes and Robert F. Raffauf. *Kava* is a model of the finest of ethnobotanical research and writing, as was the first volume of the Yale series, Wilbert's *Tobacco and Shamanism in South America* (1987). May the series continue!

A fine book on general Polynesian ethnobotany is Cox and Banack, *Islands, Plants, and Polynesians* (1991).

Ska Pastora   The number of articles on *ska Pastora* has almost doubled since the original draft of this book was written. Still, *ska Pastora* remains an obscure plant. The availability of salvinorin A will doubtless create a momentary stir among those looking for new psychonautical experiences, but besides the novelty, most people are interested in more pleasurable experiences. Hopefully, the authorities will let such experimentation run its course.

What is not needed are articles such as the one by Valdes (1994), waving red flags that "both *S. divinorum* and salvinorin A are prime candidates to become drugs of widespread use . . . more attractive than trying to synthesize LSD or phencyclidine derivatives." Valdes's paper exemplifies the problems inherent in the "hands off" approach to studying sacred plants. He is unable to make any differentiation between the plant allies of class *existentia* and class *phantastica*. He warns about emergency room visits when none have yet occurred. He thinks that because salvinorin A is a substance of great power it will necessarily become a popular drug, even though it is clear that he himself has little interest in or attraction to the experience. That said, I agree fully with Valdes when he concludes, "The extreme potency of salvinorin A could readily lead to overdosing and its associated problems." Though what the "associated problems" are is rather vague. Still, a person changing into a bear is not to be taken lightly.

The titles of the *Salvia divinorum* articles are self-explanatory. Hofmann (1980, 1990) describes his visit to Maria Sabina with his wife and Gordon Wasson. More ethnopharmacology is in Valdes (1983, 1987, 1994). The chemistry of salvinorin is in Valdes (1984, 1994), Ortega (1982), and Siebert (1994). Siebert was the first to publish on the human psychoactivity of salvinorin A. Reisfield (1993) describes the botany and taxonomy of the plant.

Marijuana   The *Cannabis* literature is extensive. General discussions are in Schultes and Hofmann (1979) and Emboden (1979). The best general history is Abel (1980). Ancient history is outlined in Aldrich (1977) and in Aldrich's article in *High Times* (1978). Sloman (1979) tells some behind-the-scenes stories of Anslinger and marijuana prohibition.

The medicinal aspects of marijuana, which we barely mentioned, are found in Grinspoon and Bakalar (1993). A sociological look at marijuana is in Novak (1980); this book also contains a good annotated bibliography. Pharmacology is discussed in Nahas (1984), but look for rebuttals and arguments to his conclusions in Brecher (1972), Conrad (1993), Goode (1993), and Petersen (1977). Nahas's relationship to Waldheim is in Conrad (1993).

Both Gold (1993) and Starks (1990) cover the chemistry, Gold focusing on chemical modifications of CBD and THC. The best book on cultivation is Frank and Rosenthal (1990).

Rubin (1976) is an excellent collection of essays on social and cultural aspects of marijuana use. The nature of the high experience is explored in Tart (1971) and Berke (1974). Ebin (1961) and Solomon (1966) are anthologies of literary writings about *Cannabis* and other psychotropic substances.

Some of the supposedly classical references to hemp often cited in the literature are doubtful. Schultes and Hofmann (1979) state, "In Thebes, Hemp was made into a drink said to have opium-like properties." After much scouring, I can only conclude that this assertion is based on a sentence in Diodorus (1:97:3) in which he is trying to prove that Homer spent time in Egypt by stating the Theban women still, in his time, drink nepenthe. So "Thebes" refers to the Egyptian city, not the Greek city, and the drug in question is nepenthe, the drink of the forgetting of sorrow, not likely to be hemp.

In the same book the authors state that Democritus refers to hemp's being "drunk with wine and myrrh." Schultes and Hofmann are probably echoing William Emboden (1979), who identifes *potamaugis* with hemp. I find the identification unlikely. The only reference I have found is in Pliny (XXIV: 164). Pliny lists a series of plants from a lost book of Democritus called *Chirocmeta*, all of which may be fabulous. *Potamaugis,* "river gleam," also called *thalassaegle,* or "sea brightness," supposedly causes men to rave, seeing weird visions. The plant is said to grow on the banks of the Indus. Nothing about it sounds like hemp to me. Emboden confused this plant with the "leaves of laughter," mentioned in a following paragraph, which, indeed, is said to be taken with myrrh and wine. If anyone can perfect this "myrrh and wine" mixture, please let me know; THC is notoriously insoluble in aqueous solutions.

Footsteps of the Green Man

Most of my information about the Green Man in Europe, and especially about the Green Man in English and Continental churches and cathedrals, is from William Anderson (1990), supplemented by Raglan (1939) and my own observations in Spain. Anderson's book, *Green Man,* is excellent, containing superb photography by Clive Hicks and a well-written and thoroughly researched text. The cloth edition is out of print, but a paperback edition is available from Harper-Collins.

More information about the "miscellaneous plants" is available from the usual gang of suspects: Duke (1985), Rätsch (1992), Ott (1993), Schultes and Hofmann (1980), Grieve (1971), and Moore (1979, 1989, 1993).

For the Dionysian thread see Otto (1973), Detienne (1989), Kerenyi (1976), Danilou (1984), and Brown (1959, 1966, 1991). And, of course, Nietzsche.

The L.S. quote about the English tavern signs is in Mortlock and Williams (1947).

Hildegard of Bingen (1985) reproduces twenty-five of her illuminations, along with commmentary by Matthew Fox.

The story of Thomas Morton and Merrymount can be found in Horowitz (1978) and other histories of the early colonial period. Merrymount is also the subject of a story by Nathaniel Hawthorne and a piece by William Carlos Williams in *In the American Grain*. Morton's own version of the story is in his book *New English Canaan*.

A striking painting of "La Serpiente de Metal" by Sebastien Bourdon (1616–1671), depicting the snake hanging from a crosslike pole, is in the Prado in Madrid.

Much more of Norman O. Brown's "Daphne" could have been quoted with relevance, but is better enjoyed in its own context (Brown 1991).

Nitrous Oxide

The best book is Shedlin, Wallechinsky, and Salyer (1992). Besides history and the editors' own wealth of experience and insights, the book contains substantial excerpts from Davy and from Blood, which are very hard to come by.

Health risks are covered in the Sharp (1992) monograph, somewhat. The bibliography is good.

Internet has proved to be a useful source of information on this topic.

The Poison Path II The koan of the "turtle-nosed snake" is in *The Blue Cliff Records;* see Cleary and Cleary (1992), case 22. Case 87 is another koan on medicine and disease. See also case 6 and case 37 in the *Mumonkan* (Aitken 1990b or Shibayama 1974). The Derrida quote is from Derrida (1981). On *pharmaka,* see Empedocles (1992): 27/23. The poem by Heine is quoted by Freud in "Narcissism." Shiqi Xinyue has been translated by Cleary (1990).

II. REFERENCES

Books Relating to ETHNO- BOTANY

Abhayadatta. 1979. *Buddha's Lions: The Lives of the Eighty-Four Siddhas.* Translated by James B. Robinson. Dharma.

Agrippa, Henry Cornelius. [1655] 1978. *Fourth Book of Occult Philosophy.* London: Askin.

Aitken, Robert. 1982. *Taking the Path of Zen.* North Point Press.

Aitken, Robert. 1984. *The Mind of Clover: Essays in Zen Buddhist Ethics.* North Point Press.

Aitken, Robert. 1990a. *The Dragon Who Never Sleeps: Verses for Zen Buddhist Practice.* Larkspur Press.

Aitken, Robert. 1990b. *The Gateless Barrier: The Wu-Men Kuan.* North Point Press.

Aldrich, Michael. 1979. *The Dope Chronicles, 1850–1950.* Edited by Gary Silver. Harper and Row.

Anderson, Edgar. 1952. *Plants, Man, and Life.* University of California Press.

Anderson, William. 1990. *Green Man: The Archetype of Our Oneness with the Earth.* Photographs by Clive Hicks. HarperCollins.

Applegate, Richard B. 1978. *Atishwin: The Dream Helper in South-Central California.* Ballena Press Anthropological Papers No. 13. Ballena Press.

Barron, Frank; Murray Jarvik; Sterling Bunnel; et al. 1972. *Altered States of Awareness: Readings from Scientific American.* W. H. Freeman.

Bataille, Georges. 1992. *On Nietzsche.* Paragon House.

Baudelaire, Charles. 1971. *Artificial Paradise: On Hashish and Wine as Means of Expanding Individuality.* Translated by Ellen Fox. Herder and Herder.

Beck, Charlotte Joko. 1989. *Everyday Zen: Love and Work.* Harper and Row.

Bergland, Richard. 1988. *The Fabric of Mind.* Penguin.

Bhaishajyaguru Vaiduryaprabha Tathagata: The Sutra of the Lord of Healing. 1936. Peiping: Society of Chinese Buddhists.

Bharati, Agehananda. 1982. *The Light at the Center: Context and Pretext of Modern Mysticism.* Ross-Erikson.

Blackwell, Will H. 1990. *Poisonous and Medicinal Plants.* Prentice-Hall.

Blake, William. 1982. *The Complete Poetry and Prose of William Blake.* Edited by David V. Erdman. Rev. ed. University of California Press.

Blosser, Bret. 1994. Lessons in Mazatec Curanderismo. Manuscript.

Blum, Richard H., et al. 1969. *Society and Drugs: Social and Cultural Observations.* Jossey-Bass.

Blumgarten, A. S. 1944. *Textbook of Materia Medica, Pharmacology and Therapeutics.* 7th ed. Macmillan.

Blunt, Wilfrid, and Sandra Raphael. 1979. *The Illustrated Herbal.* Thames and Hudson.

Bodley, John H. 1978. *Preliminary Ethnobotany of the Peruvian Amazon.* Washington State University Laboratory of Anthropology Report No. 55.

Bohm, David. 1980. *Wholeness and the Implicate Order.* Routledge & Kegan Paul.

Böhme, Jacob. 1620. *Signatura Rerum.* In *The Signature of All Things.* 1969.

Böhme, Jacob. 1958. *Six Philosophic Points.* Introduction by Nicolas Berdyaev. Ann Arbor Paperbacks, University of Michigan.

Böhme, Jacob. 1969. *The Signature of All Things.* Cambridge, England: James Clark.

Book of Lambspring: A Noble Philosopher concerning the Philosophical Stone. 1936. Los Angeles: Sacred Wisdom Science.

Bourguignon, Erika. 1977. Altered States of Consciousness, Myths, and Rituals. In *Drugs, Rituals, and Altered States of Consciousness.* Edited by B. Du Toit. Amsterdam: Balkema.

Bourguignon, Erika. 1989. Trance and Shamanism: What's in a Name? *Journal of Psychedelic Drugs* 21(1):9-15.

Braden, William. 1967. *The Private Sea: LSD and the Search for God.* Quadrangle.

Bramly, Serge. 1975. *Macumba: The Teachings of Maria-Jose, Mother of the Gods.* St. Martin's Press.

Bravo, Gary, and Charles Grob. 1989. Shamans, Sacraments, and Psychiatrists. *Journal of Psychedelic Drugs* 21(1):123-128.

Brecher, Edward M., and the editors of *Consumer Reports.* 1972. *Licit and Illicit Drugs: The Consumers Union Report on Narcotics, Stimulants, Depressants, Inhalants, Hallucinogens, and Marijuana including Caffeine, Nicotine, and Alcohol.* Little, Brown.

Brown, Norman O. 1959. *Life against Death: The Psychological Meaning of History.* Wesleyan University Press.

Brown, Norman O. 1966. *Love's Body.* Random House.

Brown, Norman O. 1991. *Apocalypse and/or Metamorphosis.* University of California Press.

Brown, Norman O. 1994. Love Hath Reason, Reason None. Manuscript.

Buchanan, Scott. 1991. *The Doctrine of Signatures: A Defense of Theory in Medicine.* 2d ed. University of Illinois Press.

Budavari, Susan, ed. 1989. *The Merck Index: An Encyclopedia of Chemicals, Drugs, and Biologicals.* 11th ed. Merck.

Budge, E. A. Wallis. [1927] 1978. *Herb-Doctors and Physicians in the Ancient World: The Divine Origin of the Craft of the Herbalist.* Chicago: Ares.

Burckhardt, Titus. 1967. *Alchemy: Science of the Cosmos, Science of the Soul.* Translated by William Stoddart. London: Stuart & Watkins.

Burkert, Walter. 1987. *Ancient Mystery Cults.* Harvard University Press.

Burland, C. A. 1967. *The Arts of the Alchemists.* London: Weidenfeld and Nicolson.

Burroughs, William. 1959. *Naked Lunch.* Grove Press/Castle Books.

Bye, Robert A., Jr. 1979. Hallucinogenic Plants of the Tarahumara. *Journal of Ethnopharmacology* 1(1).

Camporesi, Piero. 1989. *Bread of Dreams: Food and Fantasy in Early Modern Europe.* Translated by David Gentilcore. University of Chicago Press.

Cary-Yale Visconti Tarocchi Deck. 1984. U.S. Games.

Castaneda, Carlos. 1968. *The Teachings of Don Juan: A Yaqui Way of Knowledge.* University of California Press.

Castaneda, Carlos. 1971. *A Separate Reality: Further Conversations with Don Juan.* Simon & Schuster.

Castaneda, Carlos. 1972. *Journey to Ixtlan: The Lessons of Don Juan.* Simon & Schuster.

Chand, Devi, trans. 1990. *The Atharvaveda: Sanskrit Text with English Translation.* New Delhi: Munshiram Manoharlal Publishers.

Cleary, J. C., trans. 1990. *A Tune beyond the Clouds: Zen Teachings from Old China.* Asian Humanities Press.

Cleary, Thomas, trans. 1993. *The Flower Ornament Scripture: The Avatamsaka Sutra.* Shambhala.

Cleary, Thomas, and J. C. Cleary. 1992. *The Blue Cliff Record.* Shambhala.

Clulee, Nicholas H. 1988. *John Dee's Natural Philosophy: Between Science and Religion.* London: Routledge.

Cole, John N. 1979. *Amaranth: From the Past, For the Future.* Rodale Press.

Conze, Edward. 1959. *Buddhist Meditation.* London: George Allen and Unwin.

Cooke, Mordecai C. [1860] 1990. *The Seven Sisters of Sleep: A Popular History of the Seven Prevailing Narcotics of the World.* Quarterman Publications.

Cooper, Jack R.; Floyd E. Bloom; and Robert H. Roth. 1991. *The Biochemical Basis of Neuropharmacology.* 6th ed. Oxford University Press.

Copenhaver, Brian P. 1992. *Hermetica: The Greek Hermeticum and the Latin Asclepius.* Cambridge University Press.

Cowley, Abraham. [1662] 1700. *Book of Plants.* In *The Third Part of the Works of Mr. Abraham Cowley, Being His Six Books of Plants.* 2d. ed. London: Charles Harper.

Coyote Man. 1973a. *Sun, Moon, and Stars.* Berkeley: Brother William Press.

Coyote Man. 1973b. *The Destruction of the People.* Berkeley: Brother William Press.

Coyote Man, and Brother William. 1972. *Get the Buzzon.* Berkeley: Brother William Press.

Crowley, Aleister. N.d. *Magick in Theory and Practice.* Castle Books.

Crowley, Aleister. 1969. *The Book of Thoth.* Kashmarin Press/Shambhala.

Crowley, Aleister. 1973. *The Qabalah of Aleister Crowley: Three Texts.* Samuel Weiser.

Dali, Salvador. 1983. *Tarot Universal Dali Deck.* Barcelona: Talleres Graficos Soler.

Danielou, Alain. 1964. *Hindu Polytheism.* Bollingen 73. Pantheon.

Danielou, Alain. 1984. *Shiva and Dionysus: The Religion of Nature and Eros.* Translated by K. F. Hurry. Inner Traditions International.

Darwin, Erasmus. 1791. *The Botanic Garden: The Loves of the Plants.* London: J. Johnson.

Davenport, Guy, trans. 1981. *Herakleitos and Diogenes.* Grey Fox Press.

David-Neel, Alexandra. 1937. *Magic and Mystery in Tibet.* Crown.

Davidson, Gustav. 1967. *A Dictionary of Angels: Including the Fallen Angels.* Free Press, Collier/Macmillan.

De Angulo, Jaime. N.d. Unpublished papers. Special Collections. University of California, Santa Cruz.

De Angulo, Jaime. 1926. The Background of Religious Feeling in a Primitive Tribe. *American Anthropologist* 28(2):352-360.

De Angulo, Jaime. 1950. Indians in Overalls. *Hudson Review* 3(3):237-77.

De Angulo, Jaime. 1957. *Indian Tales.* Hill and Wang.

De Angulo, Jaime. 1974a. *Coyote's Bones.* Turtle Island.

De Angulo, Jaime. 1974b. *The Lariat.* Turtle Island.

DeKorne, Jim. 1994. *Psychedelic Shamanism: The Cultivation, Preparation and Shamanic Use of Psychotropic Plants.* Port Townsend: Loompanics.

Delay, J. and P. Deniker. 1961. *Méthodes Chimiothérapeutiques en Psychiatrie: Les Nouveaux Medicaments Psychotropes.* Paris: Masson

De Mille, Richard. 1976. *Castaneda's Journey: The Power and the Allegory.* Capra Press.

De Ropp, Robert S. 1976. *Drugs and the Mind.* Rev. ed. Delta.

Derrida, Jacques. 1981. *Dissemination.* Translated by Barbara Johnson. University of Chicago Press.

Detienne, Marcel. 1989. *Dionysos at Large.* Translated by Arthur Goldhammer. Harvard University Press.

Deutsch, Helene. 1969. *A Psychoanalytic Study of the Myth of Dionysus and Apollo: Two Variants of the Son-Mother Relationship.* International Universities Press.

Diamond, Stanley. 1974. *In Search of the Primitive: A Critique of Civilization.* Transaction Books/E. P. Dutton.

Díaz, José Luis. 1979. Ethnopharmacology and Taxonomy of Mexican Psychodysleptic Plants. *Journal of Psychedelic Drugs* 11(1,2):71-101.

Dick, William B. 1903. *Dick's Encyclopedia of Practical Receipts and Processes.* Dick and Fitzgerald.

Dobkin de Rios, Marlene, and Michael Winkelman. 1989. Shamanism and Altered States of Consciousness: An Introduction. *Journal of Psychedelic Drugs* 21(1):1-7.

Dodds, E. R. 1973. *The Greeks and the Irrational.* University of California Press.

Duerr, Hans Peter. 1985. *Dreamtime: Concerning the Boundary Between wilderness and Civilization.* Translated by Felicitas D. Goodman. B. Blackwell.

Duke, James A. 1985. *CRC Handbook of Medicinal Herbs.* CRC Press.

Duke, Steven B., and Albert C. Gross. 1994. *America's Longest War: Rethinking Our Tragic Crusade against Drugs.* Jeremy P. Tarcher.

Duran, Fray Diego. 1975. *Book of the Gods and Rites; and The Ancient Calendar.* Translated by Fernando Horcasitas and Doris Heyden. University of Oklahoma Press.

Durr, R. A. 1970. *Poetic Vision and the Psychedelic Experience.* Syracuse University Press.

Du Toit, B., ed. 1977. *Drugs, Rituals, and Altered States of Consciousness.* Amsterdam: Balkema.

Ebin, David, ed. 1961. *The Drug Experience: First-Person Accounts of Addicts, Writers, Scientists, and Others.* Orion.

Eddington, A. S. 1928. *The Nature of the Physical World: The Gifford Lectures, 1927.* Macmillan.

Edmonds, John Maxwell. 1959. *The Fragments of Attic Comedy.* Vol. 2. Leiden: Brill.

Efron, Daniel H., ed. 1967. *Ethnopharmacologic Search for Psychoactive Drugs.* Public Health Service Publication No. 1645.

Elferink, Jan G. R. 1988. Some Little-Known Hallucinogenic Plants of the Aztecs. *Journal of Psychedelic Drugs* 20(4):427-435.

Eliade, Mircea. 1964. *Shamanism: Archaic Techniques of Ecstasy.* Translated by Williard R. Trask. Bollingen 76. Pantheon.

Emboden, William. 1979. *Narcotic Plants: Hallucinogens, Stimulants, Inebriants, and Hypnotics, Their Origins and Uses.* Rev. ed. Macmillan.

Emerson, Ralph Waldo. 1944. *Emerson's Essays.* Illustrated Modern Library.

Empedocles. 1992. *The Poem of Empedocles: A Text and Translation.* Translated by Brad Inwood. University of Toronto.

Erfurt, Birgit Boline. *Karma Tarot Deck.* U.S. Games.

Escohotado, Antonio. 1990. *El Libro de los Venenos: Guia de Drogas, Las Licitas y las Otras.* Madrid: Omnibus Mondadori.

Escohotado, Antonio. 1992. *Historia de las Drogas.* 3d ed. Madrid: Alianza Editorial.

Estrada, Alvaro. 1981. *Maria Sabina: Her Life and Chants.* Translated by Henry Munn, with an essay by R. Gordon Wasson. Ross-Erikson.

Euripides. 1944. *Bacchae.* Edited by E. R. Dodds. Oxford: Clarendon Press.

Evans, Rod L., and Irwin M. Berent, eds. 1992. *Drug Legalization: For and Against.* La Salle: Open Court.

Evans, William Charles. 1989. *Trease and Evans' Pharmacognosy.* 13th ed. London: Bailliere Tindall.

Fabricius, Johannes. 1989. *Alchemy: The Medieval Alchemists and Their Royal Art.* Aquarian Press.

Feininger, Andreas. 1975. *Roots of Art.* Viking.

Fikes, Jay Courtney. 1993. *Carlos Castaneda, Academic Opportunism, and the Psychedelic Sixties.* Victoria: Millennia Press.

Fischer, Roland. 1971. A Cartography of the Ecstatic and Meditative States. *Science* 174:897-904.

Flaherty, Gloria. 1992. *Shamanism and the Eighteenth Century.* Princeton University Press.

Flattery, David Stophlet, and Martin Schwartz. 1989. *Haoma and Harmaline: The Botanical Identity of the Indo-Iranian Sacred Hallucinogen "Soma."* University of California Publications in Near Eastern Studies, vol. 21. University of California Press

Folkard, Richard Jr. 1884. *Plant Lore, Legends, and Lyrics: Embracing the Myths, Traditions, Superstitions, and Folklore of the Plant Kingdom.* London: S. Low.

Foster, Nelson, and Linda S. Cordell, eds. 1992. *Chilies to Chocolate: Food the Americas Gave the World.* University of Arizona Press.

Fox, Matthew. 1988. *The Coming of the Cosmic Christ: The Healing of Mother Earth and the Birth of a Global Renaissance.* Harper San Francisco.

Frazer, James George. 1923. *The Golden Bough: A Study in Magic and Religion.* Macmillan.

Freeland, L.S. 1923. Pomo Doctors and Poisoners. *University of California Publications in Archaeology and Anthropology* 20:62.

Freud, Sigmund. 1964. *Complete Works.* London: Hogarth.

Fulcanelli. 1971. *Fulcanelli, Master Alchemist: Le Mystere des Cathedrales.* Translated by Mary Sworder. London: Neville Spearman.

Fuller, Thomas C., and Elizabeth McClintock. 1986. *Poisonous Plants of California.* University of California Press.

Furniss, B.S.; A.J. Hannaford; P.W.G. Smith; A.R. Tatchell. 1991. *Vogel's Textbook of Practical Organic Chemistry.* 5th ed. Wiley.

Furst, Peter T., ed. 1972. *Flesh of the Gods: The Ritual Use of Hallucinogens.* Praeger.

Furst, Peter T. 1976. *Hallucinogens and Culture.* Chandler and Sharp.

Gallegon, Rocio Alarcon. 1988. *Etnobotánica de los Quichuas de la Amazonia Equatoriana.* Quito: Museos del Banco Central del Ecuador.

Gallegon, Rocio Alarcon. 1990. Personal communication. Jatun Sacha, Ecuador.

Gampopa. 1971. *Jewel Ornament of Liberation.* Translated by Herbert V. Guenther. Clear Light Series, Shambhala.

Gifford, Edward Winslow, and Gwendoline Harris Block. [1930] 1990. *Californian Indian Nights Entertainments.* University of Nebraska.

Gimbutas, Marija. 1974. *The Gods and Goddesses of Old Europe, 7000 to 3500 BC: Myths, Legends, and Cult Images.* University of California Press.

Ginsberg, Allen. 1961. *Kaddish and Other Poems, 1958–1960.* City Lights Books.

Ginsberg, Allen. 1966. *Reality Sandwiches.* City Lights Books.

Ginzburg, Carlo. 1991. *Ecstasies: Deciphering the Witches' Sabbath.* Pantheon.

Godwin, Joscelyn. 1991. *Robert Fludd: Hermetic Philosopher and Surveyor of Two Worlds.* Phanes Press.

Goethe, Johann Wolfgang von. 1963. *Faust.* Translated by Walter Kaufman. Anchor.

Goode, Erich. 1993. *Drugs in American Society.* 4th ed. McGraw-Hill.

Govinda, Lama Anagarika. 1960. *Foundations of Tibetan Mysticism.* E. P. Dutton.

Govinda, Lama Anagarika. 1976. *Psycho-cosmic Symbolism of the Buddhist Stupa.* Dharma Press.

Govinda, Lama Anagarika. 1981. *The Inner Structure of the I Ching: The Book of Transformations.* Wheelwright/Weatherhill.

Graves, Robert. 1948. *The White Goddess.* London: Faber and Faber.

Graves, Robert. 1956. *The Crowning Privilege.* Doubleday.

Graves, Robert. 1960. *Food for Centaurs: Stories, Talks, Critical Studies, Poems.* Doubleday.

Graves, Robert. 1971a. *Difficult Questions, Easy Answers.* Doubleday.

Graves, Robert. 1971b. Introduction to the *New Larousse Encyclopedia of Mythology.* Hamlyn.

Greene, Mott T. 1992. *Natural Knowledge in Preclassical Antiquity.* Johns Hopkins University Press.

Gregg, Richard B., and Helen Philbrick. 1966. *Companion Plants and How to Use Them.* Knopf.

Grieve, Mrs. M. 1971. *A Modern Herbal.* 2 vols. Dover.

Griffith, Ralph T. H., trans. 1976. *The Hymns of the Rig Veda.* Delhi: Motilal Banarsidass.

Guenther, Herbert V. 1969. *Yuganaddha: The Tantric View of Life.* 2d ed. Varanasi, India: Chowkhamba Publication.

Gupta, Shakti M. 1970. *Plant Myths and Traditions in India.* Leiden: Brill.

Hall, Manly P. 1978. *The Tarot: An Essay.* Philosophical Research Society.

Hanh, Thich Nhat. 1987. *The Miracle of Mindfulness: A Manual on Meditation.* Rev. ed. Beacon.

Hansen, Harold A. [1978] 1983. *The Witch's Garden.* Translated by Muriel Crofts. Unity Press.

Harner, Michael J. 1973. *Hallucinogens and Shamanism.* Oxford University Press.

Hauschka, Rudolf. 1966. *The Nature of Substance.* London: Vincent Stuart.

Heffern, Richard. 1974. *Secrets of the Mind-Altering Plants of Mexico.* Pyramid.

Heiser, Charles B. 1969. *Nightshades: The Paradoxical Plants.* W. H. Freeman.

Helfand, William H. 1980. Vin Mariani. *Pharmacy in History* (22):1.

Heninger, S. K., Jr. 1974. *Touches of Sweet Harmony: Pythagorean Cosmology and Renaissance Poetics.* The Huntington Library.

Heywood, V. H., ed. 1978. *Flowering Plants of the World.* Mayflower Books.

High Times. 1978. *High Times Encyclopedia of Recreational Drugs.* Stonehill Publishing.

Hildegard of Bingen. 1985. *Illuminations.* Edited by Matthew Fox. Santa Fe: Bear & Co.

Hildegard of Bingen. 1987. *Book of Divine Works: With Letters and Songs.* Edited by Matthew Fox. Santa Fe: Bear & Co.

Hobhouse, Henry. 1987. *Seeds of Change: Five Plants That Transformed Mankind.* Perennial.

Hodgman, Charles D., ed. 1961. *Handbook of Chemistry and Physics.* 42d ed. Chemical Rubber Company.

Hofmann, Albert. 1979. How LSD Originated. Translated by Jonathan Ott. *Journal of Psychedelic Drugs* 11(1,2):53-60.

Hofmann, Albert. 1980. *LSD: My Problem Child*. Translated by Jonathan Ott. McGraw-Hill.

Homer. 1991. *The Odyssey*. Translated by A. T. Murray. Loeb/Harvard.

Horowitz, David. 1978. *The First Frontier: The Indian Wars and America's Origins, 1607–1776*. Simon & Schuster.

Hudson, Travis, and Ernest Underhay. 1978. *Crystals in the Sky: An Intellectual Odyssey involving Chumash Astronomy, Cosmology, and Rock Art*. Ballena Press Anthropological Papers No. 10. Ballena Press.

Huxley, Aldous. 1954. *The Doors of Perception*. Harper & Bros.

Huxley, Aldous. 1956. *Heaven and Hell*. Harper & Bros.

Huxley, Aldous. [1958] 1960. *Brave New World Revisited*. London: Chatto & Windus.

Huxley, Aldous. 1962. *Island*. Harper & Bros.

Huxley, Aldous. 1977. *Moksha: Writings on Psychedelics and the Visionary Experience (1931–1963)*. Edited by Michael Horowitz and Cynthia Palmer. Stonehill Publishing.

Huxley, Laura. 1975. *The Timeless Moment: A Personal View of Aldous Huxley*. Celestial Arts.

Iamblichus. 1988. *The Theology of Arithmetic: On the Mystical, Mathematical, and Cosmological Symbolism of the First Ten Numbers*. Translated by Robin Waterfield. Phanes Press.

Jaeger, Edmund C. 1972. *A Source-Book of Biological Names and Terms*. 3d ed. Charles C. Thomas.

Jaffe, Bernard. 1957. *Crucibles: The Story of Chemistry from Ancient Alchemy to Nuclear Fission*. Fawcett/Premier.

James, William. 1902. *The Varieties of Religious Experience: A Study in Human Nature*. Longmans, Green.

Jeffers, Robinson. 1941. *Be Angry at the Sun and Other Poems*. Random House.

Johns, Timothy. 1990. *With Bitter Herbs They Shall Eat It: Chemical Ecology and the Origins of Human Diet and Medicine*. University of Arizona Press.

Julien, Robert M., M.D. 1988. *A Primer of Drug Action: A Concise, Nontechnical Guide to the Actions, Uses, and Side Effects of Psychoactive Drugs*. 5th ed. W. H. Freeman.

Jung, C. G. 1967. *Alchemical Studies*. Bollingen 20(13). Princeton University Press.

Jung, C. G. 1968. *Psychology and Alchemy*. 2d ed. Bollingen 20(12). Princeton University Press.

Jung, C. G. 1976. *Mysterium Coniunctionis: An Inquiry into the Separation and Synthesis of Psychic Opposites in Alchemy*. 2d ed. Bollingen 20(14). Princeton University Press

Junius, Manfred M. 1985. *Practical Handbook of Plant Alchemy: How to Prepare Medicinal Tinctures and Elixers*. Inner Traditions.

Kaplan, Stuart. 1980. *The Encyclopedia of Tarot*. Vol. 1. U.S. Games.

Kaplan, Stuart. 1985. *The Encyclopedia of Tarot*. Vol. 2. U.S. Games.

Kaplan, Stuart. 1990. *The Encyclopedia of Tarot*. Vol. 3. U.S. Games.

Kapleau, Philip. 1965. *The Three Pillars of Zen: Teaching, Practice, Enlightenment*. Beacon.

Kerenyi, C. 1959. *Asklepios: Archetypal Image of the Physicians's Existence*. Bollingen 65(3). Pantheon.

Kerenyi, C. 1962. *The Religion of the Greeks and Romans*. E. P. Dutton.

Kerenyi, C. 1967. *Eleusis: Archetypal Image of Mother and Daughter*. Bollingen 65(4). Pantheon.

Kerenyi, C. 1976. *Dionysos: Archetypal Image of Indestructible Life*. Bollingen 65. Princeton University Press.

Kervran, C. L. 1972. *Biological Transmutations*. Bristol: Crosby Lockwood.

Kluckhohn, Clyde. [1944] 1968. *Navaho Witchcraft*. Beacon.

Kramer, Heinrich, and James Sprenger. 1971. *The Malleus Maleficarum.* Translated by Montague Summers. Dover.

Krochmal, Arnold, and Connie Krochmal. 1979. *A Guide to the Medicinal Plants of the United States.* Quadrangle.

La Barre, Weston. 1970a. Old and New World Narcotics: A Statistical Question and an Ethnological Reply. *Economic Botany* 24:73-80.

La Barre, Weston. 1970b. *The Ghost Dance: The Origins of Religion.* Doubleday.

La Barre, Weston. 1979. Shamanic Origins of Religion and Medicine. *Journal of Psychedelic Drugs* 11(1,2):7-11.

Larsen, Stephen. 1976. *The Shaman's Doorway: Opening the Mythic Imagination to Contemporary Consciousness.* Harper and Row.

Las Casas, Bartolome. 1992. *The Devastation on the Indies: A Brief Account.* Translated by Herma Briffault. Johns Hopkins University Press.

Lee, Paul. 1994. Personal communication. Santa Cruz, California.

Lehane, Brendan. 1977. *The Power of Plants.* McGraw-Hill.

Lehner, Ernst, and Johanna Lehner. 1973. *Folklore and Odysseys of Food and Medicinal Plants: An Illustrated Sourcebook of Therapeutic, Magical, Exotic and Nutritional Uses.* Farrar, Straus, Giroux.

Lennard, Henry L., et al. 1972. *Mystification and Drug Misuse: Hazards in Using Psychoactive Drugs.* Harper and Row/Perennial.

Lenormand Astro Mythological Tarot Deck. Grimaud.

Leonard, Linda Schierse. 1989. *Witness to the Fire: Creativity and the Veil of Addiction.* Shambhala.

Leon-Portilla, Miguel. 1962. *The Broken Spears: The Aztec Account of the Conquest of Mexico.* Beacon.

Leon-Portilla, Miguel. [1963] 1970. *Aztec Thought and Culture: A Study of the Ancient Nahuatl Mind.* University of Oklahoma Press.

Leon-Portilla, Miguel. 1992. *Fifteen Poets of the Aztec World.* University of Oklahoma Press.

Lessing, Ferdinand D., and Alex Wayman. 1968. *Mkhas Grub Rje's Fundamentals of Buddhist Tantras.* Indo-Iranian Monographs Vol. 8. The Hague: Mouton.

Lewin, Louis. 1931. *Phantastica, Narcotic and Stimulating Drugs: Their Use and Abuse.* London: Kegan Paul, Trench, Trubner.

Lewis, Walter H., and Memory P. F. Elvin-Lewis. 1977. *Medical Botany: Plants Affecting Man's Health.* Wiley.

Li, Hui-Lin. 1978. Hallucinogenic Plants in Chinese Herbals. *Journal of Psychedelic Drugs* 10(1)17-25.

Loeb, E. M. 1929. Shaman and Seer. *American Anthropologist* 31:60-84.

Lommel, Andreas. 1967. *The World of the Early Hunters: Medicine-men, Shamans, and Artists.* London: Evelyn, Adams, & Mackay.

Luck, Georg. 1985. *Arcana Mundi: Magic and Occult in the Greek and Roman Worlds.* Johns Hopkins University Press.

Luna, Luis Eduardo. 1984. The Concept of Plants as Teachers among Four Mestizo Shamans of Iquitos, Northeastern Peru. *Journal of Ethnopharmacology* 11:135-156.

Luna, Luis Eduardo. 1986. *Vegetelismo: Shamanism among the Mestizo Population of the Peruvian Amazon.* Stockholm Studies in Comparative Religion 27. Almqvist & Wiksell International.

Luna, Luis Eduardo, and Pablo Amaringo. 1991. *Ayahuasca Visions: The Religious Iconography of a Peruvian Shaman.* North Atlantic Books.

MacLeod, Barbara. 1980. Sensory Isolation and Vision Quest. Manuscript.

Maier, Michael. 1989. *Atalanta Fugiens: An Edition of the Emblems, Fugues and Epigrams.* Translated by Joscelyn Godwin. Phanes Press.

Mamallacta, Mercedes. 1990. Personal communication. Jatun Sacha, Ecuador.

Martinez, Dieter, and Karlheinz Lohs. 1987. *Poison: Sorcery and Science, Friend and Foe.* Edition Leipzig.

Masson, Marcelle. 1966. *A Bag of Bones: Legends of the Wintu Indians of Northern California.* Naturegraph.

Matsunaga, Alicia. 1969. *The Buddhist Philosophy of Assimilation: The Historical Development of the Honji-Suijaku Theory.* Tuttle.

May, Gerald G. 1991. *Addiction and Grace: Love and Spirituality in the Healing of Addictions.* HarperCollins.

McLean, Adam. 1989. *The Alchemical Mandala: A Survey of the Mandala in the Western Esoteric Traditions.* Phanes Press.

Mead, G. R. S. 1964. *Thrice-Greatest Hermes: Studies in Hellenistic Theosophy and Gnosis.* Watkins.

Merivale, Patricia. 1969. *Pan the Goat-God: His Myth in Modern Times.* Harvard University Press.

Metzner, Ralph. 1974. *Maps of Consciousness.* Collier.

Meyer, Marvin W. 1987. *The Ancient Mysteries: A Sourcebook; Sacred Texts of the Mystery Religions of the Ancient Mediterranean World.* Harper and Row.

Miller, Jonathan Sparrow. 1990. Personal communication. Jatun Sacha, Ecuador.

Minty, Park. 1978. *Interpretation and Dionysos: Method in the Study of a God.* The Hague: Mouton.

Montgomery, Robert. 1990. Personal communication. Jatun Sacha, Ecuador.

Montgomery, Robert. 1991. *Botanical Preservation Corps Field Training Manual.* Sebastopol: Botanical Preservation Corps.

Mooney, James. [1896] 1973. *The Ghost-Dance Religion and Wounded Knee.* Dover.

Moore, Michael. 1979. *Medicinal Plants of the Mountain West.* Museum of New Mexico Press.

Moore, Michael. 1989. *Medicinal Plants of the Desert and Canyon West.* Museum of New Mexico Press.

Moore, Michael. 1993. *Medicinal Plants of the Pacific West.* Red Crane Books.

Morton, Thomas. 1967. *New English Canaan.* With notes by Charles Francis Adams, Jr. Burt Franklin.

Muenscher, Walter Conrad. 1951. *Poisonous Plants of the United States.* Rev. ed. Macmillan.

Munz, Philip A. 1970. *A California Flora.* University of California Press.

Murti, T. V. I. 1974. *The Central Philosophy of Buddhism: A Study of the Madhyamika System.* London: George Allen and Unwin.

Muse, Maude B. 1936. *Materia Medica, Pharmacology, and Therapeutics.* 2d ed. W. B. Saunders.

Musto, David F. 1987. *The American Disease.* Expanded ed. Oxford University Press.

Mylonas, George E. 1974. *Eleusis and the Eleusinian Mysteries.* Princeton University Press.

Nabhan, Gary Paul. 1982. *The Desert Smells Like Rain: A Naturalist in Papago Indian Country.* North Point Press.

Nabhan, Gary Paul. 1987. *Gathering the Desert.* University of Arizona Press.

Nabhan, Gary Paul. 1989. *Enduring Seeds: Native American Agriculture and Wild Plant Conservation.* North Point Press.

Nebesky-Wojkowitz, Rene de. 1956. *Oracles and Demons of Tibet.* Oxford University Press.

Nietzsche, Friedrich. 1974. *The Gay Science: With a Prelude in Rhymes and an Appendix of Songs.* Translated by Walter Kaufmann. Vintage.

Nietzsche, Friedrich. 1992. *Basic Writings.* Translated by Walter Kaufmann. Modern Library.

Noel, Daniel C. 1976. *Seeing Castadeda: Reactions to the "Don Juan" Writings of Carlos Castaneda.* Capricorn/J. P. Putnam's Sons.

O'Flaherty, W. D. 1973. *Asceticism and Eroticism in the Mythology of Shiva.* Oxford University Press.

Ortiz de Montellano, Bernard. 1990. *Aztec Medicine, Health, and Nutrition.* Rutgers University Press.

Ott, Jonathan. 1976. *Hallucinogenic Plants of North America.* Wingbow.

Ott, Jonathan. 1993. *Pharmacotheon: Entheogenic Drugs, Their Plant Sources and History.* Natural Products Co.

Otto, Walter F. 1973. *Dionysus: Myth and Cult.* Indiana University Press.

Ouspensky, P. D. 1974. *The Psychology of Man's Possible Evolution.* 2d ed. Vintage.

Ouspensky, P. D. 1976. *The Symbolism of the Tarot: Philosophy of Occultism in Pictures and Numbers.* Dover.

Ovid. 1960. *The Metamorphoses.* Translated by Horace Gregory. Mentor.

Pagels, Elaine. 1988. *Adam, Eve, and the Serpent.* Random House.

Palmer, Cynthia, and Michael Horowitz, eds. 1982. *Shaman Woman, Mainline Lady: Women's Writings on the Drug Experience.* William Morrow.

Paracelsus. 1537. Sieben Defensiones. In *Selected Writings.* Edited by J. Jacobi. (Pantheon 1958).

Paracelsus. 1958. *Paracelsus: Selected Writings.* 2d ed. Bollingen 28. Edited by Jolande Jacobi. Translated by Norbert Guterman. Pantheon.

Paracelsus. 1967. *The Hermetic and Alchemical Writings of Paracelsus.* Edited by A. E. Waite. 2 vols. University Books.

Paracelsus. 1990. *Paracelsus: Essential Readings.* Translated by Nicholas Goodrick-Clarke. England: Crucible.

Patai, Raphael. 1994. *The Jewish Alchemists: A History and Source Book.* Princeton University Press.

Pauli, Wolfgang. 1955. The Influence of Archetypal Ideas on Kepler. In *The Interpretation of Nature and the Psyche,* C. G. Jung and W. Pauli. Bollingen/Pantheon.

Pendell, Dale, ed. 1975. Jaime de Angulo Section. *Kuksu: Journal of Backcountry Writing.* No. 4.

Plato. 1928. *Euthyphro, Apology, Crito, Phaedo, Phaedrus.* Putnam/Loeb Library.

Pliny. 1968. *Natural History.* Harvard/Loeb.

Plowman, Timothy, et al. 1990. Significance of the Fungus *Balansia cyperi* Infecting Medicinal Species of Cyperus (Cyperaceae) from Amazonia. *Economic Botany* 44(4):452–462.

Porter, Bill. 1993. *Road to Heaven: Encounters with Chinese Hermits.* Mercury House.

Prusinkiewicz, Przemyslaw, and Aristid Lindenmayer. 1990. *The Algorithmic Beauty of Plants.* Springer-Verlag.

Radin, Paul. [1927] 1957. *Primitive Man as Philosopher.* Dover.

Radin, Paul. 1984. *The Trickster: A Study in American Indian Mythology.* Introduction by Stanley Diamond. Schocken Books.

Raffauf, Robert F. 1970a. *A Handbook of Alkaloids and Alkaloid-Containing Plants.* Wiley Interscience.

Raffauf, Robert F. 1970b. Some Notes on the Distribution of Alkaloids in the Plant King-
     dom. *Economic Botany* 24(1):34-38.

Raglan, Lady. 1939. The Green Man in Church Architecture. *Folklore* 50(1)45-57.

Rätsch, Christian. 1989. *Gateway to Inner Space: Sacred Plants, Mysticism, and Psychotherapy.*
     Dorset: Prism Press.

Rätsch, Christian. 1992. *The Dictionary of Sacred and Magical Plants.* Santa Barbara: ABC-
     CLIO.

Reichel-Dolmatoff, Gerardo. 1971. *Amazonian Cosmos: The Sexual and Religious Symbolism
     of the Tukano Indians.* University of Chicago Press.

Reichel-Dolmatoff, Gerardo. 1975. *The Shaman and the Jaguar: A Study of Narcotic Drugs
     among the Indians of Colombia.* Temple University Press.

Reiter, Rayna R., ed. 1975. *Toward an Anthropology of Women.* Monthly Review Press.

Renfrew, J. M. 1973. *Palaeoethnobotany: The Prehistoric Food Plants of the Near East and
     Europe.* London: Methuen/Columbia University Press.

Ricciuti, Edward R. 1978. *The Devil's Garden: Facts and Folklore of Perilous Plants.* Walker.

Riedlinger, Thomas J. 1982. Sartre's Rite of Passage. *Journal of Transpersonal Psychology*
     14(2):105-123.

Riedlinger, Thomas, ed. 1990. *The Sacred Mushroom Seeker: Essays for R. Gordon Wasson.*
     Dioscorides Press.

Rinzler, Carol Ann. 1990. *The Complete Books of Herbs, Spices, and Condiments: From Garden
     to Kitchen to Medicine Chest.* Facts on File.

Rose, Jeanne. 1983 [1972]. *Herbs and Things: A Compendium of Practical and Exotic Herbal
     Lore.* Perigee/Putnam.

Rose, Ronald. 1956. *Living Magic: The Realities Underlying the Psychical Practices and Beliefs
     of Australian Aboriginies.* Rand McNally.

Roszak, Theodore. 1986. *From Satori to Silicon Valley: San Francisco and the American
     Counterculture.* Don't Call It Frisco Press.

Rudgley, Richard. 1994. *Essential Substances: A Cultural History of Intoxicants in Society.* Ko-
     dansha.

Sanders, N. K. 1969. *The Epic of Gilgamesh.* Penguin.

Sanfield, Steve. 1983. *A New Way: Hoops and Reports: 1976–82.* Tooth of Time.

Sartre, Jean Paul. 1959. *Nausea.* Translated by Lloyd Alexander. New Directions.

Schenk, Gustav. 1955. *The Book of Poisons.* Translated by Michael Bullock. Rinehart.

Schleiffer, Hedwig. 1973. *Sacred Narcotic Plants of the New World.* Hafner/Macmillan.

Schleiffer, Hedwig. 1979. *Narcotic Plants of the Old World Used in Rituals and Everyday Life:
     An Anthology of Texts from Ancient Times to the Present.* Lubrect & Cramer.

Schneider, Albert. 1902. *Powdered Vegetable Drugs.* Pittsburgh: Calumet.

Schneiderman, Stuart. 1988. *An Angel Passes: How the Sexes Became Divided.* New York
     University Press.

Schultes, Richard Evans. 1969. Hallucinogens of Plant Origin. *Science* 163:245-254.

Schultes, Richard Evans. 1976. *Hallucinogenic Plants.* Golden Press.

Schultes, Richard Evans. 1977a. Avenues for Future Ethnobotanical Research into New
     World Hallucinogens and Their Uses. In *Drugs, Rituals, and Altered States of Conscious-
     ness.* Edited by B. Du Toit. Amsterdam: Balkema.

Schultes, Richard Evans. [1970] 1977b. The Botanical and Chemical Distribution of Hal-
     lucinogens. In *Drugs, Rituals, and Altered States of Consciousness.* Edited by B. Du Toit.
     Amsterdam: Balkema.

Schultes, Richard Evans. 1979a. Hallucinogenic Plants: Their Earliest Botanical Descrip-
     tions. *Journal of Psychedelic Drugs* 11(1,2):13-24.

Schultes, Richard Evans. 1979b. Phytochemical Gaps in Our Knowledge of Hallucinogens. In *Progress in Phytochemistry*.

Schultes, Richard Evans, and Albert Hofmann. 1979. *Plants of the Gods: Origins of Hallucinogenic Use*. McGraw-Hill.

Schultes, Richard Evans, and Albert Hofmann. 1980. *The Botany and Chemistry of Hallucinogens*. 2d ed. Charles C. Thomas.

Schultes, Richard Evans, and Robert F. Raffauf. 1990. *The Healing Forest: Medicinal and Toxic Plants of the Northwest Amazonia*. Dioscorides Press.

Scully, Virginia. 1970. *A Treasury of American Indian Herbs: Their Lore and Their Use for Food, Drugs, and Medicine*. Bonanza.

Serres, Michel. 1982. *The Parasite*. Johns Hopkins University Press.

Shakespeare, William. 1952. *Complete Works*. Edited by G. B. Harrison. Harcourt, Brace.

Shibayama, Zenkei. 1974. *Zen Comments on the Mumonkan*. Harper and Row.

Shulgin, Alexander T. 1992. *Controlled Substances: Chemical and Legal Guide to Federal Drug Laws*. 2d ed. Ronin.

Shulgin, Alexander, and Ann Shulgin. 1991. *Pihkal: A Chemical Love Story*. Berkeley: Transform Press.

Siegel, Ronald K. 1989. *Intoxication: Life in Pursuit of Artificial Paradise*. E. P. Dutton.

Snellgrove, David L., trans. 1959. *Hevajra Tantra*. Oxford University Press.

Snellgrove, David L. 1967. *The Nine Ways of Bon*. Oxford University Press.

Snyder, Gary. 1970. *Six Sections from Mountains and Rivers without End plus One*. Four Seasons.

Snyder, Gary. 1972. *Manzanita*. Four Seasons.

Snyder, Gary. 1980. *The Real Work: Interviews and Talks 1964–1979*. New Directions.

Snyder, Gary. 1990. *The Practice of the Wild: Essays by Gary Snyder*. North Point Press.

Snyder, Gary. 1992. *No Nature: New and Selected Poems*. Pantheon.

Soothill, William Edward, and Lewis Hodous. 1972. *A Dictionary of Chinese Buddhist Terms: With Sanskrit and English Equivalents and a Sanskrit-Pali Index*. Taipei: Ch'eng Wen.

Staal, Frits. 1975. *Exploring Mysticism: A Methodological Essay*. University of California Press.

Stafford, Peter. 1992. *Psychedelics Encyclopedia*. 3d ed. Ronin.

Strong, James. 1990. *The New Strong's Concordance of the Bible*. Thomas Nelson.

Stuhr, Ernest T. 1933. *Manual of Pacific Coast Drug Plants: A Consideration of the Medicinal Plants Thriving Throughout the Pacific Slope States*. Science Press Printing Co.

Suzuki, Daisetz Teitaro. [1930] 1994a. *Studies in the Lankavatara Sutra*. Taipei: SMC Publishing.

Suzuki, Daisetz Teitaro. [1932] 1994b. *The Lankavatara Sutra: A Mahayana Sutra*. Taipei: SMC Publishing.

Suzuki, Shunryu. 1970. *Zen Mind, Beginner's Mind: Informal Talks on Zen Meditation and Practice*. Weatherhill.

Swain, Tony, ed. 1975. *Plants in the Development of Modern Medicine*. Harvard University Press.

Szasz, Thomas. 1974. *Ceremonial Chemistry: The Ritual Persecution of Drugs, Addicts, and Pushers*. Doubleday/Anchor.

Szasz, Thomas. 1992. *Our Right to Drugs: The Case for a Free Market*. Praeger.

Tabor, Edward. 1970. Plant Poisons in Shakespeare. *Economic Botany* 24(1):81-94.

Tarocchi del Mantegna Deck. [1465] 1981. Edizione del Seleone.

Tart, Charles T., ed. 1969. *Altered States of Consciousness: A Book of Readings*. Wiley.

Taussig, Michael T. 1987. *Shamanism, Colonialism, and the Wild Man: A Study in Terror and Healing*. University of Chicago Press.

Taylor, Thomas. 1991. *The Theoretic Arithmetic of the Pythagoreans.* Samuel Weiser.

Thorwald, Jurgen. 1963. *Science and Secrets of Early Medicine: Egypt, Babylonia, China, Mexico, Peru.* Harcourt, Brace, and World.

Thurman, Robert A. F., trans. 1976. *The Holy Teaching of Vimalakirti: A Mahayana Scripture.* Pennsylvania State University Press.

Thurman, Robert A. F., trans. 1994. *The Tibetan Book of the Dead: Liberation through Understanding in the Between.* Bantam.

Touchstone, Joseph C., and Murrell F. Dobbins. 1983. *Practice of Thin Layer Chromatography.* 2d ed. Wiley.

Trismegistus, Hermes. [1882] 1975. *Divine Pymander, and Other Writings of Hermes Trismegistus.* Translated by John D. Chambers. Samuel Weiser.

Trungpa, Chogyam. 1973. *Cutting through Spiritual Materialism.* Shambhala.

Turner, Alice K. 1993. *The History of Hell.* Harcourt Brace.

Tyler, Varro E. 1981. *Pharmacognosy.* 8th ed. Philadelphia: Lea & Febiger.

Underhill, Ruth Murray. [1938] 1968. *Singing for Power: The Song Magic of the Papago Indians of Southern Arizona.* University of California Press.

Wagner, H.; S. Bladt; and E. M. Zgainski. 1984. *Plant Drug Analysis.* Springer-Verlag.

Waite, Arthur Edward. 1970. *Alchemists through the Ages.* Rudolf Steiner Publications.

Waite, Arthur Edward. 1990. *The Hermetic Museum.* Samuel Weiser.

Waley, Arthur. 1965. *The Way and Its Power: A Study of the Tao Teh Ching and Its Place in Chinese Thought.* London: George Allen and Unwin.

Wasson, R. Gordon. 1963. Notes on the Present Status of Ololiuhqui and the Other Hallucinogens of Mexico. *Botanical Museum Leaflets* 20(6):161–193. Harvard University.

Wasson, R. Gordon, Albert Hofmann, and Carl A. P. Ruck. 1978. *Road to Eleusis: Unveiling the Secret of the Mysteries.* Ethno-mycological Studies no.4. Harcourt Brace Jovanovich.

Wasson, R. Gordon; Stella Kramrisch; Jonathan Ott; and Carl A. P. Ruck. 1986. *Persephone's Quest: Entheogens and the Origins of Religion.* Yale University Press.

Watkins, Calvert. 1978. Let Us Now Praise Famous Grains. *Proceedings of the American Philosophical Society* 122(1):9–17.

Wasson, V. P., and R. Gordon Wasson. 1957. *Mushroom, Russia, and History.* Pantheon.

Watson, Burton. 1968. *The Complete Works of Chuang Tzu.* Columbia University Press.

Watts, Alan. 1962. *Joyous Cosmology: Adventures in the Chemistry of Consciousness.* Vintage.

Weil, Andrew. 1972. *The Natural Mind: A New Way of Looking at Drugs and the Higher Consciousness.* Houghton Mifflin.

Weil, Andrew. 1980. *The Marriage of the Sun and Moon: A Quest for Unity in Consciousness.* Houghton Mifflin.

Weil, Andrew, and Winifred Rosen. 1983. *Chocolate to Morphine: Understanding Mind-Active Drugs.* Houghton Mifflin.

Whitten, Norman E., Jr. 1976. *Sacha Runa: Ethnicity and Adaptation of Ecuadorian Jungle Quichua.* University of Illinois Press.

Whitten, Norman E., Jr. 1982. *Sicuanga Runa: The Other Side of Development in Amazonian Ecuador.* University of Illinois Press.

Wieger, L. 1965. *Chinese Characters: Their Origin, Etymology, History, Classification and Signification.* Dover.

Wind, Edgar. 1968. *Pagan Mysteries in the Renaissance.* Rev. ed. Norton.

Woiche, Istet. [1928] 1992. *Annikadel: The History of the Universe as Told by the Achumawi Indians of California.* Recorded and edited by C. Hart Merriam. University of Arizona Press.

Yates, Frances A. 1972. *The Rosicrucian Enlightenment.* London: Routledge and Kegan Paul.

Yensen, Richard. 1988. From Mysteries to Paradigms: Humanity's Journey from Sacred Plant to Psychedelic Drugs. *ReVision* 10(4):31-50.

Zaehner, R. C. 1972. *Zen, Drugs and Mysticism.* Pantheon.

Zennie, Thomas M., and C. Dwayne Ogzwalla. 1977. Ascorbic Acid and Vitamin A Content of Edible Wild Plants of Ohio and Kentucky. *Economic Botany* 31:76-79.

Zinberg, Norman E., ed. 1977. *Alternate States of Consciousness: Multiple Perspectives on the Study of Consciousness.* Free Press/Macmillan.

Zoja, Luigi. 1989. *Drugs, Addiction and Initiation: The Modern Search for Ritual.* Sigo Press.

Zubrick, James W. 1988. *The Organic Chem Lab Survival Manual: A Student's Guide to Techniques,* 2d ed. Wiley.

Zukofsky, Louis. 1987. *80 Flowers.* Pirate edition.

Books Relating to THANATO-PATHICS

Bower, Bruce. 1993. Smoke Gets in Your Brain. *Science News* 143(3):46-47.

Bramly, Serge. 1975. *Macumba: The Teachings of Maria-Jose, Mother of the Gods.* St. Martin's Press.

Dunhill, Alfred H. 1961. *The Gentle Art of Smoking.* London: Max Reinhardt.

Elferink, J. G. R. 1983. The Narcotic and Hallucinogenic Use of Tobacco in Pre-Columbian Central America. *Journal of Ethnopharmacology* 7:111-122.

Gallegon, Rocio Alarcon. 1990. Personal communication. Jatun Sacha, Ecuador.

Heller, Steve. 1994. Smoke and Mirrors. *U&lc* 21(1):34-37. International Typeface Corporation.

Janiger, Oscar, and Marlene Dobkin de Rios. 1973. Suggestive Hallucinogenic Properties of Tobacco. *Medical Anthropology Newsletter* 4:6-11.

Julien, Robert M., M.D. 1988. *A Primer of Drug Action: A Concise, Nontechnical Guide to the Actions, Uses, and Side-Effects of Psychoactive Drugs.* 5th ed. W. H. Freeman.

Klein, Richard. 1993. *Cigarettes Are Sublime.* Duke University Press.

Raloff, J. 1994. Some Cigarette Makers Manipulate Nicotine. *Science News* (146)1:7.

Schleiffer, Hedwig. 1973. *Sacred Narcotic Plants of the New World.* Hafner/Macmillan.

Sherman, Milton M. 1970. *All About Tobacco.* Sherman National.

Vickery, Hubert Bradford, et al. 1933. *Chemical Investigations of the Tobacco Plant.* Carnegie Institution of Washington.

Watson, Pamela. 1983a. The Ethnopharmacology of Pituri. *Journal of Ethnopharmacology* 8:303-311.

Watson, Pamela. 1983b. *The Precious Foliage: A Study of the Aboriginal Psycho-active Drug Pituri.* University of Sydney Press.

Wilbert, Johannes. 1987. *Tobacco and Shamanism in South America.* Yale University Press.

Books Relating to INEBRIANTS AND ALCOHOL

Abel, Ernest L. 1987. *Alcohol: Wordlore and Folklore.* Prometheus Books.

Alcohol Distiller's Handbook. 1980. Cornville, Arizona: Desert Publications.

Anderson, Edgar. 1952. *Plants, Man, and Life.* University of California Press.

Ardussi, John A. 1977. Brewing and Drinking the Beer of Enlightenment in Tibetan Buddhism: The Doha Tradition in Tibet. *Journal of the American Oriental Society* 97.2:115-124.

Austin, Gregory A. 1985. *Alcohol in Western Society from Antiquity to 1800.* ABC-CLIO Information Services.

Barrios, Virginia B. de. 1971. *A Guide to Tequila, Mezcal and Pulque.* Mexico City: Mexicana Minutae.

Barrows, Susanna, and Robin Room, eds. 1991. *Drinking: Behavior and Belief in Modern History.* University of California Press.

Berry, C. J. J. 1971. *Home Brewed Beers and Stouts.* Amateur Winemaker.

Blood, Benjamin Paul. 1874. *The Anesthetic Revelation and the Gist of Philosophy.*

Blood, Benjamin Paul. N.d. *Tennyson's Trances and the Anaesthetic Revelation.*

Blumgarten, A. S. 1944. *Textbook of Materia Medica, Pharmacology and Therapeutics.* 7th ed. Macmillan.

Bravery, H. E. 1969. *Home Brewing without Failures: How to Make Your Own Beer, Ale, Stout, and Cider.* Arc Books.

Butterfield, Roger. 1947. *The American Past: A History of the United States from Concord to Hiroshima, 1775–1945.* Simon and Schuster.

Carter, William E. 1977. Ritual, the Aymara, and the Role of Alcohol in Human Society. In *Drugs, Rituals, and Altered States of Consciousness* Edited by B. Du Toit. Amsterdam: Balkema.

Chase, Edithe Lea, and Capt. W. E. P. French. N.d. *Toasts for All Occasions.* Barse & Co.

Digby, John and Joan Digby. 1988. *Inspired to Drink: An Anthology.* William Morrow.

Doran, Roxana B. 1930. *Prohibition Punches: A Book of Beverages.* Dorrance & Co.

Du Toit, B., ed. 1977. *Drugs, Rituals, and Altered States of Consciousness.* Amsterdam: Balkema.

Edmonds, Walter D. 1968. *The Musket and the Cross: The Struggle of France and England for North America.* Little, Brown.

Emboden, William. 1977. Dionysus as a Shaman and Wine as a Magical Drug. *Journal of Psychedelic Drugs* 9(3):187-192.

Emerson, E. R. 1908. *Beverages, Past and Present.* G. P. Putnam's Sons.

Engelmann, Larry. 1979. *Intemperance: The Lost War against Liquor.* Free Press.

Faith, Nicholas. 1987. *Cognac.* Godine.

Forbes, R. J. 1948. *Short History of the Art of Distillation.* Leiden: Brill.

Gautier, Theophile, and Charles Baudelaire. 1972. *Hashish, Wine, Opium.* Translated by Maurice Stang. London: Calder & Boyars.

Gilmore, Thomas B. 1987. *Equivocal Spirits: Alcoholism and Drinking in Twentieth Century Literature.* University of North Carolina Press.

Goodwin, Donald W. 1990. *Alcohol and the Writer.* Penguin.

Greene, Mott T. 1992. *Natural Knowledge in Preclassical Antiquity.* Johns Hopkins University Press.

Hannum, Hurst, and Robert S. Blumberg. 1976. *Brandies and Liquors of the World.* Doubleday.

The Holiday Drink Book. 1951. Peter Pauper Press.

Hunt, Peter. 1961. *Eating and Drinking: An Anthology for Epicureans.* London: Ebury Press.

James, William. 1882. Subjective Effects of Nitrous Oxide. In *Altered States of Consciousness.* Edited by Charles T. Tart. (Wiley, 1969).

James, William. 1902. *The Varieties of Religious Experience: A Study in Human Nature.* Longmans, Green.

Kerenyi, Carl. 1976. *Dionysos: Archetypal Image of Indestructible Life.* Bollingen 65. Princeton University Press.

McCarthy, Raymond G., ed. 1959. *Drinking and Intoxication: Selected Readings in Social Attitudes and Controls.* Free Press/Yale Center of Alcoholic Studies.

Mortlock, Geoffrey, and Stephen Williams. 1947. *The Flowing Bowl: A Book of Blithe Spirits and Blue Devils.* London: Hutchinson.

Nashe, Thomas. 1965. *Selected Writings.* Edited by Stanley Wells. Cambridge University Press.

Pliny. 1968. *Natural History.* Harvard/Loeb.

Rae, Simon, ed. 1991. *The Faber Book of Drink, Drinkers and Drinking.* Faber and Faber.

Renfrew, J. M. 1973. *Palaeoethnobotany: The Prehistoric Food Plants of the Near East and Europe.* London: Methuen/Columbia University Press.

Roueche, Berton. 1960. *The Neutral Spirit: A Portrait of Alcohol.* Little, Brown.

Saint-Exupery, Antoine de. 1943. *The Little Prince.* Harcourt, Brace and World.

Sanfield, Steve. 1983. *A New Way: Hoops and Reports: 1976–82.* Tooth of Time.

Simmonds, P. L. 1877. *Hops: Their Cultivation, Commerce, and Uses in Various Countries.* London: E. & F. N. Spon.

Sournia, Jean-Charles. 1990. *A History of Alcoholism.* Basil Blackwell.

Sui, Shu-sen. 1991. *Wine of Endless Life: Taoist Drinking Songs.* Translated by Jerome P. Seaton. White Pine Press.

Thomas, Jerry. 1930. *The Bon Vivant's Companion; or, How to Mix Drinks.* Edited and with an introduction by Herbert Asbury. Knopf.

Toye, Nina, and A. H. Adair. 1925. *Drinks: Long and Short.* London: William Heinemann.

Trawick, Buckner B. 1978. *Shakespeare and Alcohol.* Amsterdam: Rodopi.

Vaillant, George E. 1983. *The Natural History of Alcoholism: Causes, Patterns, and Paths to Recovery.* Harvard University Press.

Wasson, Edmund Atwill. 1914. *Religion and Drink.* Burr.

Watkins, Calvert. 1978. Let Us Now Praise Famous Grains. *Proceedings of the American Philosophical Society* 122(1):9-17.

Waugh, Alec. 1959. *In Praise of Wine, and Certain Noble Spirits.* William Sloane.

Wykes, Alan. 1979. *Ale and Hearty: Gleanings from the History of Brews and Brewing.* London: Jupiter.

Younger, William. 1966. *Gods, Men and Wine.* World Publishing.

Books Relating to ETHER, INHALANTS, N$_2$O

Blood, Benjamin Paul. 1874. *The Anaesthetic Revelation and the Gist of Philosophy.* Amsterdam, N. Y.

Clark, Xenos. quoted in letter/ William James *The Varieties of Religious Experience* (Longmans, Green, 1902).

Davy Humphrey. 1799. *Researches Chemical and Philosophical.* Quoted in Michael Shedlin and David Wallechinsky, with Saunie Salyer, *Laughing Gas: Nitrous Oxide* (Ronin 1992).

Ginsberg, Allen. 1966. *Reality Sandwiches.* City Lights Books.

Hayter, Alethea. 1988. *Opium and the Romantic Imagination: Addiction and Creativity in De Quincey, Coleridge, Baudelaire, and Others.* Rev. ed. Wellingborough, England: Crucible/Thorsons.

High Times. 1978. *High Times Encyclopedia of Recreational Drugs.* Stonehill Publishing.

Irving, John. 1985. *The Cider House Rules.* William Morrow.

James, William. 1902. *The Varieties of Religious Experience: A Study in Human Nature.* Longmans, Green.

Lewin, Louis. 1931. *Phantastica, Narcotic and Stimulating Drugs: Their Use and Abuse.* London: Kegan Paul, Trench, Trubner.

Nunn, J. F. 1987. Clinical Aspects of the Interaction between Nitrous Oxide and Vitamin B12. *British Journal of Anaesthesiology.* 59(1):3-13.

Sharp, Charles W.; Fred Beauvais; and Richard Spence. 1992. *Inhalant Abuse: A Volatile Research Agenda.* National Institute on Drug Abuse Research Monograph no.129.

Sharp, Charles W., and L. Thomas Carroll. 1978. *Voluntary Inhalation of Industrial Solvents.* National Institute on Drug Abuse/Department of Health, Education, and Welfare Publ. No. (ADM)79-779.

Sharp, Charles W., and Mary Lee Brehm. 1977. *Review of Inhalants: Euphoria to Dysfunction.* National Institute on Drug Abuse Research Monograph no.15.

Shedlin, Michael, and David Wallechinsky, with Saunie Salyer. 1992. *Laughing Gas: Nitrous Oxide.* Ronin.

Books Relating to RHAPSODICA AND ABSINTHE

Albert-Puleo, Michael. 1978. Mythobotany, Pharmacology, and Chemistry of Thujone-Containing Plants and Derivatives. *Economic Botany* 32:65-74.

Arnold, Wilfred Niels. 1988. Vincent van Gogh and the Thujone Connection. *Journal of the American Medical Association* (260)20:3042-3044.

Arnold, Wilfred Niels. 1989. Absinthe. *Scientific American* June:113-117.

Castillo, J. Del, et al. 1975. Marijuana, Absinthe and the Central Nervous System. *Nature* 253:365-366.

Conrad, Barnaby, III. 1988. *Absinthe: History in a Bottle.* Chronicle Books.

Delahaye, Marie-Claude. N.d. *L'Absinthe: Histoire de la Fee Verte.* Berger-Levrault.

Dick, William B. 1903. *Dick's Encyclopedia of Practical Receipts and Processes.* Dick & Fitzgerald.

Fenaroli, Giovanni. 1971. *Handbook of Flavor Ingredients.* Edited, translated, and revised by Thomas E. Furia and Nicolo Bellanca. Chemical Rubber Co.

Flower, D., and H. Maas. 1967. *The Letters of Ernest Dowson.* London: Cassell.

Kenyon, Michael. 1990. A Bottle of Absinthe *Gourmet,* October:144.

Meilach, Dona, and Mel Meilach. 1979. *Homemade Liqueurs.* Contemporary Books.

Pal, D. C., and S. K. Jain. 1989. Notes on Lodha Medicine in Midnapur District, West Bengal, India. *Economic Botany* 43(4):464-470.

Rack, John. 1863 *The French Wine and Liquor Manufacturer.* Dick & Fitzgerald.

Snyder, Gary. 1991. Earrings Dangling and Miles of Desert. *Yale Review* 80(1 and 2) April.

Sournia, Jean-Charles. 1990. *A History of Alcoholism.* Basil Blackwell.

Vogt, Donald D. 1981. Absinthium: A Nineteenth-Century Drug of Abuse. *Journal of Ethnopharmacology* 4:337-342.

Vogt, Donald D., and Michael Montagne. 1982. Absinthe: Behind the Emerald Mask. *The International Journal of the Addictions* 17(6):1015-1029.

Zafar, M. M.; M. E. Hamdard; and A. Hameed. 1990. Screen of Artemisia Absinthium for Antimalarial Effects on *Plasmodium berghei* in Mice: A Preliminary Report. *Journal of Ethnopharmacology* 30:223-226.

Zolotow, Maurice. 1971. Absinthe. *Playboy,* June:169-174.

Books Relating to EUPHORIANTS

Addens, T. J. 1939. *The Distribution of Opium Cultivation and the Trade in Opium.* Haarlem: Joh. Enschede en Zonen.

Aldrich, Michael. 1979. *The Dope Chronicles: 1850–1950.* Edited by Gary Silver. Harper and Row.

Algren, Nelson. 1949. *The Man with the Golden Arm.* Doubleday.

Atal, C. K., and B. M. Kapur, eds. 1982. *Cultivation and Utilization of Medicinal Plants..*

Baudelaire, Charles. 1971. *Artificial Paradise: On Hashish and Wine as Means of Expanding Individuality.* Translated by Ellen Fox. Herder and Herder.

Bentley, K. W. 1954. *The Chemistry of the Morphine Alkaloids.* Monographs on the Chemistry of Natural Products. Clarendon/Oxford University Press.

Berridge, Virginia, and Griffith Edwards. 1987. *Opium and the People: Opiate Use in Ninetheenth-Century England.* Yale University Press.

Bruhn, J. G., and U. Nyman. 1982. *Papaver bracteatum* as a Source of Thebaine. In *Cultivation and Utilization of Medicinal Plants.* Edited by C. K. Atal.

Burroughs, William. 1959. *Naked Lunch.* Grove Press/Castle Books.

Cocteau, Jean. 1958. *Opium: The Diary of a Cure.* Translated by Margaret Crosland and Sinclair Road. Grove Press/Evergreen.

Cooke, Mordecai C. [1860] 1990. *The Seven Sisters of Sleep: A Popular History of the Seven Prevailing Narcotics of the World.* Quarterman.

Courtwright, David T. 1982. *Dark Paradise: Opiate Addiction in America before 1940*. Harvard University Press.

Darwin, Erasmus. 1978. *The Botanic Garden: The Loves of the Plants*. Garland Publishing.

Delgado, Jaime N., and William A. Remers, eds. 1991. *Wilson and Gisvold's Textbook of Organic, Medicinal, and Pharmaceutical Chemistry*. 9th ed. Lippincott.

De Quincey, Thomas. [1822] 1950. *Confessions of an English Opium Eater*. Heritage Press.

De Quincey, Thomas. [1856] 1982. *Confessions of an English Opium Eater*. Everyman's Library.

Detzer, Eric. 1988. *Poppies: Odyssey of an Opium Eater*. Mercury House.

Drake, William Daniel, Jr. 1974. *The International Cultivator's Handbook*. Wingbow.

Ebin, David, ed. 1961. *The Drug Experience: First-Person Accounts of Addicts, Writers, Scientists, and Others*. Orion.

Edmonds, John Maxwell. 1959. *The Fragments of Attic Comedy*. Vol. 2. Leiden: Brill.

Extraction of Alkaloids from Papaver Species. 1968. *Institut National de Recherche Chimique Appliquee Brit*. 1:128-30.

Gampopa. 1971. *Jewel Ornament of Liberation*. Translated by Herbert V. Guenther. Clear Light Series, Shambhala.

Gautier, Theophile, and Charles Baudelaire. 1972. *Hashish, Wine, Opium*. Translated by Maurice Stang. London: Calder & Boyars.

Grey-Wilson, Christopher. 1993. *Poppies: The Poppy Family in the Wild and in Cultivation*. Timber Press.

Griffith, William. 1993. *Opium Poppy Garden: The Way of a Chinese Grower*. Ronin.

Hayter, Alethea. 1988. *Opium and the Romantic Imagination: Addiction and Creativity in De Quincey, Coleridge, Baudelaire, and Others*. Rev. ed. Wellingborough, England: Crucible/Thorsons.

Hazum, E., et al. 1981. Morphine in Cow and Human Milk. *Science* 213: 1010-1012.

Hoffmann, F., La Roche & Co. 1937. Morphine and Codeine from Poppies. *Chemical Abstracts* 31:2360.

Hogshire, Jim. 1994. *Opium for the Masses: A Practical Guide to Growing Poppies and Making Opium*. Loompanics.

Husain, Akhtar, and J. R. Sharma. 1983. *The Opium Poppy*. Lucknow, India: Central Institute of Medicinal and Aromatic Plants. India: Lucknow.

Jeffers, Robinson. 1941. *Be Angry at the Sun and Other Poems*. Random House.

Kohn, Marek. 1987. *Narcomania: On Heroin*. Faber and Faber.

Krivanek, Jara. 1988. *Heroin: Myths and Reality*. Sydney: Allen and Unwin.

Latimer, Dean, and Jeff Goldberg. 1981. *Flowers in the Blood: The Story of Opium*. Franklin Watts.

Levinthal, Charles F. 1988. *Messengers of Paradise: Opiates and the Brain; The Struggle over Pain, Rage, Uncertainty and Addiction*. Anchor/Doubleday.

Lewin, Louis. 1931. *Phantastica, Narcotic and Stimulating Drugs: Their Use and Abuse*. London: Kegan Paul, Trench, Trubner.

Lydon, Susan Gordon. 1993. *Take the Long Way Home: Memoirs of a Survivor*. Harper.

Madyastha, K. Madhava, and Surendra P. Bhatnagar. 1982. Chemical and Biochemical Aspects of Opium Alkaloids. In *Cultivation and Utilization of Medicinal Plants*. , Edited by C. K. Atal and B.M. Kapur. Jammu-Tawi, India: Council of Scientific and Industrial Research.

McCoy, Alfred W. 1972. *The Politics of Heroin in Southeast Asia*. Harper and Row.

Merlin, Mark David. 1984. *On the Trail of the Ancient Opium Poppy*. Fairleigh Dickinson University Press.

Narcotics Anonymous. 1988. 5th ed. World Service Office.

O. 1979. *Opium Poppy Cultivation.* Seattle: Real Concepts.

Palmer, Cynthia, and Michael Horowitz, eds. 1982. *Shaman Woman, Mainline Lady: Women's Writings on the Drug Experience.* William Morrow.

Pepper, Art, and Laurie Pepper. 1979. *Straight Life: The Story of Art Pepper.* Schirmer.

Ramanathan, V. S. 1966. Progress in Production of Opium in India. *Sci. Cult.* 32(1)3-8.

Ramanathan, V. S. 1980. Study on the Deterioration of Morphine and Its Preservation by Chemicals in the Fresh Latex of Opium Poppy. *Indian Journal of Agricultural Research* Part 2, 13:85.

Ramanathan, V. S. 1982. Utilization of Opium and Its Alkaloids in Medicine. In *Cultivation and Utilization of Medicinal Plants.* Edited by C. K. Atal and B.M. Kapur. India: Jammu-Tawi, Council of Scientific and Industrial Research.

Ramparts editors, and Frank Browning. 1972. *Smack.* Harrow Books/Harper and Row.

Schelling, Andrew. 1984. Some Notes on Drinking a Pipe. Manuscript.

Schmid, H., and P. Karrer. 1945. On Water Soluble Substances from *Papaver s. Helv. Chim. Acta* 28:722-740.

Singh, H. G. 1982. Cultivation of Opium Poppy. In *Cultivation and Utilization of Medicinal Plants.* Edited by C. K. Atal and B.M. Kapur. Jammu-Tawi, India: Council of Scientific and Industrial Research.

Small, Lyndon F., and Robert E. Lutz. 1932. *Chemistry of the Opium Alkaloids.* U.S. Government Printing Office.

Trebach, Arnold S. 1982. *The Heroin Solution.* Yale University Press.

Westermeyer, Joseph. 1982. *Poppies, Pipes, and People: Opium and Its Use in Laos.* University of California Press.

Books Relating to PACIFICA AND KAVA

Cox, Paul Alan, and Sandra Anne Banack. 1991. *Islands, Plants, and Polynesians: An Introduction to Polynesian Ethnobotany.* Dioscorides Press.

Fackelmann, Kathy A. 1992. Pacific Cocktail: The History, Chemistry, and Botany of the Mind-Altering Kava Plant. *Science News* 141:424-425.

Glassman, Sidney F. 1950. *Ponape's National Beverage.* Research Reviews, Office of Naval Research, Department of the Navy.

Lebot, Vincent, Mark Merlin, and Lamont Lindstrom. 1992. *Kava: The Pacific Drug.* Yale University Press.

Lindstrom, Lamont. 1991. Kava, Cash, and Custom in Vanuatu. *Cultural Survival Quarterly* 15(2):28-31.

Books Relating to EXISTENTIANS AND SKA PASTORA

Blosser, Bret. 1994. Lessons in Mazatec Curanderismo. Manuscript

Blosser, Bret. 1988-1993. Personal communications.

Epling, Carl, and Carlos D. Jativa-M. 1962. A New Species of *Salvia* from Mexico. *Botanical Museum Leaflets* 20(7):75-76. Harvard University.

Hofmann, Albert. 1980. *LSD: My Problem Child.* Translated by Jonathan Ott. McGraw-Hill.

Hofmann, Albert. 1990. Ride through the Sierra Mazateca in Search of the Magic Plant *Ska Maria Pastora.* In *The Sacred Mushroom Seeker.* Edited by Thomas J. Riedlinger. Dioscorides Press.

Montgomery, Rob. 1993. Personal communications.

Nichols, David. 1993. *Screening Report: Salvinorin A.* Manuscript.

Nichols, David. 1993-1994. Personal communications.

Ortega, Alfredo; John F. Blount; and Percy S. Manchand. 1982. Salvinorin: A New Trans-Neoclerodane Diterpene from *Salvia divinorum* (Labiatae). *Journal of the Chemical Society Perkins Transactions* 1:2505-2508.

Ott, Jonathan. 1992,1994. Personal communications. Xalapa, Vera Cruz, Mexico.

Ott, Jonathan. 1993. *Pharmacotheon: Entheogenic Drugs, Their Plant Sources and History.* Natural Products Co.

Reisfield, Aaron S. 1993. The Botany of *Salvia divinorum* (Labiatae). SIDA 15(3):349-366.

Rooke, Steve. 1993. Personal communication.

Siebert, Daniel J. 1993-1994. Personal communications.

Siebert, Daniel J. 1994. *Salvia divinorum* and Salvinorin A: New Pharmacologic Findings. *Journal of Ethnopharmacology* 43:53-56.

Valdes, Leander J., III; G. M. Hatfield; M. Koreeda; A. G. Paul. 1987. Studies of S*alvia divinorum* (Lamiaceae), an Hallucinogenic Mint from the Sierra Mazateca in Oaxaca, Central Mexico. *Economic Botany* 41(2)283-291.

Valdes, Leander J., III; José Luis Díaz; Ara G. Paul. 1983. Ethnopharmacology of Ska Pastora (*Salvia divinorum*, Epling and Jativa-M). *Journal of Ethnopharmacology* 7:287-312.

Valdes, Leander J., III; W. M. Butler; G. M. Hatfield; A. G. Paul; M. Koreeda. 1984. Divinorin A, a Psychotropic Terpenoid, and Divinorin B from the Hallucinogenic Mexican Mint *Salvia divinorum. Journal of Organic Chemistry* 49:4716-4720.

Valdes, Leander J., III. 1994. S*alvia divinorum* and the Unique Diterpene Hallucinogen, Salvinorin (Divinorin) A. *Journal of Psychoactive Drugs* 26(3):277-283.

Wasson, R. Gordon. 1962. A New Mexican Psychotropic Drug from the Mint Family. *Botanical Museum Leaflets* 20(1):77-84. Harvard University.

Wasson, R. Gordon. 1963. Notes on the Present Status of Ololiuhqui and the Other Hallucinogens of Mexico. *Botanical Museum Leaflets* 20(6):161-193. Harvard University.

**Books
Relating to
EVAESTHETICA
AND
CANNABIS**

Abel, Ernest L. 1980. *Marihuana: The First Twelve Thousand Years.* London: Plenum Press.

Aldrich, Michael R. N.d. Notes on Brunner (1977). Manuscript.

Aldrich, Michael R. 1977. Tantric Cannabis Use in India. *Journal of Psychedelic Drugs* 9(3):227-233.

Aldrich, Michael R. 1979. *The Dope Chronicles: 1850–1950.* Edited by Gary Silver. Harper and Row.

Aldrich, Michael R. 1994. Personal communications.

Baudelaire, Charles. 1971. *Artificial Paradise: On Hashish and Wine as Means of Expanding Individuality.* Translated by Ellen Fox. Herder and Herder.

Baudelaire, Charles, and Theophile Gautier. 1971. *The Poem of Hashish: The Hashish Club.* Harper Perennial.

Benet, Sula. 1976. Early Diffusion and Folk Uses of Hemp. In *Cannabis and Culture.* Edited by Vera Rubin. The Hague: Mouton.

Berke, Joseph. 1974. *The Cannabis Experience: An Interpretive Study of the Effects of Marijuana and Hashish.* London: P. Owen.

Bloomquist, Edward R. 1972. *Marijuana: The Second Trip.* Glencoe Press. Boire, Richard Glen. 1993. *Marijuana Law.* Ronin. Brecher, Edward M., and the editors of *Consumer Reports.* 1972. *Licit and Illicit Drugs: The Consumers Union Report on Narcotics, Stimulants, Depressants, Inhalants, Hallucinogens, and Marijuana Including – Caffeine, Nicotine, and Alcohol.* Little, Brown.

Brunner, Theodore F. 1977. Marijuana in Ancient Greece and Rome? The Literary Evidence. *Journal of Psychedelic Drugs* 9(3):221-225.

Conrad, Chris. 1993. *Hemp: Lifeline to the Future.* Creative Xpressions.

Crowley, Aleister. 1909. The Psychology of Hashish. In *Hasheesh: The Herb Dangerous.* Edited by David Hoye. (Level Press,.1974).

De Angulo, Jaime. N.d. Unpublished papers. Special Collections. University of California, Santa Cruz.

Devane W. A., Mechoulam R., et al. 1992. Isolation and Structure of a Brain Constituent That Binds to the Cannabinoid Receptor. *Science* 258(5090):1946–1949.

Dorje, K. Tendzin. 1994. Soma, Amrita, and Dutsi: Psychotropic Plants in Indian Religions from the Vedas to Vajrayana. Manuscript.

Ebin, David, ed. 1961. *The Drug Experience: First-Person Accounts of Addicts, Writers, Scientists, and Others.* Orion.

Emboden, William. 1979. *Narcotic Plants: Hallucinogens, Stimulants, Inebriants, and Hypnotics, Their Origins and Uses.* Rev. ed. Macmillan.

Fackelmann, Kathy A. 1993. Marijuana and the Brain: Scientists Discover the Brain's Own THC. *Science News* 143:88.

Flattery, David Stophlet, and Martin Schwartz. 1989. *Haoma and Harmaline: The Botanical Identity of the Indo-Iranian Sacred Hallucinogen "Soma."* University of California Publications in Near Eastern Studies, vol. 21. University of California Press

Frank, Mel, and Ed Rosenthal. 1990. *Marijuana Grower's Guide.* Rev. ed. Red Eye Press.

Gautier, Theophile, and Charles Baudelaire. 1972. *Hashish, Wine, Opium.* Translated by Maurice Stang. London: Calder & Boyars.

Gold, D. 1993. *Cannabis Alchemy: The Art of Modern Hashmaking.* Ronin/Twentieth Century Alchemist.

Goode, Erich. 1993. *Drugs in American Society.* 4th ed. McGraw-Hill.

Grinspoon, Lester. 1971. *Marihuana Reconsidered.* Harvard University Press.

Grinspoon, Lester, and James B. Bakalar. 1993. *Marihuana: The Forbidden Medicine.* Yale University Press.

High Times. 1978. *High Times Encyclopedia of Recreational Drugs.* Stonehill Publishing.

Hoye, David, ed. 1974. *Hasheesh: The Herb Dangerous.* Level Press.

Li, Hui-Lin. 1978. Hallucinogenic Plants in Chinese Herbals. *Journal of Psychedelic Drugs* 10(1)17–25.

Li, Hui-Lin. 1976. Origin and Use of Cannabis in Eastern Asia: Their Linguistic-CulturalImplication. In *Cannabis and Culture.* Edited by Vera Rubin. The Hague: Mouton.

Ludlow, Fitz Hugh. 1979. *The Hasheesh Eater: Being Passages from the Life of a Pythagorean.* City Lights Books.

Marihuana: A Signal of Misunderstanding: First Report of the National Commission on Marihuana and Drug Abuse. 1972. U.S. Government Printing Office.

Mezzrow, Milton "Mezz," and Bernard Wolfe. 1946. *Really the Blues.* Random House.

Nahas, Gabriel G. 1984. *Marihuana in Science and Medicine.* Raven Press.

Nietzsche, Friedrich. 1954. *The Philosophy of Nietzsche.* Random House.

Novak, William. 1980. *High Culture: Marijuana in the Lives of Americans.* Knopf.

Petersen, Robert C., ed. 1977. *Marihuana Research Findings: 1976.* National Institute on Drug Abuse Research Monograph No.14.

Rosenthal, Franz. 1971. *The Herb: Hashish versus Medieval Muslim Society.* Leiden: Brill.

Rubin, Vera. 1976. *Cannabis and Culture.* The Hague: Mouton.

Sacharoff, Shanta. 1972. *Flavors of India.* 101 Productions.

Schultes, R. E.; W. M. Klein; T. Plowman; T. E. Lockwood. 1976. Cannabis: An Example of Taxonomic Neglect. In *Cannabis and Culture.* Edited by Vera Rubin. The Hague: Mouton.

Schultes, Richard Evans, and Albert Hofmann. 1979. *Plants of the Gods: Origins of Hallucinogenic Use.* McGraw-Hill.

Sloman, Larry. 1979. *Reefer Madness: The History of Marijuana in America.* Bobbs-Merrill.

Solomon, David, ed. 1966. *Marijuana Papers.* Bobbs-Merrill.

Starks, Michael. 1990. *Marijuana Chemistry: Genetics, Processing and Potency.* 2d ed. Ronin.

Szasz, Thomas. 1974. *Ceremonial Chemistry: The Ritual Persecution of Drugs, Addicts, and Pushers.* Doubleday/Anchor.

Tart, Charles T. 1971. *On Being Stoned.* Palo Alto: Science and Behavior Books.

Thompson, D'Oud. 1994. Personal communication.

Touw, Mia. 1981. The Religious and Medicinal Uses of Cannabis in China, India, and Tibet. *Journal of Psychoactive Drugs* 13(1):23-34.

Wieger, L. 1965. *Chinese Characters: Their Origin, Etymology, History, Classification and Signification.* Dover.

Yeats, W. B. 1944. *Autobiography.* Macmillan.

Zinberg, Norman E. 1979. On Cannabis and Health. *Journal of Psychedelic Drugs* 11(1,2):135-144.

CREDITS

I. AUTHOR'S ACKNOWLEDGMENTS

Many people contributed to this book, both directly and indirectly. I would like particularly to thank Norman O. Brown, Scott Clements, Antonio Escohotado, Robert Forte, R. Edward Grumbine, Gary Paul Nabhan, Merle Pendell, Andrew Schelling, Jack Shoemaker, and Gary Snyder, for critically reading the manuscript and offering valuable suggestions.

Many others gave freely of their time, knowledge, encouragement, and poetic and scientific acumen, including Robert Aitken, Alaska (Olvido Gara), Michael Aldrich, Steven Beckwitt, Jacqueline Bellon, Bret Blosser, Marina Bokelman, Jace Callaway, Peter Cerny, Philip Daughtry, Don Davies, James DeKorne, Marian Dockham, K. Tendzin Dorje, Josep Fericgla, Francisco Festi, Leo Figgs, Nelson Foster, Peter Furst, Joel Goodkind, Clark Heinrich, Nick Herbert, Gary Hillerson, Michael Horowitz, Marcia Jacobs, William Kasper, Greg Keith, Laura Kelly, Dorje Kirsten, Paul Lee, Juan Luque, Barbara MacLeod, Mercedes Mamallacta, Thomas Marshall, Robyn Martin, Dennis J. McKenna, Terence McKenna, Barbara Meier, Ralph Metzner, Jonathan Miller, Robert Montgomery, Jonathan Ott, Howard Pendell, The Peninsula Group of Santa Cruz, Just Pope, Karl Ray, Thomas Riedlinger, Steven Rooke, Giorgio Samorini, Steven Sanfield, Yerba Santa, Stacy Schaefer, Robert Schelling, Armand Schwerner, Alexander T. Shulgin, Anne Shulgin, Daniel Siebert, Will Staple, Allen Stovall, Susan Suntree, John Sweeney, Richard Thieltges, Da'oud Thompson, Manuel Torres, Steven Van Heiden, Djahel Vivaver, Anne Waldman, Bob Wallace, and Jonathan F. Winter.

I am indebted to them all.

I especially want to thank Thomas Christensen and Mercury House for the vision and expertise to transform an eccentric manuscript into a finished book.

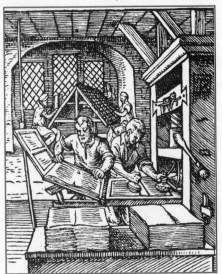

BOOKWORK, JOST AMMAN, 1568

II. ILLUSTRATIONS

We have attempted to designate artist's or owner's "official" titles by quotation marks, while titles assigned by others are indicated by initial capitals with no quotation marks (the sources we used, however, often make the distinction uncertain). Page references are provided in parentheses following titles.

The repeating decorative border (xiii, 8, 10, 23, 26, 78, 137, 208) is taken from *Mer des Hystoires,* 1488–89 (a translation of the Medieval classic of history and legend, the *Rudimentum Noviciorum*), printed by Pierre Le Rouge for Vincent Commin.

Preliminaries TITLE PAGE: Title page illustration for *De natura stirpium libri tres* (iii) by Simon de Colines, 1536. TABLE OF CONTENTS: The Lover in the Wood (ix) from *Hypnerotomachia Poliphili,* 1499 [for this, the only illustrated book from Aldus Manutius's Aldine Press, Aldus employed a font designed by Francesco Griffo; it is the model for the typeface called Bembo, which is employed in the present book]; The Fool and His Bauble (xii) from John H. Towsen, *Clowns,* 1976 (where the original source is not identified). Following the FOREWORD BY GARY SNYDER: Adam and Eve (xv) from Anthoine Vérard, *Bible en Francoys,* 1505.

Power Plants ON THE NATURE OF POISON: alchemical symbols (4) drawn by Thomas Christensen; "The Alchemist" (5), by Martin Johann Schmidt, 18th c., from *The High Times Encyclopedia of Recreational Drugs.* PLANT PEOPLE: Daphne (6) by Jacqueline Bellon; portrait of Nicholas Copernicus (7) courtesy of the author. PLANTS AS TEACHERS: "Nuestra Gente 'Namuy Misag,'" (9) Hernández, de Alba, G., Bogotá, reprinted from *Plants of the Gods,* Richard Evans Schultes and Albert Hofmann, copyright © 1992 by permission of EMB-Service for Publishers. ON THE NATURE OF THE ALLY: "Siberian Petroglyph of Shaman with Mushroom-Crowned Head" (11) from Biedermann, H., *Lexikon der Felsbildkunst,* Graz, 1976, reprinted from *Plants of the Gods,* Richard Evans Schultes and Albert Hofmann, copyright © 1992 by permission of EMB-Service for Publishers. PRUNUS EMARGINATA: "Prunus Emarginata" (14) from Willis Linn Jepson, *A Manual of the Flowering Plants of California,* 1925. THE GREAT WORK: plant and crystal woodcut (16) by Victor Hammer from Otto Reicher's *Thauernreise,* 1938; "Alchemya" (17) from *The High Times Encyclopedia of Recreational Drugs.* SUN MEDICINE/MOON MEDICINE: Tarot Cards (Sun, Moon, Two of Pentacles) (18–19) from Arthur Edward Waite, *The Pictorial Key to the Tarot* (1910), "from designs by Pamela Colman Smith"; the tao with hexagrams (20). SCIRPUS ATROVIRENS: "Scirpus Californicus" (21) from Willis Linn Jepson, *A Manual of the Flowering Plants of California,* 1925. METHODOLOGY I: Bodhidharma with Tea Plant, (24) from Ernst and Johanna Lehner, *Folklore and Odysseys of Food and Medicinal Plants,* 1962, where it is identified as "an old Chinese drawing." METHODOLOGY II:

"Le Marquis de Force-Nature en Habit de Laboratoire" (27), 1716, from *The High Times Encyclopedia of Recreational Drugs*.

Thanatopathia   THANATOPATHIA: Death on Horseback (30), 1463, from *Der Ackermann aus Böhmen*, ca. 1463. NICOTIANA TABACUM: Mayan God (32) from Palenque, Mexico; Tobbaco Flower (33 and 35) from 16th c. Aztec statue of Xochipilli, the Prince of Flowers; Nose Pipe (36) from Oviedo y Valdés, 1547 ; "Broad-Leaved Petum" (37) from Charles de l'Ecluse, 1579; Tobacco Plant (39) from Nicolas Monarde, *Joyfull Newes out of the Newe Founde Worlde*, 1577; Nicotiana, (41) from Matthias de l'Obel, *Stirpium Adversaria Nova*, 1576. DUBOISIA HOPWOODII: "Duboisia hopwoodii" (47) drawn by Carolyn Knight, reprinted from Pamela Watson, *The Precious Foliage*, by permission of the Anthropology Museum, The University of Queensland. KILLING TIME: "Calavera" (48) from José Guadalupe Posada, *El Gran Panteón Amoroso* (The Great Cemetery of Lovers, ca. 1895); Death and the Printers (49) from *La Grand Danse Macabre*, Lyon, 1500; the Dying Man's Visions (50) from *Ars Moriendi*, 1450.

Inebriantia   INEBRIANTIA: Toast, (52) Aubrey Beardsley, 1893. SACCHAROMYCES CEREVISIAE: Toast (53), from Günther Zainer, *Das Golden Spiel*, 1472; Playing Card (54) from Jost Amman, *Charta Lusoria*, 1588. VITIS VINIFERA: Wine Production (60) from Crescenzi, *Libro della Agricultura*, 1511; "Wine Grape" (61) from Mattioli, *Commentaires*, 1579; Image of Lovers and Fool in Arbor (62) redrawn by Thomas Christensen from original by Alart du Hameel, late 15th century; Grape Arbor (64) from Cresenzi, *Opus Commodorum Ruralium*, 1493. HORDEUM VULGARE: Beer Tasters, (66) from seal of Hammurabi, 1913 BC; "Hoppe-Garden" (67) from Scot, *A Perfite Platforme*, 1576; Goddess of Pulque (68) from the *Codex Laud*; "Hop Plant" (69) from Dodonaes, *Purgantium*, 1574. AQUA VITAE: Red-Figure Vase Painting (73) by "The Brygos Painter," 5th c. BC; "Gin Lane" (74), William Hogarth, 1753; "A Students' Drinking Bout" (75) from *Directorium statuum*, 1489; Etching by Anders Zorn, *The Toast*, (77) 1893. All rights reserved. The Metropolitan Museum of Art, Bequest of Blanche S. Guggenheimer, 1953. (53.628.1). THE ALCOHOLIC MUSE: Bacchus Asleep with Playing Children (79), Hans Baldung Grien, 1510, from the Christian Brothers Collection at the Wine Museum of San Francisco; THE POISON PATH II: Ten of Swords (81) from Arthur Edward Waite, *The Pictorial Key to the Tarot* (1910), "from designs by Pamela Colman Smith"; comic business (82) from from John H. Towsen, *Clowns*, 1976 (where the original source is not identified). ETHER: inhaling device and 19th c. dentistry cartoon (84, 86) from *The High Times Encyclopedia of Recreational Drugs*; FOSSIL FUEL: illustration (90) by Guy Murchie from his *The Seven Mysteries of Life: An Exploration of Science and Philosophy*, 1978, copyright © 1978 by Guy Murchie, reprinted by permission of Houghton Mifflin Co., all rights reserved; MEAD AND THE DIVINE MADNESS: Mycenaean gem (93) after V. Karger, *Maissau*; reproduced in Marija Gimbutas, *The Gods and Goddess of Old Europe 7000–3500 BC: Myths, Legends and Cult Images*, University of California Press, 1974; Renaissance bee keeping (94) from *Œuvres de Virgil*, Lyon, 1529; honey harvesting (96) from Mattioli, *Commentaires*, 1579.

Rhapsodica ON THE SEDUCTION OF ANGELS: hermaphroditic angel (100) from *Rosarium Philosophorum,* the second part of *De Alchimia Opuscula,* 1550; Turkish miniature (101) reproduced in Peter Lamborn Wilson, *Angels,* The Alchemist and the Angel (102) from *Musaeum Hermeticum Reformatum et Amplificatum . . .,* 1678. ARTE-MISIA ABSINTHIUM: Artemisia Tridentata (103) from from Willis Linn Jepson, *A Manual of the Flowering Plants of California,* 1925; Artemesia absinthium (105) from Mattioli, *Commentaires,* 1579; "George Moore at the Café de la Nouvelle Athènes" (106) Edouard Manet, 1878; "Absinthe Drinkers," (107) anonymous, 1870s; "The Drinker" ("La Buveuse") (110), Henri de Toulouse-Lautrec, 1889, Indian ink and blue chalk, Musée Toulouse-Lautrec collection, all rights reserved by Musée Toulouse-Lautrec, Albi, France; "The Absinthe Drinker" (113), Edouard Manet, 1862. CALEA ZACATECHICHI: "Calea zacatechichi" (114) drawn by I. Brady, from Schultes and Hofmann, *Botany and Chemistry of Hallucinogens,* 2nd ed., 1980, courtesy of Charles C Thomas, Publisher, Springfield, Illinois.

Euphorica EUPHORICA: The Goddess of Night (118) from Ernst and Johanna Lehner, *Folklore and Odysseys of Food and Medicinal Plants,* 1962, where it is identified as an "antique cameo." PAPAVER SOMNIFERUM: "Papaver somniferum" (121) after Kohler, *Medizal-Planzen-Atlas,* 1887; "Papaver Somniferum" (127) from Mattioli, *Commentaires,* 1579;. "Corn Poppy" (Papaver rhoeus) (134) from Mattioli, *Commentaires,* 1579. HEROIN AND THE NATURE OF ADDICTION: "Help Your Local Junky Kick," (141) Michael Myers, early 1970s.

Pacifica PIPER METHYSTICUM: Piper methysticum (150) from *Traveaux et Documents,* #205 (1986), "Les Kavas de Vanautu." Reprinted by permission of Edition de l'Orstom, Paris.

Existentia SALVIA DIVINORUM: "Salvia melliflora" (156) from Willis Linn Jepson, *A Manual of the Flowering Plants of California,* 1925; "Leaf-Primordia at the Growing-Point" (159) from George Adams and Olive Whicher, *The Plant Between the Sun and Earth,* 1980, where it is attributed "from Church," without further explanation; "Sage" (161) from Valentin, *Krauterbuch,* 1719; "Salvia divinorum" (166) drawn by I. Brady, from Schultes and Hofmann, *Botany and Chemistry of Hallucinogens,* 2nd ed., 1980, courtesy of Charles C Thomas, Publisher, Springfield, Illinois; Werewolf (173) from K. Voelkner, *Von Werwölfen und anderen Tiermenschen,* 1924; Head of Hun Hunahpu (175) from a Late Classic Maya vase, which appears in Mary Miler and Karl Taube, *The Gods and Symbols of Ancient Mexico and the Maya: An Illustrated Dictionary of Mesoamerican Religion,* 1993.

Evæsthetica ON CAMP FOLLOWERS: "Apollo and Daphne," (178) probably by Jacopo Ripanda, active between 1490 and 1530; CANNABIS SATIVA: Cannabis (183) from Leonard Fuchs, *Kreuterbuch,* 1543; Cannabis (185) from the *German Herbarius* of Peter Schöffer, 1485; Cannabis (187) from Dioscorides, *Anicia Juliana,* AD 512; Chinese ideograms (181) and Cannabis leaves (188) drawn by Thomas Christensen; two classical Chinese images of Shên-Nung (205, 206), one from the *High Times Encyclopedia of Recreational Drugs,* the artists of which are unknown to us.

DIE GIFTKUCHE: Weiditz, *An Alchemist at Work* (209) from *The High Times Encyclopedia of Recreational Drugs.*

Metaphysica REVERIES ON THE GREEN MAN: "The Green Man and French Horn," London pub sign (211) from *The Green Man: the Archetype of Our Oneness with the Earth* by William Anderson. Photograph © 1990 by Clive Hicks. Reprinted by permission of HarperCollins Publishers, Inc.; "The Author Meets the Wild Man" (212), from Diego de San Pedro, *Carcel de Amor,* 1493, "Bacchus" (214) by Gabriel Muller, 18th c.; Green Man (216) by Villard de Honnecourt, 13th c.; Green Man (217) by Hans Weiditz, 1521; the well-developed plant person (221), which actually represents a "prodigy" from the age of exploration, appeared in Hartmann Schedel's so-called *Nuremberg Chronicle,* 1493; Ornamental Sheet with a Wild Man (225) probably by the Master of the Dutuit Mount of Olives, mid-15th c. (some attribute this work to the master ES and Martin Schongauer). NITROUS OXIDE: Caricature of Sir Humphrey Davy's nitrous oxide experiments (230) from *The High Times Encyclopedia of Recreational Drugs.* THE POISON PATH II: the hub of the Buddhist wheel of life (236) is from a temple fresco of Sankar Gompa, Leh; "Poster for 'La Plume'" (239), by James Ensor, 1898, lithograph, printed in green outline, handcolored with stencils, composition 21 x 14$^{11}/_{16}$ inches, The Museum of Modern Art, New York Purchase, photograph © The Museum of Modern Art, New York, reproduced by permission.

Back Matter REFERENCES: "Playing card (248) by Amman. CREDITS: The Printer, with the Press Open (282) by Jost Amman, from *Panoplia Omnium Artium* by Hartmann Schopper, 1568. ABOUT THE AUTHOR: Portrait of the Author (289) by Just Pope.

III. TEXT CREDITS

For more information about text sources, see the "Commentary" section of *References,* pp. 248–260, along with the bibliography that follows it, 260–281. Should oversights or errors occur, they will be corrected in the following printings upon written notification to the publisher. Page references in parenthesis.

The author and publisher are grateful to those who have given permission for their work to be cited, among them: Aitken, Robert (7) from *The Dragon Who Never Sleeps: Verses for Zen Buddhist Practice,* Larkspur Press, Monterey, Kentucky, and Parallax Press, Berkeley; by permission of the author. Brown, Norman O. (220) from "Love Hath Reason, Reason None," unpublished paper, by permission of the author. Brown, Norman O. (225) From *Apocalypse and/or Metamorphosis.* Reprinted by permission. Copyright © 1991, the Regents of the

ABOUT THE AUTHOR

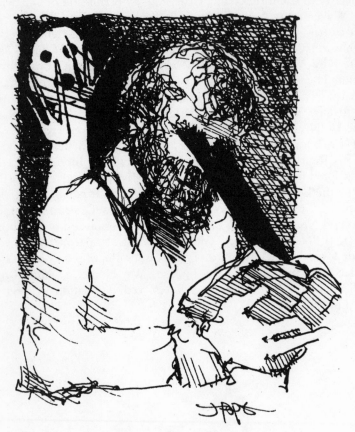

THE AUTHOR AS DRAWN BY JUST POPE

DALE PENDELL is a poet, software engineer, and longtime student of ethnobotany. His poetry has appeared in many journals, and he was the founding editor of *KUKSU: Journal of Back-country Writing*. He has led workshops on ethnobotany and ethnopoetics for the Naropa Institute and the Botanical Preservation Corps.

GARY SNYDER is the author of numerous books of poetry and collections of essays. In 1975, he received a Pulitzer Prize for his book *Turtle Island*. He has long taken an anthropological and poetic approach to the relation between nature and human culture.